Understanding
WOMEN
with AD/HD

Understanding
WOMEN
with AD/HD

UPDATED EDITION

Edited by Kathleen G. Nadeau, Ph.D.
and Patricia O. Quinn. M.D.

Advantage Books

Cover Design: Karen Monaco

Library of Congress Cataloging-in-Publication Data

Understanding Women with AD/HD / edited by Patricia O. Quinn and Kathleen G. Nadeau.

    p. cm.

    Includes bibliographical references and index.

    ISBN 0-9660366-4-6 (alk. paper)

    1. Attention-deficit disordered adults.

    2. Attention-deficit hyperactivity disorder

    3. Attention-deficit disorder in adults. 4. Women-Mental health

    I. Title: Understanding women with AD/HD II. Nadeau, Kathleen G.

    III. Quinn, Patricia O.

    RJ506.H9 G464 2002

    616.85'89—dc21   2001053669

Case histories in this book are either composites of several patients' histories or are stories submitted by actual patients or their families. Identities have been changed to protect patient confidentiality.

The term AD/HD is used in this book in order to conform with current nomenclature. It is intended to include all aspects of the disorder, including non-hyperactive type, and is at times interchangeable with the terms ADD, ADHD, or ADD-H.

The material presented in this book is intended for informational purposes only and should not be considered a substitute for medical advice.

Published by
Advantage Books
3268 Arcadia Place NW
Washington, DC 20015

10 9 8 7 6 5 4 3

Printed in the U.S.A.

DEDICATION

To our daughters

Langdon, whose courage, honesty, and tenacity has
taught me much about the talents and strengths
of women with AD/HD. KN

and

Tara, who has grown into a beautiful, strong woman
with many talents and unlimited potenial. PQ

Acknowledgements

We thank the many girls and women that we have worked with over the years, who have taught us about the unique challenges of being a female with AD/HD. Our appreciation also goes to researchers and clinicians in the field of AD/HD, whose work has been repeatedly cited in this text. Their pioneering work has led to the recognition of AD/HD in females as an important, under-recognized population in need of treatment. Our appreciation, especially, to Sari Solden, author of the first book on women with AD/HD, whose writings have led countless women to feel understood for the first time, after repeated misdiagnoses or dismissals of their concerns.

We would also like to acknowledge the important work of Miranda Gaub and Caryn Carlson, whose ground-breaking meta-analysis of gender-related research on AD/HD brought coherency to the limited amount of data that was available at the time of their work and highlighted the importance of gender issues in AD/HD research. We also want to recognize Julia Rucklidge and Bonnie Kaplan for their work exploring the demoralizing negative effects upon women of living for many years with undiagnosed AD/HD as well as the healing power of diagnosis and understanding. All of these female researchers have been highly influential in broadening the field of AD/HD inquiry to include important gender-related issues.

And, finally, our thanks go to Barbara Michaluk and Karen Monaco for their endless patience with us as this book has grown, evolved, and changed. We would never have reached the end of this long road without your creativity, hard work, and willingness to persevere.

Kathleen G. Nadeau, Ph.D. and Patricia O. Quinn, M.D.

Preface

Countless women with undiagnosed Attention Deficit/Hyperactivity Disorder (AD/HD) have grown up suspecting that something was wrong, but never knowing that they had a common, highly treatable condition. These women have suffered unnecessarily, under-functioning at school and in the workplace, struggling in their daily lives, believing that they were lazy or unmotivated.

Historically, AD/HD (as it is currently known) was considered to be a behavior disorder that only affected young boys who were hyperactive, impulsive and distractible. Only recently have we come to realize that AD/HD affects people throughout their lives and that many are not hyperactive or impulsive at all, but struggle more with problems related to inattention.

Now, we are undergoing another revolution in our understanding of AD/HD. Increasing evidence suggests that many females, perhaps as many as males, are affected by AD/HD. However, although AD/HD is the most highly researched childhood psychiatric disorder, over 99% of all published research has studied populations that are predominantly or exclusively male.

Since 1996, we have devoted our careers to the advancement of the recognition of AD/HD in women and girls, to increasing the focus on gender issues in AD/HD research, and in advocating for a paradigm shift in our concept of AD/HD that will allow for the development of diagnostic criteria that are more appropriate for females.

The chapters that you will read in this groundbreaking volume are written by those in the vanguard—researchers and clinicians who have treated women with AD/HD, who have carefully observed women with AD/HD, and who report their observations and findings so that more women may be accurately diagnosed and treated.

This volume begins with a re-assessment of the current diagnostic criteria for AD/HD from a gender perspective. It is our ardent with that, before the next diagnostic manual is created, that a task-force including significant numbers of AD/HD authorities with a strong interest in gender issues will develop new, more gender-sensitive diagnostic criteria. Perhaps this chapter will serve as a catalyst for this process.

Next, several chapters review the existing research on gender differences. Our hope is that such research will grow exponentially in the near future. Later chapters focus on treatment, coexisting conditions, and a broad range of life issues affected by AD/HD.

We hope that this volume represents an important beginning that will further the understanding of AD/HD in women, but much remains to be done. Although many mothers of children are also affected, parenting programs do not take the mothers' AD/HD into account. Although women with AD/HD are at risk to develop serious psychiatric disorders if they go untreated, most affected women remain undiagnosed. Currently, the professional training of most mental health service providers overlooks this important disorder that affects the lives of so many women and their families.

This book as been compiled to help women with AD/HD, their friends, family members, and members of the general public to understand how this disorder affects women and how they can be helped. We encourage all who read this volume to help spread the word. Share this book with professionals, with educators, with employers. AD/HD is a disorder that affects many women. Women deserve diagnosis and treatment, and most importantly, deserve an opportunity to lead better, more fulfilling lives.

Kathleen G. Nadeau, Ph.D. and Patricia O. Quinn, M.D.

TABLE OF CONTENTS

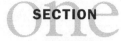

SECTION one

DIAGNOSIS
OF AD/HD
IN WOMEN

CHAPTER 1

Rethinking DSM-IV*

Kathleen G. Nadeau, Ph.D.
Patricia O. Quinn, M.D.

A D/HD, as it is defined today, is a product of its history. Most of our understanding of AD/HD, to date, is based on the study of males, or more accurately, on the study of boys. However, after years of taking male subject studies as the norm, professionals are beginning to question whether findings based on young males are truly representative of the broader population of individuals with AD/HD.

Efforts are now being made to understand how AD/HD affects girls, and even less is understood about how AD/HD impacts the lives of women. One thing, however, is clear—the number of females with AD/HD has been greatly underestimated. Recent studies suggest that the number of women with AD/HD may be nearly equal to that of men with this disorder (Walker, 1999; Faraone et al., 2000).

* American Psychiatric Association. (1994). *Diagnostic and statistical manual for mental disorders* (4th ed.). Washington, DC: Author.

Those who are predominantly inattentive, which is true for the majority of girls, are more difficult to identify (Epstein et al., 1991). Because they are less disruptive, and less difficult for parents and teachers to manage, they are referred less often for evaluation and treatment. Gaub and Carlson (1997) suggest that those few girls who *are* referred may be the most severely affected, and are not representative of most girls with AD/HD. The underreferral of girls has important implications, not only for girls, but for women as well. When diagnosis and treatment are delayed, the potentially damaging impact of undiagnosed AD/HD, including low self-esteem, underachievement, and secondary anxiety and depression, compounds over the course of many years (Rucklidge & Kaplan, 1997). Beiderman and his colleagues voice similar concerns, writing that, "The under-identification and under-treatment of females with AD/HD may have substantial mental health and education implications, . . . research is needed to develop a better understanding of clinical indicators of AD/HD in females" (Biederman et al., 1994, p. 27).

A Clear Need for Diagnostic Instruments Designed for Girls and Women

In November, 1994, a meeting of many well-known AD/HD researchers was convened at the National Institutes of Health to consider gender issues and AD/HD. Conference participants agreed that there was a need to develop rating scales more sensitive to AD/HD in girls (Arnold, 1996). But to date, despite this recommendation, the most commonly used parent and teacher questionnaires continue to emphasize behaviors more typical of males, patterns of hyperactivity and impulsivity. The first self-report questionnaire specifically designed for girls was published in 1999 (Nadeau, Littman, & Quinn, 1999). A similar questionnaire for women with AD/HD has been designed by Nadeau and Quinn (see Chapter 2). More work is needed to develop diagnostic instruments that address the different presentations of AD/HD in females at different stages of their lives.

AD/HD in Women

There is increasing agreement among experts in the field that the DSM-IV criteria used to diagnose AD/HD are not entirely appropriate for adults, and are perhaps even less appropriate for women. However, before beginning a detailed discussion of the gender-related diagnostic issues, the following three vignettes are offered as examples of the range of ways that women's AD/HD symptoms can be manifested.

AD/HD, Predominately Hyperactive/Impulsive Type

"Marie" contacted a psychologist requesting that her twin seven-year-old girls be evaluated for AD/HD. As she discussed their behavior, she commented parenthetically that she had behaved in very similar ways when she was a girl. A few months later, Marie requested an evaluation for herself, saying that she strongly believed that she also had AD/HD, and hoped that receiving the proper treatment would help her to better manage her life.

Marie recounted a history of having been a very "difficult" girl, argumentative and frequently in conflict with her mother. She did not enjoy school and earned mediocre grades despite an above average IQ. Unlike her "perfect" older sister, Marie always tested the limits. Tell her not to do something and she just had to give it a try. Talkative and social in class, Marie entered her teen years as a bit of a rebel, not afraid to defy teachers or parents, and always looking for fun. She began smoking and drinking in her mid-teens, climbed out the window at night to meet boyfriends, and argued over curfews when she was finally allowed to date.

Marie's mother was college educated, unusual for a woman of her generation, and very status conscious. While Marie's older sister met her mother's standards of behavior and achievement, Marie rebelled against the pressure and disapproval she felt. She deliberately dated boys of whom she knew her mother would disapprove. Rather than going to college, as her sister had, Marie's only goal was to "get out of the house" after high school. She hopped from one low-paying job to the next, spending her paycheck on clothes and "fun." She entered a very short-lived marriage in her early twenties—she had eloped after knowing her husband only a couple of months—and left the marriage just as precipitously when their chronic arguments became explosive.

By her mid-twenties, Marie met her next husband—a calmer, more patient young man who seemed to enjoy her spirit and to tolerate her angry outbursts. They married when Marie was 25. A year later, Marie was the mother of twin girls. Just as she had never planned her life prior to marriage, she continued to live day-to-day, using birth control erratically and with ambivalence due to her Catholic upbringing. Two years after the twins' arrival, she gave birth to a son, and three years later gave birth to a second set of twins!

By the time that Marie sought an evaluation for AD/HD, she had created a permanently overwhelming life for herself. By living impulsively, without planning ahead, and making decisions without considering the consequences, Marie had unwittingly created a very AD/HD-unfriendly life for herself—a life that held few options for change.

AD/HD, Predominately Inattentive Type

"Elizabeth's" case is typical of women with primarily inattentive AD/HD. Relatively shy as a young girl, she had attended a small school, an ideal setting for her. By devoting many hours to after-school studies, she was able to make A's. By the time she graduated from eighth grade, she had even won a few academic awards.

Upon entering high school, however, her AD/HD challenges were more evident. She managed to get by, however her class notes were disorganized and she needed help to understand what was said in lecture classes. When long-term projects were assigned, she had difficulty choosing a topic and getting started on the research. *Frequently starting assignments the night before they were due, she would work all night to complete them. Elizabeth "got by" in high school, working very hard to earn a B average. She had few friends and was often unhappy.*

Her college experience proved even more difficult. She attended a large public university where she continued to have trouble writing papers, tending to procrastinate until the last minute. Her procrastination was not due to more pleasurable pursuits, but was the result of her difficulty with putting her thoughts on paper in any cohesive fashion.

After her marriage, midway through college, her husband helped her with all of her papers. Upon graduation from college, Elizabeth decided not to pursue further education. Completion of college had been so difficult, she concluded that she had "had enough."

Elizabeth became a housewife and mother, giving birth to three children over the next five years. The unstructured aspects of housekeeping were difficult for her. She injected structure into her life through the schedules of her husband and children.

Gradually, however, the structure provided by her family decreased. Her children were older and in school all day, while her husband's hours became less predictable after going into business for himself. She now had many hours of unstructured time, and found that she had increasing difficulty maintaining schedules and routines. At a point when she felt her life should be easier, instead she felt frustrated and ineffective. With little structure in her life, Elizabeth found that she was unable to pursue activities she had dreamed of having time for when the children were older. When her son was diagnosed with AD/HD, she began to entertain the possibility of the diagnosis for herself as well.

AD/HD, Combined Type

"Jesse" was the youngest child in a family with three older brothers, two of whom had AD/HD. A precocious child, she learned to talk and walk early. Her parents joked that she had been "born talking and hadn't stopped since." Jesse was strong-willed and very insistent upon having her own way. Although her parents were more

tolerant of her behaviors, adults outside the family sometimes described Jesse as "bossy" or "spoiled." As a preschooler, Jesse had frequent temper tantrums and was overly reactive to fatigue or frustration. She had difficulty tolerating any change in her daily routine and had intense, exaggerated reactions to even the slightest physical injury.

In elementary school, Jesse did well academically, although she typically talked too much in class. An extrovert, Jesse approached other girls easily, but had difficulty keeping friends due to her tendencies to be bossy and argumentative. Jesse excelled in athletics and played on many sports teams with the boys. As a teenager, Jesse was a "risk taker" and got into trouble for smoking and driving a friend's car before she had her license. Although her grades began to suffer in high school, her achievements in sports earned her an athletic scholarship to college.

In college, Jesse just "got by." She always felt that she could do better, and often started the semester planning to work hard. These good intentions never seemed to last for long. With grades ranging from A's to D's, Jesse became more concerned as she entered her junior year. Her boyfriend was planning to attend law school after graduation and encouraged her to do the same. Because her own efforts to buckle down and apply herself had never lasted, she finally decided to seek help at the college counseling center. Jesse had always believed, deep down, that she was smart, but something kept getting in the way. Her counselor, after talking with her for a while and taking a family history, suggested an evaluation for AD/HD.

As can be gleaned from their stories, all of these women appear on the surface to be successful. Two attended college and all would seem, at a cursory glance, to be functioning without impairment. None of them would meet the DSM-IV "age-of-onset" criterion requiring that symptoms must be evident prior to age seven. They were all bright and "got by" in school. However, good grades were earned only with great effort and many hours of work. Their grades were typically well below what they were capable of earning based on their overall intelligence. They had difficulty with time management and organization. They had difficulty completing assignments and often needed other individuals (a parent, husband, or boyfriend) to keep them on track. They had difficulty with social relationships with peers, and were either shy or bossy around others. Marie was overwhelmed by the situation she had created for herself through lack of planning; Elizabeth reported feeling unhappy most of the time; and Jesse could be considered somewhat oppositional.

None of these women ever considered the diagnosis of AD/HD until adulthood, even though one of them had two brothers with AD/HD. Yet, all of these women suffered from clinically significant symptoms of AD/HD, and needed appropriate treatment in order to function better and make needed changes in their lives.

Looking at DSM-IV from a Gender Perspective

Results of a recent study suggest that current DSM-IV diagnostic criteria are perceived as more descriptive of males than females (Ohan & Johnston, 1999). All too often, women seeking an evaluation for AD/HD do not receive this diagnosis because their histories do not fit the stereotypic AD/HD patterns of young, hyperactive males. Clinicians who expect a report of poor academic functioning and behavioral problems in elementary school will overlook many, if not most women with AD/HD. Clinicians who equate AD/HD with those who have never attended college, or who have failed to graduate from college, will misinterpret signs of AD/HD in highly intelligent women who may have earned a Ph.D., law, or medical degree. Women with primarily inattentive type AD/HD who present with a low arousal level may be diagnosed with dysthymia, while women of the combined or hyperactive/impulsive types, who have a high energy level, impulsivity, and verbal aggression, may be diagnosed with bipolar disorder. While depression or bipolar disorder may be present, coexisting with AD/HD, in many cases, female patterns of AD/HD are being misinterpreted.

DSM-IV did much to focus the world on the fact that AD/HD is a disorder of both attention and hyperactivity, and that one or the other pattern may predominate in individuals. However, it did little to clarify the diagnostic picture for adults, especially women. When the DSM was revised in 1994, experts engaged in AD/HD research had developed their clinical experience treating children (specifically elementary school-aged boys). Those symptoms proposed for the disorder specifically listed in Criterion A (Hyperactive/Impulsive symptoms), reflect this child focus, often referring to behaviors that are developmentally inappropriate for an adult (e.g., schoolwork, climbing activities, leaving seat, etc.) In addition, the requirement that six or more of these symptoms must be present to make the diagnosis does little to address the possibility that an older individual may have as few as three or four symptoms of hyperactivity or impulsivity, yet, at the same time, may experience significant AD/HD-related impairment in other areas more typical of adults, for example, problems with organization, time management, and forgetfulness.

The wording in DSM-IV allows for the occurrence of fewer DSM-IV symptoms in adults by stating that all symptoms may not be present in adulthood. In such a case, impairment may still be noted, however, the disorder should be labeled "in partial remission." Clearly, the DSM-IV, like its predecessors, remained focused on childhood symptomatology, viewing adults as having only "partial" AD/HD.

Barkley (1995) proposed that AD/HD is developmental in nature, and manifests itself differently, albeit with equal impairment, at different life stages. There is growing evidence that AD/HD not only varies by age, but also by gender, with females showing different symptom patterns and differences in age of onset and life course. Furthermore, a range of protective factors, including high IQ, can mask evidence of AD/HD until the demands of the environment increase and symptoms can no longer remain hidden. In the following sections, these age, gender, and environmental influences on the expression of AD/HD will be explored further.

Age Differences

If one looks at the age-appropriateness of DSM-IV criteria, one begins to appreciate the problem of documenting the persistence of the disorder over the life-span. These criteria, developed exclusively through the observation of children, prove increasingly problematic when attempting to diagnose adolescents and adults. Symptoms of inattention seem fairly stable across the life-span, while hyperactive symptoms decrease with age (Hart, Lahey, Loeber, Applegate, & Frick, 1995), and problems of executive functioning become more prominent as the environmental expectations for such functions increase (Barkley, 1997a). Using the DSM-IV criteria across the life-span make it seem that individuals gradually outgrow AD/HD, when they are simply outgrowing the child-based criteria set (Barkley, 1997b, p 4).

Environmental Differences

DSM-IV acknowledges (under Criterion C) that there are certain circumstances that may mitigate the symptoms of the disorder. "Signs of the disorder may be minimal or absent when the individual is under very strict control, is in a novel setting, is engaged in especially interesting activities, in a one-to-one situation . . . , or while the person experiences frequent rewards for appropriate behavior" (p. 79). What is not addressed, however, is that such mitigating conditions may differ for males and females. For example, "strict control" may have to be very overt and active in dealing with a hyperactive/impulsive boy, while a verbal correction or critical comment may constitute "strict control" for a shy, withdrawn girl with AD/HD. Likewise, "especially interesting activities" are well-known to vary according to gender. While boys with AD/HD may show excellent focus and protracted concentration when playing an electronic game, girls may find that social interactions or verbal communication, such as being read to, are "especially interesting."

In the same vein, what constitutes a "frequent reward" for a girl may be quite different than for a boy who is more hyperactive or oppositional. A recent study suggests that predominantly inattentive students (the subtype in which the majority of girls with AD/HD are found) are primarily motivated by teacher approval, whereas hyperactive and impulsive children are more motivated by winning in a competitive activity (Booth, Carlson, Shin, & Canu, 2001). When such gender differences are considered, it becomes clearer why AD/HD in girls may be misunderstood or overlooked.

Criterion A

The symptoms listed under Criterion A for diagnosis of AD/HD not only create problems with age-based norms, but also are not always as appropriate for delineating the diagnosis in females, and may represent a significant gender bias. In a study conducted by Ohan and Johnston, the perception of gender appropriateness of diagnostic criteria was examined. When mothers of children with AD/HD, seven to 14 years of age, were questioned, they rated most DSM-IV symptoms as more typical of males. In general, mothers rated the task oriented symptoms of DSM-IV (i.e., "often loses things necessary for tasks . . . often does not finish schoolwork, etc.") as descriptive of males, and the socially oriented DSM-IV symptom ("talks excessively") as descriptive of females (Ohan & Johnston, 1999).

Two recent studies of adults with AD/HD (Stein et al., 1995; Arcia & Conners, 1998) found gender differences in the responses to adult AD/HD questionnaires. Women reported more problems with dysphoria (moodiness, depressed feelings), disorganization, and low self-esteem, while men reported problems with conduct, attention, stress intolerance and poor social skills. Thus, there is growing evidence at all life stages that females with AD/HD demonstrate behavioral differences as well as differences in their experiences related to AD/HD.

Associated Features

While the symptoms listed under Criterion A of DSM-IV remain the official diagnostic description, other associated features are listed. These associated features may vary according to age and developmental level. While these features are currently not seen as primary, they may be more salient when addressing gender differences.

Associated features listed in DSM-IV (p. 80) include low frustration tolerance, bossiness, stubbornness, excessive temper outbursts, and excessive and frequent insistence that demands be met—associated features seen more often in individuals with combined type or predominantly hyperactive/impulsive AD/HD. In addition, mood lability, dysphoria, rejection by peers, demoralization, and poor self-esteem are listed (p. 80). Research suggests that the inattentive group may have more "associated features" such as anxiety, mood disorders, and more often be rated socially withdrawn or shy (Lahey & Carlson, 1992; Morgan, Hynd, Riccio, & Hall, 1996). These associated features may further contribute to the invisibility of an individual's AD/HD status because they may be interpreted as primary symptoms of other conditions unrelated to AD/HD. In Sari Solden's book, *Women with Attention Deficit Disorder*, these same features of low self-esteem, anxiety, and mood disorders are reported to be common in women with AD/HD. One needs only to review the cases presented earlier to see the prominence of these features in the lives of women and girls with AD/HD.

Criterion B

Some hyperactive-impulsive or inattentive symptoms that caused impairment were present before the age of seven years.

Early onset of AD/HD symptoms seems to be associated with hyperactivity, more severe symptoms, reading problems, and poorer school performance (McGee et al., 1992). Inattentive symptoms, more often reported for girls, tend to have a later onset (Lahey et al., 1994) making it important to address this age-of-onset criterion necessary for the diagnosis of AD/HD. Even when symptoms of inattention *are* present at an early age, children without hyperactivity often go undiagnosed. As one study points out (Epstein, Shaywitz, Shaywitz, & Woolston, 1991), clinicians correctly diagnose nonhyperactive AD/HD only about half of the time. Even as late as adolescence, girls' AD/HD patterns are less likely to be identified in the classroom because, despite their attentional and organizational difficulties, they tend to escape notice because they are less disruptive (Faraone et al., 1998).

When protective influences such as a high IQ, a supportive family, relatively good social skills, and no symptoms of conduct disorder, are present the diagnosis of AD/HD-combined type has been reported to be delayed (Tzelepis, Schubiner, & Warbasse, 1995). Thus, girls with multiple "protective factors" and/or predominantly inattentive AD/HD may not be diagnosed until later childhood or adolescence (Faraone, Biederman, Weber, & Russell, 1998), if even then.

Later diagnosis of AD/HD in some females may simply be the reflection of insensitivity of the DSM-IV criteria to the early signs of the disorder in girls. However, in certain instances there seems to be an actual difference among females in the course of the disorder based on primary symptomatology. Hucssy (1990) has pointed out that there appears to be a worsening of symptoms of AD/HD with the onset of puberty in girls.

Girls who did not call attention to themselves through externalizing or hyperactive behaviors, and who could do well in school through great effort and long hours, would not be identified during the early years. Often it is not until the onset of puberty and the demands of middle school that these girls demonstrate impairment. Indeed, individuals with AD/HD with superior IQs may be able to compensate academically for many years, thus running the risk of late diagnosis (Brown, 1998).

The findings of these studies, taken together, strongly suggest that Criterion B is often not appropriate for females, with the result that many girls and women with AD/HD are not diagnosed and treated.

Criterion C

Some impairment from the symptoms is present in two or more settings (e.g., at school [or work] and at home).

Females may work harder than males to compensate for or hide symptomatology in their efforts to meet parent and/or teacher expectations (Booth et al., 2001). As discussed earlier, "approval" is the most salient reward for many girls with AD/HD, leading them, despite clinically significant symptoms of AD/HD, to work hard to overcome their difficulties. Thus, good grades and positive teacher reports in grade school may simply be a measure of effort rather than level of impairment. Furthermore, Ohan and Johnston's (1999) findings that DSM-IV AD/HD symptoms are considered more descriptive of boys, leaves open the possibility that impairment exists that is not accurately described using these criteria.

In adulthood, using broad measures such as educational achievement, employment level, or marital status as signs of impairment or lack thereof doesn't take into account the enormous daily struggle experienced by many women with AD/HD to cope as environmental demands increase. Just as girls work intensely to compensate for AD/HD in the classroom, so do women with AD/HD put forth exhausting efforts to function at home and in the workplace. Solden (1995) and others have written of feelings of shame and inadequacy experienced by women with AD/HD as they struggle to meet the gender role expectations of wives, homemakers, and mothers. If one compares the degree of difficulty or the amount of time and effort that a woman with AD/HD needs to invest to maintain even a semblance of normalcy, as compared to women without AD/HD, her impairments in functioning may be more readily determined.

Criterion D

There must be clear evidence of clinically significant impairment in social, academic, or occupational functioning.

"Evidence of clinically significant impairment" is a new criterion, appearing for the first time in DSM-IV, reflecting a blurring of the concepts of *diagnosis* and *disability*. In DSM-III-R, there were no impairment requirements, nor were there requirements for evidence of impairment in more than one setting. Degrees of impairment, from mild to severe were recognized in DSM-III-R. However, when the DSM-IV was published, not long after acrimonious public debates about AD/HD began, the concept of AD/HD had changed. For the first time, there were requirements for evidence of "clinically significant impairment," demonstrated in "two or more settings"—a close paraphrasing of disability law that requires a "substantial impairment" in "a major life function" in order to make a disability determination.

As a result of this added impairment criterion, the process of diagnosis has become limited by guidelines more appropriate for disability determination. As for many, if not most, psychiatric or developmental disorders, AD/HD symptoms exist along a continuum. This fact was clearly recognized in DSM-III-R guidelines that acknowledged "mild, moderate, and severe" degrees of "ADD." Such degrees of severity are readily acknowledged for other disorders, as are distinctions between diagnosis and disability. In depression, for example, the degree of depression necessary for diagnosis and treatment is clearly distinct from the degree of depression necessary to qualify for disability benefits. No one would argue that a diagnosis of depression was invalid if the individual were not "disabled" by depression.

Whatever the reasons for their adoption, current DSM-IV restrictions have come at the expense of the individual suffering with AD/HD, particularly for females. Even with the less restrictive DSM-III-R criteria, many females did not receive a diagnosis, despite significant attentional difficulties, because they did not fit the male-derived diagnostic criteria. Now, with more stringent DSM-IV criteria that require evidence of significant impairment in two or more settings, females whose symptoms are less noticeable, who are less disruptive, who exhibit fewer behavioral problems, and who work hard to compensate for their attention-related difficulties, are even less likely to receive a diagnosis and much-needed treatment.

Criterion E

The symptoms . . . are not better accounted for by another mental disorder (e.g., Mood Disorder, Anxiety Disorder, Dissociative Disorder, or a Personality Disorder).

The inclusion of this criterion is meant to prevent the misdiagnosis of AD/HD when another disorder is responsible for the symptomatology. However, AD/HD, particularly for adults, is often accompanied by several other conditions. Biederman and his colleagues (Biederman, Newcomb, & Sprich, 1991; Biederman, Faraone, & Lapey, 1992; Biederman, Faraone, Spencer, & Wilens, 1993) have presented evidence indicating that the majority of persons with AD/HD have a least one and sometimes more than one additional psychiatric disorder. These disorders include depression, tics, Tourette syndrome, behavior disorders, substance abuse, obsessive-compulsive disorder, anxiety disorder, and learning disabilities. Barkley, summarizing a number of studies, indicates that as many as 75 percent of individuals with AD/HD show depression in adulthood, and as many as 27 percent may abuse alcohol (Barkley, 1990).

For adults with AD/HD, and particularly for women, it is more often these coexisting conditions that are diagnosed, while the AD/HD goes unnoticed. A study conducted by Katz, Goldstein, and Geckle published in 1998 addressed coexisting conditions in 49 males and 26 females with AD/HD. They write:

The findings of higher rates of depressive and anxiety symptoms among women suggest that women, as a group, may be under-diagnosed (with AD/HD) . . . (Their) elevated personality measurement scores may lead clinicians to diagnose depression more readily than AD/HD . . . Findings of this study suggest that women have greater psychological distress than men with AD/HD. Particularly, because of this latter finding, they may be diagnosed, correctly or incorrectly, as depressed, and AD/HD as a sole or comorbid diagnosis may be missed. (Katz et al., 1998, p. 245)

All too often, and especially in women, a clinician is too quick to diagnose these coexisting conditions as primary, while missing the diagnosis of AD/HD altogether. Women with AD/HD are commonly misdiagnosed with depression or bipolar disorder. While the symptoms specific to these coexisting disorders may respond to appropriate pharmacologic interventions, the patient continues to struggle with multiple issues of life functioning if her AD/HD is not also treated.

Looking Ahead to DSM-V

In the process of reconsidering the complex and controversial diagnosis of AD/HD, it is hoped that following issues will be considered in any future revisions:

Criteria for AD/HD in Adults

There is increasing agreement among experts in the field that many of DSM-IV criteria are not appropriate for adults (Barkley, 1997b). Several authorities have noted that adults experience significant difficulty with executive functions, but far fewer problems with impulsivity and hyperactivity. Barkley has called for new, age-appropriate diagnostic criteria across the life-span.

Criteria for AD/HD in Females

Current criteria are not equally appropriate for girls, due to numerous factors discussed earlier in this chapter. There is widespread and growing consensus that AD/HD diagnostic criteria need to become more gender sensitive (Arnold, 1996), and that, in particular, the requirement that AD/HD be evident prior to age seven is inappropriate for females (Weiss & Jain, 2000).

Given the growing questions regarding the appropriateness of current diagnostic criteria for both adults and females, one can make a reasonable assumption that current diagnostic criteria are perhaps least of all appropriate for women.

Differentiation of Diagnosis and Disability

Clearly, there needs to be a distinction between diagnosis and disability. Currently, many clinicians are forced to operate in a "gray zone" in which they cannot make a diagnosis of AD/HD, even in cases where there are clinically significant symptoms of AD/HD that would benefit from treatment. While an adult with learning disabilities is not considered to "lose" his learning disability if he or she is successful in a career, we are required by current diagnostic criteria to declare that an adult with AD/HD no longer has this disorder if he achieves career success. "Dysfunction" requirements (criteria C and D) place the mental health profession in an absurd position—

one that supposes that a genetically transmitted neurobiological condition is proclaimed to "exist," then disappear, and possibly reappear at a later point in life—depending upon mitigating factors in the environment.

The dysfunction requirements contained in Criteria C and D have greater consequences for women. Several studies suggest that the patterns of females are less readily recognized and that females may work harder and more effectively to mask their struggles, making it less likely that females will meet current diagnostic criteria.

It is hoped that mental health service providers can return to a standard whereby the sole purpose of diagnosis is to understand and appropriately treat conditions that negatively impact an individual's life. A woman with clinically significant symptoms of AD/HD deserves diagnosis and treatment so that she can function at her best.

Conclusion

The problems that DSM-IV presents in the diagnosis of women with AD/HD cannot be overemphasized. In order to properly diagnose AD/HD in adults, and especially in women, it is important to provide clinicians with a new set of criteria that are more relevant to females and more developmentally appropriate across the life-span. AD/HD, once properly diagnosed, is a very treatable condition. But without revised diagnostic guidelines, diagnosis and effective treatment for women are at risk.

References

American Psychiatric Association. (1987). *Diagnostic and statistical manual for mental disorders* (3rd ed., rev.). Washington, DC: Author.

American Psychiatric Association. (1994*). Diagnostic and statistical manual for mental disorders* (4th ed.). Washington, DC: Author.

Arcia, E., & Conners, C.K. (1998). Gender differences in AD/HD? *Journal of Developmental and Behavioral Pediatrics, 19*, 77-83.

Arnold, L. (1996). Sex differences in AD/HD: Conference summary. *Journal of Abnormal Child Psychology, 24*, 555-569.

Barkley, R.A. (1990). *Attention deficit hyperactivity disorder: A handbook for diagnosis and treatment.* New York: Guilford Press.

Barkley, R.A. (1995). A closer look at the DSM-IV criteria for AD/HD: Some unresolved issues. *AD/HD Report, 3(3),* 1-5.

Barkley, R.A. (1997a). *AD/HD and the nature of self-control.* New York: Guilford Press.

Barkley, R.A. (1997b). Age dependent decline in AD/HD: True recovery or statistical illusion. *The AD/HD Report, 5,* 1-5.

Biederman, J., Faraone, S.V., Spencer, T., Wilens, T., Mick, E., & Lapey, K.A. (1994). Gender differences in a sample of adults with attention deficit hyperactivity disorder. *Psychiatry Research, 53*, 13-29.

Biederman, J., Newcomb, J., & Sprich, S. (1991). Comorbidity of AD/HD with conduct, depressive, anxiety and other disorders. *American Journal of Psychiatry, 148*, 564-577.

Biederman, J., Faraone, S., Spencer, T., & Wilens, T. (1993). Patterns of psychiatric comorbidity, cognition, and psychosocial functioning in adults with AD/HD. *American Journal of Psychiatry, 150,* 1792-1798.

Biederman, J., Faraone, S.V., & Lapey, K. (1992). Comorbidity of diagnosis in attention-deficit hyperactivity disorder. In G. Weiss (Ed.). *Attention-deficit hyperactivity disorder, Child & Adolescent Psychiatric Clinics of North America.* Philadelphia: Saunders.

Booth, J., Carlson, C.L., Shin, M., & Canu, W. (2001). Parent, teacher, and self-rated motivational styles in the AD/HD subtypes. *AD/HD Report, 9(1),* 8-11.

Brown, T.E. (1998). *AD/HD in persons with superior IQs: Unique risks.* Presented at the 10th Annual CHADD International Conference, New York.

Epstein, M.A., Shaywitz, B.A., Shaywitz, J.L., & Woolston, J.L. (1991). Boundaries of attention deficit disorder. *Journal of Learning Disabilities, 24,* 78-86.

Faraone, S.V., Biederman, J., Weber, W., & Russell, R.L. (1998). Psychiatric, neuropsychological, and psychosocial features of DSM-IV subtypes of attention-deficit/hyperactivity disorder: Results from a clinically referred sample. *Journal of the American Academy of Child and Adolescent Psychiatry, 37,* 185-193.

Faraone, S.V., Biederman, J., Mick, E., Williamson, S., Wilens, T.E., Spencer, T., Weber, W., Jetton, J., Kraus, E., Pert, J., & Zallen, B. (2000). Family study of girls with attention deficit hyperactivity disorder. *American Journal of Psychiatry, 157,* 1077-1083.

Gaub, M., & Carlson, C. (1997). Gender differences in AD/HD: A meta-analysis and critical review. *Journal of the American Academy of Child and Adolescent Psychiatry, 36,* 1036-1045.

Hart, E.L., Lahey, B.B., Loeber, R., Applegate, B., & Frick, P.J. (1995). Developmental changes in attention-deficit hyperactivity disorder in boys: A four-year longitudinal study. *Journal of Abnormal Child Psychology, 23,* 729-750.

Huessy, H.R. (1990). *The pharmacotherapy of personality disorders in women.* Paper presented at the 143rd annual meeting of the American Psychiatric Association (symposia), New York.

Katz, L.J., Goldstein, G., & Geckle, M. (1998). Neuropsychological and personality differences between men and women with AD/HD. *Journal of Attention Disorders, 2,* 239-247.

Lahey, B.B., Applegate, B., McBurnett, K., Biederman, J., Greenhill, L., Hynd, G.W., Barkley, R. A., Newcorn, J., Jensen, P., Richters, J., Garfinkel, B., Kerdyk, L., Frick, P.J., Ollendick, T., Perez, D., Hart, E. L., Waldman, I., & Shaffer, D. (1994). DSM-IV field trials for attention deficit disorder in children and adolescents. *American Journal of Psychiatry, 151*, 1673-1685.

Lahey, B.B., & Carlson, C.L. (1992). Validity of the diagnostic category of attention deficit without hyperactivity: A review of the literature. In S.E. Shaywitz, & B.E. Shaywitz (Eds.). *Attention deficit disorder comes of age: Toward the twenty-first century.* Austin, TX: Pro-Ed.

McGee, R., Williams, S., & Feehan, M. (1992). Attention deficit disorder and age of onset of problem behaviors. *Journal of Abnormal Child Psychology, 20,* 487-502.

Morgan, A.E., Hynd, G. W., Riccio, C.A., & Hall, J. (1996). Validity of DSM-IV AD/HD predominately inattentive and combined types: Relationship to previous DSM diagnosis/subtype difference. *Journal of the American Academy of Child and Adolescent Psychiatry, 35,* 325-333.

Nadeau, K., Littman, E., & Quinn, P. (1999). *Understanding girls with AD/HD.* Silver Spring, MD: Advantage Books.

Ohan, J.L., & Johnston, C. (1999). Gender appropriateness of diagnostic criteria for the externalizing disorders. In M. Moretti (Chair), *Aggression in girls: Diagnostic issues and interpersonal factors.* Symposium conducted at the biennial meeting of the Society for Research in Child Development, Albuquerque, NM.

Rucklidge, J.J., & Kaplan, B.J. (1997). Psychological functioning in women identified in adulthood with attention-deficit/hyperactivity disorder. *Journal of Attention Disorders, 2,* 167-176.

Solden, S. (1995). *Women with attention deficit disorder: Embracing disorganization at home and in the workplace.* Grass Valley, CA: Underwood Books.

Stein, M.A., Sandoval, R., Szumowski, E., Roizen, N., Reinecke, M., Blondis, T., & Klein, A. (1995). Psychometric characteristics of the Wender Utah Rating Scale (WURS): Reliability and factor structure for men and women. *Psychopharmacology Bulletin, 31,* 423-431.

Tzelepis, A., Schubiner, H., & Warbasse, L.H. (1995). Differential diagnosis and psychiatric co-morbidity patterns in adult attention deficit disorder. In K.G. Nadeau (Ed.). *A comprehensive guide to attention deficit disorder in adults (pp. 35-57).* New York: Brunner/Mazel.

Walker, C. (1999). *Gender and genetics in AD/HD: Genetics matter; gender does not.* Paper presented at the ADDA Regional Conference, Chicago.

Weiss, M., & Jain, U. (2000). Clinical perspectives on the assessment of AD/HD in adolescence. *AD/HD Report, 8(6),* 4-7, 10.

CHAPTER 2

Women's AD/HD Self-Assessment Symptom Inventory

Kathleen G. Nadeau, Ph.D.
and Patricia O. Quinn, M.D.

The following set of self-assessment questions has been developed informally, over time, reflecting the authors' clinical experience in treating women and girls with AD/HD. Normative data has not yet been collected using this inventory, either to compare women diagnosed with AD/HD to undiagnosed women, or to compare responses of men and women diagnosed with AD/HD. Such studies, however, would both provide valuable information and lend greater validity to this inventory as a diagnostic tool.

Some of the items included in the Inventory reflect issues more typical of women with Combined Type AD/HD, while others are representative of women with Primarily Inattentive Type AD/HD. The following questions are appropriate for use as a

24

detailed, structured self-assessment of a broad range of concerns typically reported by women with AD/HD. The authors hope that this Self-Assessment Symptom Inventory will prove to be an important step in the process of exploring important gender differences in adult AD/HD and in developing a consensus on more gender and age-appropriate diagnostic criteria for women.

(The following self-assessment inventory is fully protected by copyright laws and may not be reproduced for personal or professional use. Questionnaires for clinical use can be ordered by contacting Advantage Books at 1-888-238-8588.)

Women's AD/HD Self-Assessment
Symptom Inventory (SASI)

Kathleen Nadeau, Ph.D. and Patricia Quinn, M.D.

(This scale should not be used for diagnostic purposes, but should be used as a structured interview, in conjunction with other diagnostic tools when evaluating women for possible AD/HD.)

Directions:

Rate each statement below from 0-3 to indicate how much that feeling or behavior is part of your personal experience.

0 =   That's not at all like me; that almost never happens to me.

1 =   That's a little like me; that happens to me, but not very often.

2 =   That's a lot like me; that happens to me often.

3 =   That's just like me; that happens to me almost all the time.

When an item does not pertain to you, leave that item blank.

When you encounter an item that pertains to you, but requires information you can't recall or about which you have no knowledge, respond with a question mark (?).

Part I   CHILDHOOD AD/HD PATTERNS

Answer this first group of questions retrospectively, as you recall your childhood experiences.

Inattention

_____ 1. I daydreamed in school.

_____ 2. My mind wandered, even when I *tried* to listen to the teacher.

_____ 3. In class, I didn't hear the teacher's instructions.

_____ 4. I made careless mistakes on tests.

_____ 5. I lost or misplaced things.

_____ 6. I was teased for being "spacey."

Hyperactivity

_____ 1. I "got in trouble" for talking in class.

_____ 2. I was a tomboy.

_____ 3. It was hard for me to sit still in class.

_____ 4. I felt best when I was moving around— playing sports or dancing.

_____ 5. It was hard to fall asleep at bedtime because thoughts were bouncing around in my brain.

_____ 6. I doodled or fidgeted when I had to sit still.

_____ 7. My friends called me "hyper."

_____ 8. When sitting, I tended to "tip" my chair or jiggle my legs.

Impulsivity

_____ 1. I interrupted others, even when I tried not to.

_____ 2. When upset, I said things I didn't mean.

_____ 3. I acted silly or "crazy" with my friends.

_____ 4. I acted on the spur of the moment, never thinking of the trouble I'd get into.

_____ 5. As a teenager, I drove too fast or took other risks while driving.

Productivity

_____ 1. In school, I didn't finish seat work as quickly as the rest of the class.

_____ 2. The demands of high school felt overwhelming to me.

_____ 3. I had to work much harder than my classmates to do well in school.

_____ 4. I studied or did homework late into the night.

Problems with initiation

_____ 1. I had trouble getting started on my homework.

_____ 2. It was hard for me to begin working on a project unless someone was there to keep me on track.

_____ 3. I worked better with others than alone.

Problems with follow-through/perseverance

_____ 1. It was hard for me to complete long-term school projects.

_____ 2. I dabbled in many hobbies or activities, but never really persevered in my efforts.

_____ 3. Although I took music lessons, I rarely, or never, practiced.

Problems with under-arousal

_____ 1. I felt sleepy when sitting in class, but became energetic as soon as I stood up and moved.

_____ 2. It was difficult to get up in the morning.

_____ 3. I didn't feel alert until late in the morning.

_____ 4. I didn't seem to have as much energy as my friends.

Procrastination problems

_____ 1. I was smart, but got by doing everything at the last minute.

_____ 2. I handed in my homework late, and sometimes didn't do it at all.

_____ 3. The only way I could study for a test was to stay up very late the night before.

Low motivation/underachievement

_____ 1. I didn't do as well in school as I felt I should.

_____ 2. I got by on my intelligence, and didn't really try hard in school.

_____ 3. My parents and teachers told me I could do better if I tried.

_____ 4. I start each grading period with good intentions, but never sustained them.

Organizational difficulties

_____ 1. My room was very messy.

_____ 2. My backpack/bookbag/desk was messy.

_____ 3. I had trouble being organized.

_____ 4. I had trouble keeping track of assignments, long-term projects, and due dates.

Poor time management

_____ 1. I arrived late for scheduled activities.

_____ 2. I lost track of the time.

_____ 3. I stayed up late, then had trouble getting up in the morning.

Problems with fine/gross motor control

_____ 1. My handwriting was messy.

_____ 2. I was physically awkward and did poorly in sports.

_____ 3. I tended to bump into things—corners of tables, door frames, etc.

LEARNING ISSUES

Reading problems

_____ 1. I was a slow reader.

_____ 2. When reading, my mind wandered.

_____ 3. Typically, after reading a textbook, I could not answer the questions at the end of the chapter.

_____ 4. I needed to reread information to be sure that I understood it.

_____ 5. I didn't read for pleasure.

Writing problems

_____ 1. Writing assignments were difficult for me.

_____ 2. I had lots of ideas, but couldn't organize them well when writing a paper.

_____ 3. I could explain what I knew verbally, but just couldn't get it down on paper.

Memory problems

_____ 1. I had trouble remembering the directions for assignments.

_____ 2. Even when I studied, I couldn't recall the information on a test.

_____ 3. I was forgetful and absentminded.

SOCIAL/INTERPERSONAL ISSUES

Shyness, social withdrawal

_____ 1. I felt shy and self-conscious around my classmates.

_____ 2. Even when I had something to say, I rarely raised my hand to volunteer in class.

_____ 3. I had only a few friends during school years.

_____ 4. I didn't date, or rarely dated, in high school.

Interpersonal/verbal problems

_____ 1. Other girls called me "mean" or "bossy."

_____ 2. I felt different from other girls.

_____ 3. Other girls didn't like me, but I didn't understand why.

      4.   It was hard for me to keep up with the conversation of a group of girls.

      5.   I fought and argued with my friends.

      6.   In conversation, I'd say something really "stupid," or couldn't think of anything to say.

      7.   I was very sensitive to teasing.

PSYCHOLOGICAL ISSUES

Moodiness/anxiety

      1.   I felt worried and anxious.

      2.   I felt moody and depressed for no reason.

      3.   I dreaded being called on by the teacher.

      4.   I didn't like going to school.

      5.   I became very anxious before examinations.

      6.   I was irritable as a teenager.

      7.   I cried easily.

Feeling criticized, misunderstood

      1.   I wish my parents had understood how hard high school was for me.

      2.   It felt as if my parents criticized me a lot.

      3.   My mother and I were in conflict during my high school years.

      4.   I was repeatedly humiliated or criticized by teachers or others in the school setting.

Low self-esteem

      1.   I feel a sense of shame or regret, as I look back on things I did in high school.

      2.   I wasn't really good at anything.

      3.   I didn't feel good about myself during my school years.

PROBLEMATIC BEHAVIORS

Impatience/low frustration tolerance/anger

_____ 1. I was impatient and easily frustrated.

_____ 2. Although I controlled myself at school, I had screaming arguments at home with my family.

_____ 3. I quit a task if I encountered difficulty.

_____ 4. I lost my temper when frustrated.

Risk-taking behavior

_____ 1. I took risks and acted impulsively.

_____ 2. I started smoking at a younger age than many of my friends.

_____ 3. I was sexually active earlier than other girls.

_____ 4. I drank and experimented with drugs in high school or earlier.

_____ 5. I abused alcohol or other substances in high school or earlier.

Oppositional/defiant behavior

_____ 1. I got in trouble as a teenager.

_____ 2. I rebelled against my parents.

_____ 3. My parents didn't like the kids I hung out with in high school.

_____ 4. I skipped classes in high school.

_____ 5. I fought with my parents over rules and curfews.

_____ 6. My parents didn't approve of my boyfriend in high school.

_____ 7. I was very argumentative.

_____ 8. I couldn't take "no" for an answer.

Problems with disordered eating

    _____   1. I ate compulsively as a child or teenager.

    _____   2. I developed a pattern of bulimia.

    _____   3. I became overweight after puberty.

    _____   4. I repeatedly "dieted" without success.

    _____   5. I binged on certain foods until I felt stuffed, even sick.

Part II   ADULT AD/HD PATTERNS

Inattention

    _____   1. I tend to overlook details.

    _____   2. Forms are difficult for me to complete correctly—I usually miss something.

    _____   3. It is hard for me to listen for long periods of time—in a lecture, seminar, or training class, for example.

    _____   4. My mind tends to wander when I'm reading, or when I'm listening to something that is not very interesting to me.

Distractibility

    _____   1. I am easily sidetracked, and wander from one task to the next as something catches my attention.

    _____   2. I jump from topic to topic in conversation, forgetting what I started to say.

    _____   3. I have difficulty concentrating when there is noise or conversation near me.

    _____   4. It is very difficult for me to get back on task after an interruption.

Tendency to hyperfocus

    _____   1. I tend to "hyperfocus" for long periods of time on certain activities.

_____ 2. When engaging in certain activities, I completely
          lose track of the passage of time.

_____ 3. When I'm really concentrating, I don't hear
          what people say to me.

Difficulty making transitions

_____ 1. It is difficult for me to stop an activity when
          it's time to shift to something else.

_____ 2. I can't tear myself away from an activity
          when I'm really engrossed.

Hyperactivity

_____ 1. I tend to fidget or doodle.

_____ 2. I talk so fast that others "can't get a word in."

_____ 3. I hate to sit still for long periods, and find an excuse
          to move around.

_____ 4. I seem to need less sleep than many other women.

_____ 5. I have a high energy level compared to many
          women.

_____ 6. My activity level makes the people around me
          uncomfortable.

Impulsivity

_____ 1. I buy on impulse.

_____ 2. I interrupt others in conversation, even
          when I try not to.

_____ 3. I have impulsively jumped from one job to another.

_____ 4. I have impulsively quit a job, without
          considering the consequences.

_____ 5. I have made major life decisions with little
          planning or forethought.

_____ 6. I tend to "blurt out" whatever I'm thinking,
          though I may later regret it.

Productivity

_____ 1. I just can't seem to keep up the number of
          activities and commitments that my friends
          seem to manage.

_____ 2. I have felt overwhelmed by responsibilities at certain times in my life.

_____ 3. It seems much harder for me than for others to take care of the tasks of daily living.

_____ 4. Keeping up with job demands has been difficult for me.

Problems with initiation

_____ 1. Despite my best intentions, it is often hard for me to get started on a project.

_____ 2. Getting started is much easier when I work with someone else.

Problems with task completion and perseverance

_____ 1. I tend not to finish doing the laundry— it's always "in progress."

_____ 2. I have many unfinished projects that I intend to "get around to."

_____ 3. I pick up and drop hobbies or interests.

_____ 4. I don't meet the long-term goals I set for myself.

Problems making decisions

_____ 1. I have difficulty deciding what to discard and what to keep.

_____ 2. I have difficulty making selections in large department or grocery stores.

_____ 3. Prioritizing is difficult for me   everything seems equally important.

_____ 4. Decision-making is easier if my choices are limited.

_____ 5. I have missed out on opportunities because I couldn't make a decision.

Difficulties in planning

_____ 1. Meal planning is difficult for me.

_____ 2. I rarely plan my day and typically react to events as they occur.

_____ 3. In doing a project, I figure it out as I go along.

_____ 4. I have difficulty planning ahead.

_____ 5. I rarely engage in social activities that require advance planning.

Sensitivity to over-stimulation

_____ 1. Loud noises irritate me.

_____ 2. I don't like to be in large crowds of people.

_____ 3. Shopping centers and large "superstores" feel overwhelming to me.

_____ 4. Fluorescent lighting tends to bother me.

Need for stimulation

_____ 1. I am easily bored.

_____ 2. I enjoy new projects and dislike routine activities.

_____ 3. I have a wide range of interests and activities.

_____ 4. I enjoy making changes in my life.

_____ 5. I thrive on stimulation.

Problems with under-arousal

_____ 1. I am not fully awake and alert for several hours after I rise in the morning.

_____ 2. Getting up in the morning is difficult for me.

_____ 3. I use sugar and/or caffeine to keep myself going during the day.

_____ 4. If my life circumstances allowed it, I would take a daily afternoon nap.

_____ 5. On weekends, I sleep late or nap to catch up on my sleep.

Procrastination

_____ 1. I procrastinate and resist doing tasks that are difficult or unappealing.

_____ 2. I put off tasks until the last minute.

Low motivation/ problems with self-discipline

_____ 1. I tend to do what I like before what I "ought."

_____ 2. I tend not to stick with a goal or project that takes effort.

_____ 3. Many things seem like "too much trouble" to me.

Organizational difficulties

_____ 1. My home is cluttered and messy.

_____ 2. I keep things organized at work, but my personal life is in shambles.

_____ 3. I try to get organized, but I never seem to accomplish my goal.

_____ 4. I have difficulty organizing my thoughts when writing.

_____ 5. I can't seem to manage my paperwork—either at home or at work.

Poor time management

_____ 1. I tend to run late and end up feeling frantic.

_____ 2. I overcrowd my schedule and overcommit myself.

_____ 3. I run late because I try to squeeze in "one last thing."

_____ 4. I run late because I dawdle and lose track of time.

_____ 5. I tend to underestimate how much time an activity will take.

_____ 6. My lateness is a source of irritation to others.

DIFFICULTIES RELATED TO LEARNING DISABILITIES

I was diagnosed with learning disabilities in school.

☐ yes   ☐ no

Reading difficulties

_____ 1. I rarely read for pleasure.

_____ 2. When reading, I can concentrate only if the material is very interesting to me.

_____ 3. I have difficulty recalling information that I have read.

_____ 4. I read slowly.

_____ 5. I must reread text in order to fully comprehend it.

Writing difficulties

_____ 1. Writing papers was my main area of difficulty in school.

_____ 2. I have difficulty organizing my thoughts in writing, even when I am familiar with the subject.

_____ 3. I am more comfortable explaining something verbally than in writing.

_____ 4. Difficulty with writing has caused problems for me at work.

_____ 5. Spelling is difficult for me.

_____ 6. Punctuation and grammar are difficult for me.

Memory problems

_____ 1. I need to speak the moment I think of something in order not to forget it.

_____ 2. I misplace personal belongings.

_____ 3. I have difficulty recalling the names of people and common objects.

_____ 4. I am absentminded.

_____ 5. I have to write things down to remember them.

_____ 6. I forget to do things I intend to do.

_____ 7. I have difficulty remembering multistep-directions or multi-item lists.

_____ 8. My recall is variable and unpredictable.

Problems with motor control

_____ 1. I have poor handwriting.

_____ 2. The legibility of my handwriting is variable.

_____ 3. I tend to bump into or trip over things.

_____ 4. I have poor motor coordination.

DIFFICULTIES IN AREAS OF ADULT RESPONSIBILITY

Parenting

_____ 1. My parenting is inconsistent.

_____ 2. I can't develop routines for myself, much less establish them for my child(ren).

_____ 3. I have difficulty controlling my temper toward my child(ren).

Workplace

_____ 1. I have received unsatisfactory performance ratings at work.

_____ 2. I have quit a job in order to avoid being fired.

_____ 3. I have changed jobs many times, never finding the "right" job.

Life maintenance activities

_____ 1. I don't keep up with housekeeping tasks in a regular, consistent manner.

_____ 2. My home/office are filled with disorganized piles of papers.

_____ 3. Laundry is done at the last possible moment.

_____ 4. My wardrobe is disorganized and in disarray.

_____ 5. I typically neglect making routine medical and/or dental appointments.

_____ 6. I neglect to take care of routine automobile maintenance.

_____ 7. I wait until I'm nearly out of gas before filling my tank.

_____ 8. My life is filled with numerous, avoidable crises.

Financial management

_____ 1. I have difficulty managing my money.

_____ 2. I have a large credit card debt.

_____ 3. I have difficulty balancing my checkbook.

_____ 4. I tend to file my taxes late.

_____ 5. My financial record-keeping is chaotic.

_____ 6. Some years, I have not filed my income tax.

_____ 7. I have a poor credit rating.

PSYCHOLOGICAL ISSUES

I have been diagnosed and treated for:

_____ Depression

_____ Anxiety/panic disorder

_____ Bipolar disorder

_____ Posttraumatic stress disorder

_____ Obsessive-compulsive disorder

Low self-esteem

_____ 1. I tend to hide many aspects of my life from others, fearing that I'll be judged negatively.

_____ 2. People think too highly of me and I fear that I'll be "found out."

_____ 3. I have often felt "stupid" because I couldn't seem to accomplish things that others could.

Moodiness/anxiety

_____ 1. I have felt demoralized by my failures.

_____ 2. I have felt depressed for "no reason."

_____ 3. I am anxious and worry a lot.

_____ 4. I have fears and phobias.

_____ 5. I tend to be irritable and overreact to frustration.

_____ 6. My moods vary day to day.

_____ 7. I suffer from panic attacks.

Obsessive/compulsive tendencies

_____ 1. I have perfectionist tendencies.

_____ 2. Even in unimportant tasks, I feel compelled to do a perfect job.

_____ 3. My perfectionism prevents me from completing tasks in a timely manner.

_____ 4. In my efforts to do a good job, I seem to make things more complicated than they need to be.

_____ 5. There have been periods when I've become obsessed by a particular thought or concern.

Social/interpersonal problems

_____ 1. My lateness and disorganization have caused problems in relationships.

_____ 2. I am separated and/or divorced.

_____ 3. I have been married more than once.

_____ 4. I don't tend to maintain friendships over the long term.

_____ 5. I tend to keep to myself.

_____ 6. I withdraw from other women for fear they will judge me.

_____ 7. I have always felt "different" from other women.

_____ 8. Sometimes I misread people.

_____ 9. I am not a good listener and interrupt or think about other things while someone is talking.

Low frustration tolerance

_____ 1. I hate to wait.

_____ 2. I become frustrated or angry in traffic.

_____ 3. I lose my temper if my children are noisy or argumentative.

_____ 4. I quit tasks out of frustration.

Feelings of underachievement

_____ 1. I should have done better in school.

_____ 2. I have not achieved up to my potential in my career.

_____ 3. I haven't reached the life goals I set for myself.

_____ 4. I feel disappointed in my achievements.

Feeling criticized/misunderstood

_____ 1. I am sensitive to criticism.

_____ 2. I feel that I am viewed negatively by others.

_____ 3. The people close to me don't understand my struggles to manage my life.

OTHER DIFFICULTIES

Hormonal issues

_____ 1. I have PMS symptoms, including moodiness, irritability, and low frustration tolerance.

_____ 2. My PMS symptoms have become worse over the years.

_____ 3. My AD/HD symptoms decreased during pregnancy.

_____ 4. Right before my period, my AD/HD symptoms become worse.

_____ 5. I did well in elementary school, but started having difficulty in middle or high school.

Sleep problems

_____ 1. I am a "night owl" and don't go to sleep at a reasonable hour.

_____ 2. I have difficulty falling asleep because my mind is racing.

_____ 3. If I could sleep on my schedule, I'd sleep from 3 AM to 11 AM.

Fibromyalgia

_____ 1. I have been diagnosed with fibromyalgia,

_____ 2. I have chronic muscle and/or joint pain.

Problem eating patterns

_____ 1. I eat to calm myself.

_____ 2. I tend to overeat.

_____ 3. I have had an eating disorder at sometime in my life.

_____ 4. I have abused laxatives to lose weight.

Substance abuse/addiction
_____ 1. I have a history of substance abuse.
_____ 2. I have abused alcohol.
_____ 3. I smoke cigarettes and have been unable to quit.

Patterns of "self-medication"
_____ 1. I keep myself going throughout the day with coffee, tea, and colas.
_____ 2. I have used cigarettes to improve my concentration.
_____ 3. I have regularly used marijuana, alcohol and/ or other substances to calm myself.

Abuse/trauma
_____ 1. I was repeatedly humiliated or psychologically abused in the classroom as a girl.
_____ 2. I have been in an abusive relationship as an adult.
_____ 3. I have been physically or emotionally abused.
_____ 4. I have been sexually abused.
_____ 5. I have nightmares, flashbacks, and/or extreme anxiety as a result of traumatic event(s).

SECTION

two

MEDICAL ISSUES
FOR WOMEN
WITH AD/HD

CHAPTER 3

Pharmacologic Treatment

Jefferson B. Prince, M.D.
and Timothy E. Wilens, M.D.

Pharmacotherapy should be part of a treatment plan in which consideration is given to all aspects of the patient's life. The administration of medication to women with AD/HD should be undertaken as a collaborative effort between the patient and her physician regarding the use and management of efficacious anti-AD/HD agents. The use of medication should follow a careful evaluation including medical, psychiatric, social, and cognitive assessments. If the patient is engaged in psychotherapy to address the psychological issues and life-management challenges associated with AD/HD, the clinician should also enter into collaboration with the psychotherapist who may be able to provide valuable input regarding a woman's response to medications.

In women with AD/HD, clinicians are challenged with disentangling symptoms of AD/HD from associated comorbid anxiety, mood, and substance use disorders, as well as learning disabilities (Biederman et al., 1993; Biederman et al., 1995; Biederman, 1998). Since alcohol and drug use disorders are frequently encountered in women with AD/HD and may begin at an earlier age (Wilens, Spencer, & Biederman, 1995a), a careful history of substance use is important.

Stimulants in the Treatment of AD/HD in Women

Children and adolescents with AD/HD treated with stimulants consistently demonstrate response rates around 70 percent (Wilens & Spencer, 2000), but adults have responded more equivocally, with response rates ranging from 25 percent (Mattes, Boswell, & Oliver, 1984) to 78 percent (Spencer et al., 1995). Variability in response rate among adults does not seem to be related to gender. Several studies that compared responses to stimulants of men and women found no gender differences in response or side effects (Spencer et al., 1995; Patterson, Douglas, Hallmayer, Hagan, & Krupenia, 1999; Wilens et al., 1999; Spencer et al., 2001). However, higher stimulant dose seems to increase the rate of response. For example, doses of 1.0 mg per kg of body weight per day resulted in more robust responses (Spencer et al., 1995; Iaboni, Bouffard, Minde, & Hechtman, 1996; Spencer et al., 2001) than lower stimulant doses (<0.7 mg/kg/day) (Wender, Reimherr, & Wood, 1981; Mattes et al., 1984). It is therefore important to avoid undermedication in adults.

Initiation of Therapy and Dosing Guidelines

Given the relative paucity of controlled data on the use of stimulants in women with AD/HD, dosing guideline parameters are limited. FDA guidelines for dosing reflect general cautiousness and should not be the only guide for clinical practice. For instance, absolute dose limits (in mg) do not adequately consider the requirements of adults, and may result in underdosing and less than optimal symptom response. Therefore, dosage recommendations should always be individually titrated based on therapeutic efficacy and tolerability.

The overall clinical picture, taking into account all the variables of the patient's current symptom presentation, should guide selection of the initial stimulant. Many patients respond equally well to methylphenidate or amphetamine compounds (Greenhill & Osman, 1999). When using short-acting stimulants, treatment should be started at the lowest possible dose. Initiation of treatment with once-daily dosing in the morning is advisable until an acceptable response is noted. Treatment generally starts at five mg of methylphenidate, dextroamphetamine, or amphetamine compound once daily and is titrated upward every three to five days until an effect is noted or adverse effects emerge. Repeat dosing through the day is dependent on duration of effectiveness, wear-off, and side effects. Typically, the half-life of the short-acting stimulants necessitates at least twice-daily dosing with the addition of similar or reduced afternoon doses depending on breakthrough symptoms. Typical adult dosing of methylphenidate is up to 30 mg three to four times daily, amphetamine 15 to 20 mg three to four times a day, and pemoline 75 to 225 mg daily. If an adult with AD/HD symptoms is unresponsive, or if significant side effects to the initial stimulant are experienced, consideration of an alternative stimulant or class of agents is recommended.

New Stimulant Preparations

At the present time, treatment with stimulants appears to be moving in the direction of longer acting delivery systems. Recently, the OROS system (an "osmotic pump") has been used in the development of Concerta™ to release methylphenidate for approximately eight to nine hours, thus affecting symptoms for between 10-14 hours. Concerta™ is started at 18 mg and increased in weekly 18 mg increments, as tolerated, to an effective dose level. The clinician should be aware that 18 mg of Concerta™ is bioequivalent to 15 mg total daily dose of immediate release MPH. This once a day delivery system offers the potential advantage of improving adherence to prescribed regimens. Similarly, Metadate® was recently approved as an extended release preparation. This medication consists of two types of beads with different polymer coatings that deliver MPH in a bi-phasic pattern, providing at least eight to nine hours of coverage. At this time, Metadate® is only available in 20 mg strength and is bubble packaged, enabling careful monitoring of the amount of medication taken in order to promote better compliance. Other longer-acting stimulant preparations and patches are expected to be available soon.

Monitoring Treatment with Stimulants

Once pharmacotherapy is initiated, monthly contact with the patient is recommended during the initial phase of treatment to carefully monitor response and adverse effects. Given that many adults with AD/HD have coexisting conditions, once a successful regimen of medications is identified, the clinician should monitor continued response, as well as the emergence or worsening of other symptoms. For instance, some concerns have been raised that Adderall® may cause an increase in anxiety, thus patients with coexisting anxiety disorder should be closely monitored on Adderall® (Horrigan & Barnhill, 2000). Likewise, for patients with mood disorders, long-term use of stimulants necessitates regular careful monitoring for reemergence of depression and/or mania. Patients need to be educated to recognize the symptoms of mood disturbances and how they differ from their AD/HD symptomatology.

Although not formally investigated, women with AD/HD have described variability in the efficacy of the stimulants over the course of their menstrual cycle. This anecdotal observation may be understood as we continue to investigate estrogen's influence on attention, memory, and mood (McEwen & Alves, 1999).

The Use of Stimulants in Patients with a History of Substance Abuse

Despite the theoretical abuse potential of the stimulants, there have been no reports of any cases of stimulant abuse in controlled or retrospective studies of adults with AD/HD (Langer, Sweeney, Bartenbach, Davis, & Menander, 1986). The clinician should be cautious when using stimulants in a substance abusing/using population and should monitor for substance use/abuse. If substance abuse in the patient with AD/HD is being considered, the clinician should conduct urine screens or hair sampling, keeping in mind that methylphenidate will not be identified on the urine screen under the amphetamine category, since it is metabolized primarily to ritalinic acid (Wilens & Spencer, 1998). Additionally, if patients are actively using substances, it is prudent to address issues of substance abuse before trying to address issues of AD/HD. However, if the substance use/abuse coexists with mood disorders, clinicians may need to address the mood issues concurrently with substance abuse treatment. After these issues are stable, then the clinician may reevaluate and address the AD/HD.

Side Effects of Stimulants

Adults with AD/HD generally tolerate stimulants well. However, the most frequently reported side effects are insomnia, edginess, diminished appetite, weight loss, dysphoria, obsessiveness, tics, and headaches (Wilens & Spencer, 2000). At therapeutic doses, no cases of stimulant-related psychosis have been reported in adults (Wilens & Spencer, 2000). The addition of low-dose beta-blockers (i.e., propanolol at 10 mg up to three times daily or buspirone, five to 10 mg up to three times daily) may be helpful in reducing the edginess/agitation associated with stimulant administration (Ratey, Greenberg, & Lindem, 1991).

Although concerns about cardiovascular adverse effects of stimulants have been raised (Werry & Aman, 1975), the effects of stimulants appear minimal, with slight elevations of heart rate and blood pressure that are only weakly correlated with dose (Brown, Wynne, & Slimmer, 1984; Kelly, Rapport, & DuPaul, 1988). In adults with normal blood pressure, stimulants increase systolic and diastolic blood pressure approximately four mm Hg and increase heart rate less than 10 beats per minute (Spencer et al., 1995; Wilens et al., 1997; Spencer et al., 1999). While these studies are reassuring, long-term data is lacking, as is data in adults with borderline hypertension. Clinicians should inquire about familial hypertension, regularly follow the patient's blood pressure, and proceed with caution for patients with borderline hypertension.

Medication Interactions

The interactions of the stimulants with other prescription and nonprescription medications are generally mild and not a source of concern (Wilens & Spencer, 2000). Taking sympathomimetics (i.e., pseudoephedrine) with stimulants may potentiate the effects of both medications. Antihistamines, on the other hand, may diminish the stimulant's effectiveness. Patients should be cautioned to limit the amount of citrus juices they drink since acidification of the urine increases excretion of amphetamines, reducing their effectiveness.

The use of stimulants with antidepressants is common, due to the high rate of coexistence of AD/HD and depression. A recent study (Cohen et al., 1999) showed minimal drug interaction between stimulants and tricyclic antidepressants, bupropion, or the SSRIs. Extreme caution is called for when combining stimulants and antidepressants of the monoamine oxidase inhibitor (MAOI) type due to the potential for hypertensive reactions.

Non-Stimulant Medications in the Treatment of AD/HD in Women

Despite the increasing use of stimulants for adults with AD/HD, studies have shown that up to 50 percent do not respond. A meta-analysis of data on these lower response rates suggests that lower responses are likely due to methodological limitations, i.e., varying diagnostic criteria and use of stimulant doses that are too low (Wilens & Spencer, 2000). Recent studies using stringent diagnostic criteria and more robust dosing show response rates consistent with response rates in children (Wilens & Spencer, 2000). For adults who have untoward side effects or experience an increase in coexisting symptoms such as anxiety, there are a number of non-stimulant options including antidepressants and antihypertensives, among others.

Atomoxetine

Atomoxetine is a selective norepinephrine reuptaker inhibitor, which is indicated for the treatment of AD/HD in children, adolescents, and adults. Its mode of action in the treatment of AD/HD is currently not known. However, it is the only medication that affects the regulation of norepinephine by acting as an of the presynaptic norepinerhrine transporter. It is not associated with an appreciable abuse potential and is not a controlled substance.

Dosing of atomoxetine depends on body weight. Children up to 70 kg body weight should begin with 0.5 mg/kg/day; the dose should be increased to 1.2 mg/kg/day after a minimum of 3 days on the initial dose. The maximum dose should be the lesser of 1.4mg/ kg/day or 100 mg/day. Individuals over 70 kg body weight should begin with 40 mg/day; with an increase to 80 mg/day after a minimum of 3 days.

After 2 to 4 additional weeks, the dose may be increased to a maximum of 100 mg/day in patients who have not reached optimal response. Side effects include initial weight loss, gastrointestinal distress, somnolence, and some dizziness.

Tricyclic Antidepressants (TCAs)

Over the past twenty years, the tricyclic antidepressants (TCAs) have been used as alternatives to the stimulants for AD/HD in pediatrics (Spencer et al., 1996). Despite extensive experience in children and adolescents (Spencer et al., 1996), there are only two studies of these agents in treating adult AD/HD. Compared to the stimulants, TCAs have negligible abuse potential, convenient single daily dosing, and efficacy for coexisting anxiety and depression. TCAs, however, are a less optimal choice than stimulants in addressing AD/HD symptomatology for several reasons—response rates are less robust than for stimulants, and side effects are more difficult to tolerate, with more lethal potential in overdose compared to stimulants.

Bupropion

The atypical antidepressant bupropion appears to enhance both noradrenergic and dopaminergic neurotransmission (Ascher et al., 1995). Bupropion is reported to be moderately helpful in reducing AD/HD symptoms in children (Casat, Pleasants, & Fleet, 1987) and moderately effective in comparison to methylphenidate (Barrickman et al., 1995). Given bupropion's lower response rate and delayed therapeutic effect compared to the stimulants and desipramine, it should be considered a second-line medication for the treatment of uncomplicated AD/HD. However, bupropion's tolerability, lack of cardiac adverse effects, and lack of need to monitor blood levels, also make it an attractive second-line agent. For patients with coexisting substance use disorders and/or mood lability, or in adults with cardiac abnormalities (Gelenberg, Bassuk, & Schoonover, 1991), bupropion may be considered a first-line treatment. For patients with improvement, but lack of full response to bupropion, clinicians may empirically consider addition of a low dose of stimulant. In addition, given the high rates of smoking in adults with AD/HD, as well as the ability of bupropion to facilitate smoking cessation, bupropion may be a first-line treatment for those patients with AD/HD who are smokers (Hurt et al., 1997; Shiffman et al., 2000).

Selective Serotonin Reuptake Inhibitors (SSRIs)

Although one small open trial suggests the benefit of fluoxetine for the treatment of AD/HD in children (Barrickman, Noyes, Kuperman, Schumacher, & Verda, 1991), the selective serotonin reuptake inhibitors (SSRIs) have not been systematically studied in the treatment of AD/HD. Given the SSRIs' lack of noradrenergic/dopaminergic effects, they do not appear to be effective medications for the treatment of the core symptoms of AD/HD (Spencer et al., 1996). However, venlafaxine, an antidepressant with both serotonergic and noradrenergic properties, may have anti-AD/HD efficacy. Venlafaxine may be combined with stimulants for treatment of AD/HD in adults, with ongoing blood pressure monitoring recommended.

Antihypertensives

The antihypertensives, clonidine and guanfacine, have been used in childhood AD/HD, in cases with a marked hyperactive or aggressive component (Spencer et al., 1996). However, because of a lack of efficacy data and concerns of their sedative and hypotensive effects, use in adults remains dubious. Beta-blockers may be helpful in adult AD/HD, but have not been studied under controlled conditions (Mattes, 1986; Ratey et al., 1991).

Cholinergic Agents

The relationship of nicotine and AD/HD has attracted significant attention including findings of higher than expected overlap of cigarette smoking and AD/HD in children (Milberger, Biederman, Faraone, Chen, & Jones, 1997) and higher rates of nicotine use in adults with AD/HD (Pomerleau, Downey, Stelson, & Pomerleau, 1995). One small study of two days duration showed a significant reduction in AD/HD symptoms in adults wearing standard size nicotine patches (Conners et al., 1996). Moreover, the authors have observed the efficacy of the nicotine patch in reducing AD/HD symptoms in smokers who report the emergence of AD/HD symptoms with cigarette cessation.

Wake-promoting Agents

Modafanil is a wake-promoting agent indicated for the treatment of daytime sleepiness associated with narcolepsy. Unlike stimulants, modafinil appears to indirectly activate the frontal cortex through the hypothalamus and/or tuberomam millary nucleus rather than via central dopaminergic and/or noradrenergic pathways (Eastbrooke, Chou, Miller, Saper, & Scammell, 1999). At this time, modafinil's role is generally limited to patients with refractory AD/HD.

Clinical Strategies for the Pharmacotherapy of AD/HD in Women

Having established the diagnosis of AD/HD as the primary current problem, patients should be familiarized with the risks and benefits of pharmacotherapy, the availability of alternative treatments, the likelihood of adverse effects, as well as the prognosis both with and without medications (Brown, 2000). Patient expectations need to be explored and realistic goals of treatment defined. Likewise, the clinician should educate the patient that each medication trial requires adherence to the dosing regimen, as well as use clinically meaningful doses of the medication for a reasonable duration of time. Psychological issues secondary to AD/HD, such as interpersonal difficulties, low self-esteem, and self-sabotaging patterns in their personal and professional lives, respond best to psychotherapeutic treatment concomitant with medication prescribed to address AD/HD symptomatology

(Bemporad & Zambenedetti, 1996; Ratey, Hallowell, & Miller, 1997; McDermott, 2000).

Stimulant medications are considered the first-line therapy for AD/HD in women. Given the variability in effective dose, stimulants are typically started at low doses (e.g., Ritalin 5 mg; Concerta™ 18 mg; Metadate® 20 mg; Adderall® 5 mg; Dexedrine® 5 mg) in the morning and gradually titrated upwards. Tolerability of the medication, as well as duration of effect, should be noted by the patient. Although women with AD/HD are acceptable reporters of their own conditions, it is often clinically useful to get input from the patient's significant other(s) (Murphy & Schachar, 2000). However, if no one is available to provide independent observation, data from patients can be relied upon (Murphy & Schachar, 2000). Decisions on how many doses a day and how many days of the week to take the medication should be tailored for each patient (Zametkin & Ernst, 1999). If the patient is not responding to one stimulant, it is reasonable to prescribe an alternative type of stimulant (Elia, Borcherding, Rapoport, & Keysor, 1991). The response to the stimulants is generally rapid (Wood, Reimherr, Wender, & Johnson, 1976; Spencer et al., 1995).

For patients who do not respond to an initial stimulant trial or who experience intolerable side effects, second-line agents should be considered. In addition, clinicians should consider if another coexisting disorder is primary. Typically, clinicians must distinguish anxiety and depressive disorders from core AD/HD. Anxiety and depressive disorders may also obfuscate underlying AD/HD in women. Although not formally studied, this trend may lead to under-recognition of AD/HD in women and result in under-treatment. Once the issue of coexisting anxiety and depression is adequately addressed, it will be necessary to reevaluate AD/HD symptomatology. In addition, given recent data on the ability of 17ß-estradiol (estrogen replacement therapy) to improve both mood and somatic symptoms in perimenopausal women, consideration must be given to the patient's hormonal state (de Novaes Soares, Almeida, Joffe, & Cohen, 2001). Life events where hormones are naturally in flux (i.e., menarche, delivery, and menopause) may also adversely impact mood and cognition. Treatment with exogenous estrogen may be indicated.

TCAs and bupropion may improve stimulant side effects as well as address coexisting anxiety or depression. It must be kept in mind that the response to antidepressants is slower compared to stimulants (Wilens et al., 1996). Although some adults may respond to relatively low doses of the TCAs (Ratey, Greenberg, Bemporad, & Lindem, 1992), the majority of adults appear to require solid antidepressant dosing of these agents (i.e., desipramine >150 mg daily). The SSRIs and other antidepressants have more utility for coexisting depression, anxiety, or obsessive-compulsive disorder than for treating core AD/HD symptoms. The effects of age, long-term adverse effects, gender, and stimulant use in substance abusing subgroups of AD/HD remains unstudied. The monitoring of routine side effects, vital signs, and the misuse of the medication is appropriate. The antihypertensive may be useful in adults with AD/HD and aggressive outbursts (Mattes, 1986), tic disorders, impulse control disorders, bipolar disorder, or those with adverse reactions to first and second line medications. The amino acids have not been shown to be effective, and the cholinergic enhancing compounds have yet to be studied comprehensively in AD/HD adults.

Women with ongoing substance abuse or dependence should generally not be treated until appropriate addiction treatments have been undertaken and the patient has maintained a drug and alcohol free period. The authors' experience attempting to treat adults with AD/HD and ongoing substance use disorders indicates the necessity of addressing the coexisting substance use first, and then reassessing and treating the AD/HD. Combining pharmacotherapy and psychotherapy may be particularly necessary for women with AD/HD and coexisting substance use disorders. These patients face the difficulty of overcoming their AD/HD-associated poor impulse control which may compromise their ability to successfully use effective strategies to cope with cravings and reactions to triggers (Aviram, Rhum, & Levin, 2001).

Other concurrent psychiatric disorders may also require evaluation. In subjects with AD/HD plus bipolar mood disorder, for example, the risk of mania needs to be addressed and closely monitored during the treatment of AD/HD. In cases such as these, the conservative introduction of AD/HD medications along with mood stabilizing agents should be considered.

Since learning disabilities do not respond to pharmacotherapy, it is important to identify these deficits to help define remedial interventions. For instance, this evaluation may assist in the design and implementation of an educational plan for the adult who may be returning to school, or serve as an aid for structuring the current work environment. Appropriate remedial strategies should be employed to address the morbidity of these factors at work and in school.

Combined Pharmacotherapy

Although systematic data assessing the efficacy and safety profile of combining agents for AD/HD in women are lacking, empiric use of combination treatment may be necessary in patients with residual symptomatology on single agents or with psychiatric conditions. For example, in a recent naturalistic report on TCAs for adults with AD/HD, 84 percent of adults were receiving additional psychoactive medications with 59 percent receiving adjunctive stimulants (Wilens et al., 1995b). These findings are similar to controlled data in juvenile AD/HD in which the combination of methylphenidate and desipramine improved response more than either agent used singly (Rapport, Carlson, Kelly, & Pataki, 1993). The use of methylphenidate conjointly with fluoxetine has been reported to be well tolerated and useful in improving depression in AD/HD adolescents (Gammon & Brown, 1993) and appears useful in adults with the same conditions. While the stimulants appear to be well tolerated with TCAs and SSRIs (Cohen et al., 1999), clinicians should consider potential drug interactions as have been described between TCAs and some SSRIs (Aranow et al., 1989).

Managing Sub-optimal Responses

Despite the availability of various agents for adults with AD/HD, there appears to be a number of individuals who either do not respond, or are intolerant of adverse effects of medications used to treat their AD/HD. In managing difficult cases, several therapeutic strategies are available. If adverse psychiatric effects develop concurrent with a poor medication response, alternate treatments should be pursued. Severe psychiatric symptoms that emerge during the acute phase can be problematic, irrespective of the efficacy of the medications for AD/HD. These symptoms may require reconsideration of the diagnosis of AD/HD and careful reassessment of the presence of coexisting disorders. For example, it is common to observe depressive symptoms in AD/HD adults independent of the AD/HD or its treatment. If reduction of dose or change in preparation (i.e., regular, slow-release, or long-acting) do not resolve the problem, consideration should be given to alternative treatments. Neuroleptic medications should be considered as part of the overall treatment plan in the face of coexisting bipolar disorder or extreme agitation. Concurrent nonpharmacologic interventions such as behavioral or cognitive therapy may assist with symptom reduction.

STRATEGIES IN DIFFICULT CASES OF ADULT AD/HD

(Adapted from Wilens and Spencer, 2000)

Symptoms	Interventions
Worsening or unchanged AD/HD symptoms (inattention, impulsivity, hyperactivity)	▶ Change medication dose (increase or decrease) ▶ Change timing of dose ▶ Change preparation, substitute stimulant ▶ Evaluate for possible tolerance ▶ Consider adjunctive treatment (antidepressant, alpha-adrenergic agent, cognitive enhancer) ▶ Consider adjusting non-pharmacologic treatment (cognitive/behavioral therapies, coaching, or reevaluating neuropsychological profile for executive functioning)
Intolerable side effects	▶ Evaluate if side effect is drug-induced ▶ Assess medication response vs. tolerability of side effect ▶ Aggressive management of side effect (change timing of dose; change preparation of stimulant; adjunctive or alternative treatment)
Symptoms of rebound	▶ Change timing of dose ▶ Supplement with small dose of short-acting stimulant or alpha-adrenergic agent one hour prior to symptom onset ▶ Change preparation ▶ Increase frequency of dosage

Symptoms	Interventions
Development of tics or TS, or use with comorbid tics or TS	▶ Assess persistence of tics or TS If tics abate,rechallenge ▶ If tics worsen with stimulant treatment, discontinue ▶ Consider stimulant use with adjunctive anti-tic treatment (haldol, pimozide) or use of alternative treatment (antidepressants, alpha-adrenergic agents)
Emergence of dysphoria, irritability, acceleration, agitation	▶ Assess for toxicity or rebound ▶ Evaluate development or exacerbation of comorbidity (mood, anxiety, and substance use including nicotine and caffeine) ▶ Change stimulant preparation ▶ Assess sleep and mood ▶ Consider alternative treatment
Emergence of major depression, mood lability, or marked anxiety symptoms	▶ Assess for toxicity or rebound ▶ Evaluate development or exacerbation of comorbidity ▶ Reduce or discontinue stimulant ▶ Consider use of antidepressant or antimanic agent ▶ Assess substance use ▶ Consider nonpharmacologic interventions
Emergence of psychosis or mania	▶ Discontinue stimulant ▶ Assess comorbidity ▶ Assess substance use ▶ Treat psychosis or mania

Summary

In summary, while research is limited, the literature supports pharmacotherapy as an effective treatment for women with AD/HD. Effective pharmacological treatments for AD/HD in women include the stimulants, antidepressants, and a variety of other medications. Most controlled investigations in adults with AD/HD have studied the stimulants. There tends to be a dose-related improvement in AD/HD symptoms with the stimulant medications in adults that is not gender specific. This literature supports the stimulants as the most effective available treatment for AD/HD symptoms in women. Several nonstimulant alternatives have been investigated. Although these data are limited, medications with catecholaminergic activity appear to have efficacy, whereas those with predominately serotonergic properties appear ineffective in the treatment of core AD/HD symptomatology. In cases with coexisting psychiatric conditions, residual symptoms, or adverse effects, clinical experience coupled with some literature support combining medications such as the stimulants and antidepressants. Often, cognitive/behavioral-based psychotherapies are necessary in conjunction with medication in order to fully address executive function deficits, dynamic issues (within individual and family), and residual symptomatology, as well as comorbid psychopathology in adults with AD/HD. Future controlled studies applying stringent diagnostic criteria and outcome methodology are necessary to enhance the range of pharmacotherapeutic options for women with AD/HD.

References

American Psychiatric Association. (1994). *Diagnostic and statistical manual of mental disorders (4th ed., rev.).* Washington, DC: Author.

Aranow, R. B., Hudson, J. L., Pope, H. G., Grady, T. A., Laage, T. A., Bell, I. R., & Cole, J. O. (1989). Elevated antidepressant plasma levels after addition of fluoxetine. *American Journal of Psychiatry, 146,* 911-913.

Ascher, J. A., Cole, J. O., Colin, J., Feighner, J. P., Ferris, R. M., Fibiger, H. C., Golden, R. N., Martin, P., Potter, W. Z., Richelson, E., & Sulser, F. (1995). Bupropion: A review of its mechanism of antidepressant activity. *Journal of Clinical Psychiatry, 56,* 395-401.

Aviram, R. B., Rhum, M., & Levin, F. R. (2001). Psychotherapy of adults with comorbid attention-deficit/hyperactivity disorder and psychoactive substance use disorder. *Journal of Psychotherapy Practice and Research, 10,* 179-186.

Barrickman, L., Noyes, R., Kuperman, S., Schumacher, E., & Verda, M. (1991). Treatment of AD/HD with fluoxetine: A preliminary trial. *Journal of the American Academy of Child and Adolescent Psychiatry, 30,* 762-767.

Barrickman, L., Perry, P., Allen, A., Kuperman, S., Arndt, S., Herrmann, K., & Schumacher, E. (1995). Bupropion versus methylphenidate in the treatment of attention-deficit hyperactivity disorder. *Journal of the American Academy of Child and Adolescent Psychiatry, 34,* 649-657.

Bemporad, J., & Zambenedetti, M. (1996). Psychotherapy of adults with attention deficit disorder. *Journal of Psychotherapy, 5,* 228-237.

Biederman, J. (1998). Attention-deficit/hyperactivity disorder: A life-span perspective. *Journal of Clinical Psychiatry, 59,* 4-16.

Biederman, J., Faraone, S. V., Spencer, T., Wilens, T., Norman, D., Lapey, K., Mick, E., Krifcher-Lehman, B., & Doyle, A. (1993). Patterns of psychiatric comorbidity, cognition and psychosocial functioning in adults with attention deficit hyperactivity disorder. *American Journal of Psychiatry, 150,* 1792-1798.

Biederman, J., Wilens, T., Mick, E., Milberger, S., Spencer, T., & Faraone, S. (1995). Psychoactive substance use disorder in adults with attention deficit hyperactivity disorder: Effects of AD/HD and psychiatric comorbidity. *American Journal of Psychiatry, 152,* 1652-1658.

Bressa, G. M. (1994). S-adenosyl-L-methionine (SAM-e) as antidepressant: Meta-analysis of clinical studies. *Acta Neurological Scandinavia Supplement, 154,* 7-14.

Brown, R. T., Wynne, M. E., & Slimmer, L. W. (1984). Attention deficit disorder and the effect of methylphenidate on attention, behavioral, and cardiovascular functioning. *Journal of Clinical Psychiatry, 45,* 473-476.

Brown, T. E. (Ed.). (2000). *Attention-deficit disorders and comorbidities in children, adolescents, and adults.* Washington, DC: American Psychiatric Press.

Brown, R., Colman, C., & Bottiglieri, T. (1999). *Stop depression now: SAM-e, the breakthrough supplement that works as well as prescription drugs in half the time...with no side effects.* New York: Putnam Publishing Group.

Casat, C. D., Pleasants, D. Z., & Fleet, J. V. W. (1987). A double-blind trial of bupropion in children with attention deficit disorder. *Psychopharmacology Bulletin, 23,* 120-122.

Cohen, L., Biederman, J., Wilens, T., Spencer, T., Mick, E., Faraone, S., Prince, J., & Flood, J. (1999). Desipramine clearance in children and adolescents: Absence of effect of development and gender. *Journal of the American Academy of Child & Adolescent Psychiatry, 38,* 79-85.

Conners, C., Levin, E. D., Sparrow, E., Hinton, S., Erhardt, D., Meck, W., Rose, J., & March, J. (1996). Nicotine and attention in adult attention deficit hyperactivity disorder. *Psychopharmacology Bulletin, 32,* 67-73.

de Novaes Soares, C., Almeida, O. P., Joffe, H., & Cohen, L. S. (2001). Efficacy of estradiol for the treatment of depressive disorders in perimenopausal women. *Archives of General Psychiatry, 58,* 529-534.

Eastbrooke, I., Chou, T., Miller, M., Saper, C., & Scammell, T. (1999). Modafinil activates arousal and autonomic regions. *Society for Neuroscience Abstracts, 25,* 1134.

Elia, J., Borcherding, B. G., Rapoport, J. L., & Keysor, C. S. (1991). Methylphenidate and dextroamphetamine treatments of hyperactivity: Are there true nonresponders? *Psychiatry Research, 36,* 141-155.

Gammon, G. D., & Brown, T. E. (1993). Fluoxetine and methylphenidate in combination for treatment of attention deficit disorder and comorbid depressive disorder. *Journal of Child and Adolescent Psychopharmacology, 3,* 1-10.

Gelenberg, A. J., Bassuk, E. L., & Schoonover, S. C. (1991). *The practitioner's guide to psychoactive drugs* (3rd ed.). New York: Plenum Medical Book Company.

Greenhill, L. L., & Osman, B. B. (1999). *Ritalin: Theory and practice.* New York: Mary Ann Liebert, Inc.

Horrigan, J. P., & Barnhill, L. J. (2000). Low-dose amphetamine salts and adult attention-deficit/hyperactivity disorder. *Journal of Clinical Psychiatry, 61,* 414-417.

Hurt, R. D., Sachs, D. P., Glover, E. D., Offord, K. P., Johnston, J. A., Dale, L. C., Khayrallah, M. A., Schroeder, D. R., Glover, P. N., Sullivan, C. R., Croghan, I. T., & Sullivan, P. M. (1997). A comparison of sustained-release bupropion and placebo for smoking cessation. *New England Journal of Medicine, 337,* 1195-1202.

Iaboni, F., Bouffard, R., Minde, K., & Hechtman, L. (1996). The efficacy of methylphenidate in treating adults with attention-deficit/hyperactivity disorder. In *Scientific Proceedings of the 43rd Annual Meeting of the American Academy of Child and Adolescent Psychiatry,* Philadelphia, PA.

Kelly, K. L., Rapport, M. D., & DuPaul, G. J. (1988). Attention deficit disorder and methylphenidate: A multistep analysis of dose-response effects on children's cardiovascular functioning. *International Clinical Psychopharmacology, 3,*167-181.

Langer, D. H., Sweeney, K. P., Bartenbach, D. E., Davis, P. M., & Menander, K. B. (1986). Evidence of lack of abuse or dependence following pemoline treatment: Results of a retrospective survey. *Drug and Alcohol Dependency, 17,* 213-227.

Mattes, J. A. (1986). Propanolol for adults with temper outbursts and residual attention deficit disorder. *Journal of Clinical Psychopharmacology, 6,* 299-302.

Mattes, J. A., Boswell, L., & Oliver, H. (1984). Methylphenidate effects on symptoms of attention deficit disorder in adults. *Archives of General Psychiatry, 41,*1059-1063.

McDermott, S.P. (2000). Cognitive therapy for adults with attention-deficit/hyperactivity disorder. In T.E. Brown, (Ed.). *Attention-deficit disorders in children, adolescents, and adults.* Washington, DC: American Psychiatric Press.

McEwen, B. S., & Alves, S. E. (1999). Estrogen actions in the central nervous system. *Endocrine Reviews, 20,* 279-307.

Milberger, S., Biederman, J., Faraone, S., Chen, L., & Jones, J. (1997). AD/HD is associated with early initiation of cigarette smoking in children and adolescents. *Journal of the American Academy of Child and Adolescent Psychiatry, 36,* 37-43.

Murphy, P., & Schachar, R. (2000). Use of self-ratings in the assessment of symptoms of attention deficit hyperactivity disorder in adults. *American Journal of Psychiatry, 157,* 1156-1159.

Patterson, R., Douglas, C., Hallmayer, J., Hagan, M., & Krupenia, Z. (1999). A randomized, double-blind, placebo-controlled trial of dextroamphetamine in adults with attention deficit hyperactivity disorder. *Australian and New Zealand Journal of Psychiatry, 33,* 494-502.

Pomerleau, O., Downey, K., Stelson, F., & Pomerleau, C. (1995). Cigarette smoking in adult patients diagnosed with attention deficit hyperactivity disorder. *Journal of Substance Abuse, 7,* 373-378.

Rapport, M. D., Carlson, G. A., Kelly, K. L., & Pataki, C. (1993). Methylphenidate and desipramine in hospitalized children: Separate and combined effects on cognitive function. *Journal of the American Academy of Child and Adolescent Psychiatry, 32,* 333-342.

Ratey, J., Greenberg, M., & Lindem, K. (1991). Combination of treatments for attention deficit disorders in adults. *Journal of Nervous and Mental Diseases, 176,* 699-701.

Ratey, J., Hallowell, E., & Miller, A. (1997). Psychosocial issues and psychotherapy in adults with attention deficit disorder. *Psychiatric Annals, 27,* 228-237.

Ratey, J. J., Greenberg, M. S., Bemporad, J. R., & Lindem, K. J. (1992). Unrecognized attention-deficit hyperactivity disorder in adults presenting for outpatient psychotherapy. *Journal of Child and Adolescent Psychopharmacology, 2,* 267-275.

Shekim, W. O., Antun, F., Hanna, G. L., McCracken, J. T., & Hess, E. B. (1990). S-adenosyl-L-methionine (SAM-e) in adults with AD/HD, RS: Preliminary results from an open trial. *Psychopharmacology Bulletin, 26,* 249-253.

Shiffman, S., Johnston, J. A., Khayrallah, M., Elash, C. A., Gwaltney, C. J., Paty, J. A., Gnys, M., Evoniuk, G., & Devaugh-Geiss, J. (2000). The effect of bupropion on nicotine craving and withdrawal. *Psychopharmacology, 148,* 33-40.

Spencer, T., Biederman, J., Wilens, T., Faraone, S., Prince, J., Girard, K., Doyle, R., Parekh, A., Kagan, J., & Bearman, S. K. (2001). Efficacy of a mixed amphetamine salts compound in adults with attention-deficit/hyperactivity disorder. *Archives of General Psychiatry.*

Spencer, T., Biederman, J., Wilens, T., Harding, M., O'Donnell, D., & Griffin, S. (1996). Pharmacotherapy of attention deficit disorder across the life cycle. *The Journal of the American Academy of Child and Adolescent Psychiatry, 35,* 409-432.

Spencer, T., Biederman, J., Wilens, T., Prince, J., Girard, K., Parekh, A., Doyle, R., Kagan, J., & Bearman, S. K. (1999). Efficacy and tolerability of Adderall in adults with AD/HD. In *Scientific Proceedings of the 46th Annual Meeting of the American Academy of Child and Adolescent Psychiatry,* Chicago.

Spencer, T., Wilens, T. E., Biederman, J., Faraone, S. V., Ablon, S., & Lapey, K. (1995). A double-blind, crossover comparison of methylphenidate and placebo in adults with childhood-onset attention deficit hyperactivity disorder. *Archives of General Psychiatry, 52,* 434-443.

Wender, P. H., Reimherr, F. W., & Wood, D. R. (1981). Attention deficit disorder ('minimal brain dysfunction') in adults: A replication study of diagnosis and drug treatment. *Archives of General Psychiatry, 38,* 449-456.

Werry, J. S., & Aman, M. G. (1975). Methylphenidate and haloperidol in children. *Archives of General Psychiatry, 32,* 790-795.

Wilens, T., Biederman, J., Prince, J., Spencer, T., Schleifer, D., Harding, M., Linehan, C., & Hatch, M. (1996). A double-blind, placebo-controlled trial of desipramine for adults with AD/HD. *American Journal of Psychiatry, 153,* 1147-1153.

Wilens, T., Biederman, J., Spencer, T., Frazier, J., Prince, J., Bostic, J., Rater, M., Soriano, J., Hatch, M., Sienna, M., Millstein, R., & Abrantes, A. (1999). A controlled trial of high-dose pemoline for adults with attention-deficit/hyperactivity disorder. *Journal of Clinical Psychopharmacology, 19,* 257-264.

Wilens, T., Frazier, J., Prince, J., Spencer, T., Bostic, J., Hatch, M., Abrantes, A., Sienna, M., Soriano, J., Millstein, R., & Biederman, J. (1997). A double-blind comparison of pemoline in adults with AD/HD. In *Scientific proceedings of the 44th Annual Meeting of the American Academy of Child and Adolescent Psychiatry*, Toronto.

Wilens, T., & Spencer, T. (1998). Pharmacology of amphetamines. In R. Tarter, R. Ammerman, & P. Ott (Eds.). *Handbook of substance abuse: Neurobehavioral pharmacology.* New York: Plenum Press.

Wilens, T., Spencer, T., & Biederman, J. (1995a). Are attention-deficit hyperactivity disorder and the psychoactive substance use disorders really related? *Harvard Review of Psychiatry, 3,* 260-262.

Wilens, T. E., Biederman, J., Mick, E., & Spencer, T. (1995b). A systematic assessment of tricyclic antidepressants in the treatment of adult attention-deficit hyperactivity disorder. *Journal of Nervous and Mental Diseases, 184,* 48-50.

Wilens, T. E., & Spencer, T. J. (2000). The stimulants revisited. In *Child and adolescent psychiatric clinics of North America.* Philadelphia: Saunders Press.

Wood, D. R., Reimherr, F. W., Wender, P. H., & Johnson, G. E. (1976). Diagnosis and treatment of minimal brain dysfunction in adults. *Archives of General Psychiatry, 3*3, 1453-1460.

Zametkin, A. J., & Ernst, M. (1999). Problems in the management of attention deficit hyperactivity disorder. *The New England Journal of Medicine, 340,* 40-46.

CHAPTER 4

Medication Use during Pregnancy:
A Concern for Women with AD/HD

David W. Goodman, M.D.
and Patricia O. Quinn, M.D.

The recent recognition of AD/HD as a lifelong disorder affecting three to five percent of the adult population has left thousands of women of childbearing age asking questions about the safety of taking medications used to treat this disorder and its related conditions during pregnancy. Because women with AD/HD are often treated with multiple medications, it is important to understand the benefits and risks of each of these medications when used during pregnancy.

In evaluating the safety of any medication during pregnancy, several concerns must be addressed. Will the medication have a negative effect on the developing fetus, resulting in physical deformities or causing neurological, behavioral or cognitive deficits? Does the use of medication predispose women to premature delivery or undersized infants? Does taking medication throughout the pregnancy result in withdrawal symptoms in the newborn? Might there be other long-term problems associated with exposure before birth?

The answers to these questions are not always clear. Human studies present ethical limitations and results from animal studies are not always applicable to humans. Doses given to laboratory animals usually far exceed those customarily used in adults, thus not allowing for generalizations to pregnant women.

When considering the use of medication during pregnancy, benefits and risks exist for mother and fetus/infant during four phases: 1) Pregnancy, 2) Delivery, 3) Breastfeeding, and 4) Infancy/toddlerhood. These latter include the risk of developing changes in mood, cognition, behaviors and intelligence during the life of the child due to the exposure of a specific medication during the pregnancy. The traditional and prudent medical recommendation has been to avoid all medication during pregnancy. Certainly this approach eliminates any risk to the fetus. What this traditional approach had not considered is the risk to the mother of eliminating necessary medications during pregnancy. One such risk may be a relapse of medical or psychiatric illness. A growing body of medical research has demonstrated that many medications can be taken safely during pregnancy.

To date, stimulants remain the treatment of choice for AD/HD. These include methylphenidate (Ritalin® Concerta™, Methylin®, Metadate®), the amphetamines (Dexedrine®, Dextrostat®, and Adderall®), and pemoline (Cylert®). In addition, antihypertensives (Clonidine and Tenex®) and the tricyclic antidepressants (desipramine and imipramine) have been used for the treatment of AD/HD. Other antidepressants, either alone or in combination with a stimulant, may also be prescribed for AD/HD or related conditions, including the Selective Serotonin Reuptake Inhibitors (SSRIs) such as Prozac®, Zoloft®, and Paxil®, and Wellbutrin®, a non-SSRI antidepressant. These are discussed more fully in the next section on psychotropic medications.

Risk during Pregnancy

Stimulants

Amphetamines

There have been no controlled studies specifically designed to investigate the safe use of the stimulants during pregnancy. However, the question of whether amphetamines cause damage to offspring has been looked at in animal studies and in several published case histories of women who were addicted to amphetamines as well as other drugs during pregnancy (Eriksson et al., 1978, 1981).

In animal studies, cardiac defects were reported in the offspring of mice injected with 41 times the usual human dose of amphetamine. However, no negative effects were found in the offspring of rabbits given the drug at seven times the human dose or in rats given 12.5 times the maximum human dose (Nora et al., 1965).

Numerous outcome studies have looked at the infants of women who have taken amphetamines, either during the first trimester or throughout the pregnancy. Women in these studies were usually taking amphetamines as appetite suppressants or were addicted to methamphetamine (Briggs, Freeman, & Yaffe, 1994).

One of these studies looked at 52 mothers with documented exposure to dexedrine and 50 non exposed mothers (Nora et al., 1967). No cardiac abnormalities were found in either group initially. However, when the dexedrine-exposed children were seen at three-year follow-up, investigators reported a relationship to heart defects in this population (Nora et al., 1970).

As a result of all available evidence, the prevailing recommendation is that amphetamines should be used during pregnancy only if the benefit to the mother justifies the potential risk to the fetus (PDR, 2002, p. 1512).

Methylphenidate

It is not known at this time whether methylphenidate (MPH) causes harm to the fetus when taken by pregnant women. Several studies have, however, reported on newborns exposed to methylphenidate before birth. In one study, the Collaborative Perinatal Project, involving 3082 mother-infant pairs, 11 women were found who were exposed to MPH without adverse outcome in their infants (Heinonen et al., 1977). A second group of women were identified in 1993. Of the 13 newborns in this group, one had a cardiovascular defect (F. Rosa, personal communication, FDA, 1993). In addition, there has been a case report of IV MPH abuse during pregnancy. In this case, the abuse of the drug was associated with premature birth, growth retardation and neonatal withdrawal, but not with any defects or developmental delay in the infant (DeBooy et al., 1993).

Antihypertensives

Clonidine

Studies performed giving clonidine to rabbits at doses up to three times the oral maximum recommended doses in humans produced no evidence of damage to the offspring. There have been no well-controlled studies conducted in pregnant women. However, because animal studies are not always predictive of human response, this drug is not recommended for use during pregnancy (PDR, 2002).

Antidepressants

Antidepressants are the most widely prescribed among the psychiatric class of medications and the second most prescribed among all classes of medications. In 1989, up to 14 percent of the western world's population was taking an antidepressant (Dennerstein, 1989). Antidepressants fall into several categories based on chemical structure (i.e., tricyclics) or effect on neurotransmitters (i.e., serotonergic antidepressants).

A recent study by Lee Cohen M.D. and his colleagues at Harvard (Cohen et al., 1998) suggests that the decrease or discontinuation of antidepressants during pregnancy leaves mothers extremely vulnerable to depressive relapses. The study included 24 women whose antidepressant was decreased or discontinued. During the first trimester, 59 percent of the women relapsed after a dose change in their antidepressant. In the second trimester, 13 percent relapsed. In the third trimester, three percent relapsed. The preliminary conclusion is that the decrease or elimination of an antidepressant during pregnancy leaves a woman at high risk for recurrent depression.

Tricyclic Antidepressants

Tricyclics are no longer considered a risk during pregnancy as studies have shown no significant association between in-utero exposure and morphologic/behavioral changes (Nulman, Rovet, Steward, Wolpin, Gardner, Theis, Kulin, & Koren, 1997).

Nortriptyline, an antidepressant widely used because of its therapeutic blood level monitoring, is considered quite safe during pregnancy. However, there is a small concern about possible transient withdrawal symptoms in newborns, including restlessness, increased respiratory rate, increased muscle tone, and tremors. These symptoms occur hours after birth and can last from four to ten days. As a result, it is recommended that tricyclics be discontinued two weeks prior to childbirth and resumed after delivery, if necessary (Misri & Sivertz, 1991).

Selective Serotonin Reuptake Inhibitors

Serotonergic antidepressants (SSRIs) have been studied over the past several years (Partuszak et al., 1993; Chambers et al., 1996; Kulin et al., 1998). Fluoxetine (Prozac®) has a larger database on pregnancy exposure than any other SSRI, collected during eight years of monitoring. No significant association between in-utero exposure and morphologic exposure/behavioral changes has been found based on a review of 796 pregnancies with first trimester exposure (Goldstein, 1997; Nulman et al., 1997).

Results of the first prospective study on the effects of the SSRIs (Luvox, Paxil, and Zoloft) on the fetus were only recently released (Kulin et al., 1998). In this study, 267 women from nine medical centers who were taking one of these drugs when they learned that they were pregnant were compared to 267 women who were not exposed to any medication known to cause birth defects. No differences were found between women who took these antidepressants throughout their pregnancies and those that took them only during the first trimester. It was concluded that there was no increased risk of major malformations from these drugs when used at recommended doses. There was also no increased risk of miscarriage, stillbirth, or premature delivery noted. These findings agree with previous studies and animal research on Prozac. The Swedish Medical Birth Registry reviewed the exposures of 2129 infants (2105 women) to Citalopram (Celexa®) and several antidepressants. Outside of the curious finding of significantly reduced rate of twinning for SSRI exposures, the safety data was similar to the U.S. studies (Kallen, 1987).

Other Antidepressants

Bupropion (Wellbutrin®) does not have enough pregnancy data to establish safety (Data on file, GlaxoSmithKline).

Mood Stabilizers

Dr. Viguera and colleagues (Viguera et al., 2000) recently published a retrospective analysis of relapse rates in 32 bipolar pregnant women. Sixty-seven percent of women who discontinued mood stabilizers before or during the first trimester had a mood relapse, either depression or mania. None of nine treated women relapsed during pregnancy. In the postpartum period, 16 of 32 women relapsed. Looking at risk factors for postpartum relapse, it was found that 69 percent of these women had had relapses during pregnancy compared to 12.5 percent who did not relapse during pregnancy. Dr. Viguera concludes that patients who remained well during the postpartum period were more commonly treated with a mood stabilizer during pregnancy and postpartum. Again, discontinuation of mood stabilizing medication leaves the mother at risk for mood relapse.

Use of lithium during pregnancy has been thought to be associated with Epstein Anomaly, a specific cardiac malformation (Frakenberg & Lipinski, 1983; Kallen & Tandberg, 1983; Weinstein & Goldfield, 1975). Results from this research have been reassessed and now the risk seems to be significantly less than once thought. A recently published expert consensus guideline suggests that lithium is the preferred mood stabilizer in the second to third trimester (Altshuler et al., 2001). The lithium dose may need to be reduced after delivery as lithium level may rise, causing side effects of toxicity. In this case, the risks and benefits need to be reviewed with a psychiatrist familiar with this literature.

Anticonvulsants

The use of the anticonvulsants Depakote® and Tegretol® is contraindicated during pregnancy. Both these agents create significant risks for spinal cord malformations arising from first trimester exposure and should not be prescribed during pregnancy (Lindhout & Schmidt, 1986; Cohen & Rosenbaum, 1998).

Tranquilizers

Benzodiazepines, used to treat anxiety, have been associated with cleft palate (Saxen & Saxen, 1975; Safra & Oakley, 1975). This finding has been debated recently in light of a large study that concluded that there was no increased risk

(McElhatton, 1994). These findings are also supported in a large Hungarian study of 10,698 infants with congenital abnormalities, where there was no significant association found between clonazepam and abnormalities (Czeizedl et al., 1992). However, it is still recommended that the *regular* use of benzodiazepines be avoided during pregnancy. As mentioned earlier, tricyclics and SSRIs are safe during pregnancy and can be considered as a second-line approach for treating anxiety.

Risk of Exposure during Delivery

During the delivery and shortly thereafter, there may be concern about withdrawal symptoms and signs. The infant experiences withdrawal as a result of no longer being exposed to the psychotropic agent. As mentioned, tricyclic antidepressants may leave the neonate in a withdrawal state. Although the withdrawal state may be of concern, it is transient and not life-threatening. If benzodiazepines have been used before delivery, the newborn may appear floppy with reduced arousal. High-dose exposure may produce withdrawal symptoms lasting a few days (Fisher et al., 1985). A study of fluoxetine reported no withdrawal symptoms in 35 newborns.

Risk during Breastfeeding

Breastfeeding is critically important to the bonding experience of mother and infant. With the growing trend to promote breastfeeding, decisions to breastfeed ought to be made with the most current information concerning psychiatric medications.

Stimulants

Amphetamines

Current information indicates that the amphetamines are concentrated in breast milk and may cause symptoms of addiction and withdrawal in the infant. However, in a study that followed 103 nursing infants whose mothers were taking various amounts of amphetamine, no neonatal insomnia or stimulation was observed (Ayd, 1973). Nonetheless, the American Academy of Pediatrics, in 1989, considered amphetamines to be contraindicated during breastfeeding (AAP, 1989). It is therefore recommended that these drugs not be used while nursing.

Alternative Treatments for AD/HD

Wellbutrin is secreted into the milk and should not be taken by nursing mothers because of the "potential serious reactions in nursing infants." Clonidine (Catapres) is also excreted in human milk, and caution is recommended when administering this medication to nursing mothers.

Antidepressants

Tricyclics

Two studies reviewed nortriptyline in a total of 12 mother-infant pairs. Ten of 12 infants had no detectable nortriptyline, while the remaining two infants had only a low concentration of a nortriptyline metabolite. No adverse effects were detected in any of the infants (Wisner & Perel, 1991). In a series of 60 mother-infant pairs, breast milk and infant blood was assayed for medication concentrations (tricyclics, SSRIs, and benzodiazepines). There was no evidence of medication accumulating in the infants. The study concluded that psychotropic medication use during breastfeeding is associated with extremely low infant exposure.

Selective Serotonin Reuptake Inhibitors

As of 1999, there were 82 cases reported in the literature of women breastfeeding on different SSRIs. Literature now exists on all of the serotonin antidepressants. The overall conclusion is that breastfeeding while on these agents poses no substantial risk. Within the serotonergic antidepressant category, each antidepressant seems to be found in different concentrations in breast milk. Higher concentrations have been noted for citalopram versus paroxetine. Four studies that reviewed sertraline and breastfeeding found very low levels in infant blood. The same result has been found for fluoxetine. However, despite the differences in breast milk concentrations, there still seems to be no identifiable risk to the infant. More important than breast milk concentration is the concentration of medication in the infant blood. Often, these studies include both breast milk medication concentrations and infant blood levels. There are now two studies looking at paroxetine in infant blood. Both studies have found small to undetectable blood levels.

Ultimately, one is concerned about any neurodevelopmental abnormalities that arise as a result of breast milk exposure. An Emory University study of 16 mother-infant pairs revealed no adverse effect at 24 months in infants who breastfed while the mother was taking sertraline (Stowe, 1997). Another recent study has shown that breast-fed infants of mothers taking Paxil had no detectable trace of that medication in their blood, although low concentrations were found in the milk. These infants experienced no adverse events reported by their parents or pediatricians (Stowe et al., 2000).

Mood Stabilizers

Lithium

It is generally recommended that breastfeeding be avoided for women on lithium. Infants are exposed to high levels in breast milk, which can cause clinical symptoms (Weinstein & Goldfield, 1969; Skousig & Schou, 1997).

Carbamazepine

A review of 94 infants exposed to carbamazepine during breastfeeding revealed no evidence of risk. It appears carbamazepine may be safe during nursing. However, there are two case reports of significant liver abnormalities, so caution is still wise (Merlop, Mor, & Litwin, 1992).

Risk of Later Developmental Problems

The principle concern of parents with fetal or infant exposure to psychiatric medications is the impact on neurodevelopment. Misri (1991) conducted a study following children who had been exposed to tricyclics in-utero until they were eight years old. In this study, no neurobehavioral sequelae were observed. The fluoxetine database has been collected for eight years. In 1997, Nulman and colleagues published a study of children up to age seven who had been exposed to fluoxetine or TCA in-utero. His conclusion was that there was no observed effect on global IQ, language or behavioral development in these children. Developmental milestones were achieved at the same age as non-exposed children. Preliminary conclusions suggest that exposure to fluoxetine or TCAs does not cause observable adverse neurodevelopmental effects. The other SSRIs also have such databases in development, and their findings will be reported over the next few years.

A study of lithium exposure conducted by Schou (1976) found no behavioral problems in children born without malformations. Prospective studies have, likewise, not found significant differences on behavioral or cognitive measures in those children exposed to carbamazepine during pregnancy (van der Pol et al., 1991; Scolnik et al., 1994). While no prospective studies exist for the benozdiazepines, it is thought that these agents do not contribute to adverse neurodevelopmental outcomes.

Conclusion

More information is clearly needed in the area of the safety of stimulant medication use during pregnancy. At the present time, Dr. Lee Cohen's group at Harvard, in coordination with Dr. Joseph Biederman's group, is conducting a study of women who become pregnant while on psychotropic medications including the stimulants. The publication of their findings will be a valuable addition to our understanding of how best to treat women with AD/HD during pregnancy.

Over the last five years, there has been substantial literature more clearly defining the risks associated with psychiatric medications during pregnancy. Studies have demonstrated that antidepressants (tricyclics and SSRIs) may be safely used during pregnancy, when clearly indicated. Wellbutrin®, however, has not established a safety record in published research.

Anticonvulsants clearly have definable risks and should be avoided. Lithium has moderate risk and may be used during second or third trimester for exceptional cases. Lithium dose should be reduced immediately after delivery and the lithium level of the mother should be closely monitored. Thereafter, breastfeeding should be avoided.

In the absence of medication, congenital abnormalities occur in two to four percent of births in the general population. The presence of a medication during pregnancy does not, necessarily, bear responsibility for any subsequent congenital abnormality. As with all medication regimens, the pros and cons of treatment should be thoroughly discussed with the prescribing physicians and their patients before embarking on a course of treatment. In cases where the patient is or may become pregnant, the health risk to the developing fetus must also be taken into consideration. It is strongly recommended that both parents be included in discussions with the physician, as the decisions may have lifelong consequences. Decisions should be made only after considering all available information about maternal risk and possible risk to the fetus.

This chapter is intended to assist women to make better informed medication decisions during pregnancy and lactation. In consultation with their physicians, it is hoped that the information in this chapter will help them weigh the benefits of taking psychostimulants and other psychotropic medications against the potential risks to their child in-utero, at birth, and during lactation.

DISCLAIMER

The material presented in this chapter is intended for informational purposes only and should not be considered a substitute for medical advice. The decision to use medication during pregnancy and lactation may have serious consequences and should be made only in consultation with the treating physician, who can offer advice based on knowledge of a woman's history and current circumstances.

References

Altshuler, L. L., Cohen, L.S., Moline, M.L., Kalen, D.A., Carpenter, D., & Docherty, J.P. (2001). Treatment of depression in women. *Postgraduate Medicine, Special Report,* 51-52.

American Academy of Pediatrics, Committee on Drugs (1989). Transfer of drugs and other chemicals into human milk. *Pediatrics, 84,* 924-936.

Ayd, F.J. (1973). Excretion of psychotropic drugs in human breast milk. *International Drug Bulletin, 8,* 33-40.

Briggs, G.G., Freeman, R.K., & Yaffee, S.J. (1994). *Drugs during pregnancy and lactation, (4th ed.).* Baltimore, MD: Williams and Wilkins.

Chambers, C.D., Johnson, K.A., Dick, L.N., Felix, R.J., & Jones, K.L. (1996). Birth outcomes in pregnant women taking fluoxetine. *New England Journal of Medicine, 335,*1010-1015.

Cohen, L.S., & Rosenbaum, J.F. (1998). Psychotropic drug use during pregnancy: Weighing the risks. *Journal of Clinical Psychiatry, 59 (*suppl 2), 18-28.

Czeizedl, A.E., Bod, M., & Halasz, P. (1992). Evaluation of anticonvulsant drugs during pregnancy in a population-based Hungarian study. *European Journal of Epidemiology, 8,* 122-127.

DeBooy, V.D., Seshia, M.K., Tenenbein, M., & Casiro, O.G. (1993). Intravenous pentazocine and methylphenidate abuse during pregnancy. *American Journal of Diseases of Children, 147,* 1062-1065.

Dennerstein, L., Lehert, P., & Riphagen, F. (1989). Postnatal depression: Risk factors. *Journal of Psychosomatic Obstetrics and Gynaecology, 10,* 53-67.

Ericksson, M., Larsson, G., Winbladh, B., & Zetterstrom, R. (1978). The influence of amphetamine addiction on pregnancy and the newborn infant. *Acta Paedritrica Scandinavia, 67,* 95-99.

Ericksson, M., Larsson, G., & Zetterstrom, R. (1981). Amphetamine addiction and pregnancy. *Acta Obstetrica & Gynecologica Scandinavia, 60,* 253-259.

Fisher, J.B., Edgren, B.E., Mammel, M.C., & Coleman, J.M. (1985). Neonatal apnea associated with maternal clonazepam therapy: A case report. *Obstetrica Gynecologica, 66,* 34S-35S.

Frankenberg, F.R., & Lipinski, J.F. (1983). Congenital malformations. *New England Journal of Medicine, 309,* 311-312.

Goldstein, D.J. (1997). Effects of first trimester fluoxetine exposure on the newborn. Presented at the 150th Annual Meeting of the American Psychiatric Association, San Diego. *New Research,* 191.

Heinonen, O.P., Slone, D., & Shapiro, S. (1997). *Birth defects and drugs in pregnancy.* Littleton, CO: Publishing Sciences Group.

Kallen, B. (1987). Search for teratogenic risks with the aid of malformation registries. *Teratology, 35,* 47-52.

Kallen, B., & Tandberg, A. (1983). Lithium and pregnancy. *Acta Psychiatrica Scandinavia, 309,* 311-312.

Kulin, N.A., Pastuszak, A., Sage, S.R., Schick-Boschetto, B., Spivey, G., Feldkmp, M., Ormond, K., Matsui, D., Stein-Schechman, A.K., Cook, L., Brochu, J., Rieder, M., & Koren, G. (1998). Pregnancy outcome following maternal use of the new selective serotonin reuptake inhibitors. *Journal of the American Medical Association, 279,* 609-610.

Lindhout, D., & Schmidt, D. (1986). In utero exposure to valproate and neural defects. *Lancet, 1,* 329-333.

Merlop, P., Mor, N., & Litwin, A. (1992). Transient hepatic dysfunction in an infant of an epileptic mother treated with carbamazepine during pregnancy and breastfeeding: A review. *Annals of Pharmacotherapy, 26,* 1563-1565.

Misri, S., & Sivertz, K. (1991). Tricyclic drugs in pregnancy and lactation: A preliminary report. *International Journal of Psychiatric Medicine, 21,* 157-171.

McElhatton, P. R. (1994). The effects of benzodiazepine use during pregnancy and lactation. *Reproductive Toxicology, 8,* 461-475.

Nora, J.J., Trasler, D.G., & Fraser, F.C. (1965). Malformations in mice induced by dexedrine sulfate. *Lancet, 2,* 1021-1022.

Nora, J.J., McNamara, D.G., & Fraser, F.C. (1967). Dextroamphetamine sulphate and human malformations. *Lancet, 1,* 570-571.

Nora, J.J., Vargo, T.A., Nora, A.H., Love, K.E., & McNarmara, D.G. (1970). Dextroamphetamine: A possible environmental trigger in cardiovascular malformations. *Lancet, 1,* 1290-1291.

Nulman, I., Rovet, J., Steward, D.E., Wolpin, J., Gardner, H.A., Theis, J.G.W., Kulin, N., & Koren, G. (1997). Neurodevelopment of children exposed in utero to antidepressant drugs. *New England Journal of Medicine, 336,* 258-262.

Partuszak, A., Schick-Boshetto, B., Zuber, C., Feldkamp, M., Pinelli, M., Sihn, S., Donnenfeld, A., McCormack, M., Leen-Mitchell, M., Woodland, C., Gardner, G., Horn, M., & Koren, G. (1993). Pregnancy outcome following first-trimester exposure to fluoxetine (Prozac). *Journal of the American Medical Association, 269,* 2246-2248.

Physicians Desk Reference, 2002. Montvale, NJ: Medical Economics Company.

Rosa, F. (1993). Personal communication.

Safra, M. J., & Oakley, G.P. (1975). Association between cleft lip with or without cleft palate and prenatal exposure to diazepam. *Lancet, 2,* 478-480.

Saxen, I., & Saxen, L. (1975). Association between maternal intake of diazepam and oral clefts. *Lancet, 2,* 921.

Schou, M. (1976). What happened later to the lithium babies: A follow-up study of children born without malformations. *Acta Psychiatrica Scandinavia, 54,* 193-197.

Scolnik, D., Nulman, I., Rovet, J., Gladstone, D., Czuchta, D., Gardner, H.A., Gladstone, R., Ashby, P., Weksberg, R., Einarson, T., et al. (1994). Neurodevelopment of children exposed in-utero to phenytoin and carbamazepine monotherapy [published erratum appears in *JAMA,*1994; 271, 1745]. *Journal of the American Medical Association, 271,* 767-770.

Skausig, O.B., & Schou, M. (1997). Breastfeeding during lithium therapy. *Ugeskr Laeger, 14, 139,* 400-401.

Stowe, Z.N., Llewellyn, A.M., Owens, M.J., Ritchie, J.C., Kilts, C., & Nemeroff, C.B. (1997). *Antidepressants in pregnancy and lactation.* Presented at the 150th Annual Meeting of the American Psychiatric Association, San Diego.

Stowe, Z.N., Cohen, L.S., Hostetter, A., Ritchie, J.C., Owens, M.J., & Nemeroff, C.S.B. (2000). Paroxetine in human breast milk and nursing infants, *American Journal of Psychiatry, 157,* 185-9.

van der Pol, M.C., Hadders-Algra, M., Huisjes, H.J., & Touwen, B.C. (1991). Antiepileptic medication in pregnancy: Late effects on the children's central nervous system development. *American Journal of Obstetrics and Gynecology, 164,* 121-128.

Viguera, A.C., Nonacs, R., Cohen, L.S., Tondo, L., Murray, A., & Baldessarini, R.J. (2000). Risk of recurrence of bipolar disorder in pregnant and nonpregnant women after discontinuing lithium maintenance. *American Journal of Psychiatry, 157,* 179-184.

Weinstein, M.R., & Goldfield, M.D. (1969). Lithium carbonate treatment during pregnancy: Report of a case. *Diseases of the Nervous System, 30,* 828-832.

Weinstein, M.R., & Goldfield, M.D. (1975). Cardiovascular malformations with lithium use during pregnancy. *American Journal of Psychiatry, 132,* 529-531.

Wisner, K.L., & Perel, J.M. (1991). Serum nortriptyline levels in nursing mothers and their infants. *American Journal of Psychiatry, 148,* 1234-1236.

CHAPTER 5

Hormonal Influences on Women with AD/HD

Patricia O. Quinn, M.D.

AD/HD affects the lives of millions of women, yet few receive the comprehensive treatment needed to alleviate the impact of its symptoms and to optimize functioning. Why is this the case?

First, a significant problem exists for women in obtaining an accurate and comprehensive diagnosis. Repeatedly, women report being misdiagnosed as having a primary depressive illness or bipolar disorder. While these disorders may coexist or share common features of AD/HD, they in no way account for the whole picture in many women. Dealing with undiagnosed AD/HD can certainly lead to demoralization or outright depression, but treating these secondary complications does not get to the root of the problem in these women. To date, the tendency of the medical profession has been to focus on a woman's depressive or bipolar symptomatology and not to look beyond them to consider the possibility of underlying AD/HD.

Second, even if a woman is fortunate enough to be correctly diagnosed with AD/HD, treatment regimes are usually made up of recommendations established from the experience of treating elementary school-aged boys. Hormonal fluctuations and the influence of estrogen on the brain are not even considered, much less addressed. No wonder many adolescent girls and adult women with AD/HD report only partial remission of symptoms. In addition, treatment approaches that work for boys with AD/HD may not work for girls or women. For example, when boys' symptoms worsen, it often helps to increase the level of stimulant medication, but this approach frequently fails when applied to women in perimenopause or girls who have started menstruating.

Adele is a case in point:

"I was diagnosed with AD/HD at the age of 10. In my history, the severity of my symptoms has at times been mild, and at others rendered me useless. Looking back it seems as though the severity of my AD/HD symptoms increased during times when my hormones were going through a major change, during puberty and after giving birth, for example. I keep wondering if there could be a link. I am now 37 years old, and at the very least, perimenopausal. I have gone from being a fun-loving, outgoing person to being very antisocial, wanting to stay home all the time, and feeling very much overwhelmed. Recently, my attention and memory problems seem to be worsening. Sleep does not come easy, even with medication. My doctor keeps increasing the level of my stimulant medication, but this doesn't seem to help. At present, I take 30 mg Adderall, twice a day and 75-150 mg Triazidone for sleeping."

The Estrogen Connection

Women with AD/HD must live in their bodies, and those bodies, or more specifically those brains, are subjected to monthly fluctuations of hormone levels. Recent research has confirmed that the brain is a target organ for estrogen and that estrogen's neuronal effects have important functional consequences. Specifically, estrogen has been found to stimulate certain populations of dopamine and serotonin receptors in the brain, to stimulate a significant increase in dopamine2 (D2) receptors in the striatum (Fink, Rosie, Grace, & Quinn, 1996), and to have effects throughout the brain, including midbrain catecholamine and serotonin pathways. Although the mechanism is not fully understood, further studies have established that estrogen regulates dopaminergic neurons in the basal ganglia (Van Hartesvelt & Joyce, 1986). At the neuronal synapse, estrogen increases the concentration of neurotransmitters such as serotonin, dopamine, and norepinephrine (Archer, 1999). Estrogen also seems to inhibit presynaptic dopaminergic neurons and to decrease postsynaptic excitability through a variety of mechanisms (Zakon, 1998). Thus, the cyclical production of estrogen may increase symptoms of AD/HD by down-regulating dopamine activity.

Hormones and Stimulant Medication

Little is known about the interactions between hormones and the stimulant medications. As has been pointed out previously, estrogen and progesterone seem to have both direct and indirect central nervous system effects. In addition, it is becoming clearer that these hormones can also affect response to psychostimulants. Two recent studies by Justice and deWit (1999, 2000) looked at the effect of pretreatment with estrogen on the response to amphetamine and the acute effects of amphetamine during the follicular and luteal phases of the menstrual cycle. In the first study, 10 mg of amphetamine was administered during the early follicular phase of the menstrual cycle, both with and without pretreatment with estradiol patches. The results indicated that the stimulating effects of amphetamine were increased with acute estradiol pretreatment.

In the second study, the effects of 15 mg of amphetamine were assessed at two hormonally distinct phases of the menstrual cycle in women. During the follicular phase, estrogen is initially low and then gradually rises. In the luteal phase, both estrogen and progesterone are present, with a decrease prior to menstruation. Results of this study indicated that the effect of the amphetamine was greater during the follicular phase than the luteal phase. Women reported feeling more "energetic" and more "intellectually efficient."

The results of these studies demonstrated that during the follicular phase, but not the luteal phase, responses to amphetamines were related to the levels of estrogen. These findings suggest that estrogen may enhance the response to stimulants in women, and that the effect is not seen in the presence of progesterone or in low-estrogen states. Cyclical variations of hormones (both estrogen and progesterone) during the menstrual cycle may need to be factored in when it comes to the proper dose of medication for women. From the results of these studies and clinical reports, it would seem that adolescent girls and women may experience differing clinical responses to stimulants depending on the phase of their menstrual cycle.

Estrogen, Mood, and Other Disorders

For years, marked gender differences have been observed in the prevalence of mood and anxiety disorders (Leibenluf, 1999). Only recently has estrogen been increasingly seen as playing a role in the treatment of these disorders. Estrogen appears to blunt anxiety symptoms and autonomic reactivity to stress. Recent studies confirm that estrogen alone may have modest effects as a treatment for major depression and that estrogen patches have successfully lessened psychosis in schizo-phrenic women.

According to Dr. Jayashri Kulkarni, women may be more vulnerable to relapses of schizophrenia when estrogen levels drop in menopause or during the postpartum period. She also theorizes that estrogen may serve as a protective factor, ex-plaining why women are older than men at the first episode of schizophrenia. In her study, women already receiving stan-dard antipsychotic medication were treated with an estrogen or placebo patch. Improvement was noted at day four or five of estrogen treatment, and by the end of 28 days, the results were quite striking. The women who received the 100-mcg-transdermal patch as well as antipsychotic drugs were signifi-cantly better than those treated with an antipsychotic alone (Kulkarni, J., in press).

Women with AD/HD, by definition, have dysfunction in neurotransmitter systems of their brain. With estrogen enhanc-ing release of these neurotransmitters at the synapse (Archer, 1999), one would expect improved functioning in women dur-ing high-estrogen states such as pregnancy. Remission of panic disorder has been observed during pregnancy with improve-ment noted during each trimester, with relapses after delivery (Altemus, 1999). Breastfeeding, because of its ability to keep the estrogen levels elevated, can delay this response. Could this pattern of sensitivity to high estrogen levels, resulting in improved functioning during pregnancy, be true for AD/HD in woman as well? In the following case, a mother reports on her daughter's experience:

"I have a 19-year-old daughter who was diagnosed with ADD at age 16. She became pregnant at 17. The curious thing is that all through her pregnancy, and the first six months of breastfeeding, her severe ADD symptoms vanished! She did well during her first semester of college, and she was like a completely different person. However, during her

second semester, she began to cut back drastically on the breastfeeding in preparation for weaning her son, and I suddenly realized all her ADD symptoms were returning. Over the next six months, she gradually became the person she was before pregnancy."

This case is not unique. When questioning women with AD/HD, they invariably report that they felt their best and had the least interference from AD/HD symptoms while pregnant. Huessy (1990) first addressed the issue of hormones and their relationship to AD/HD by noting that girls with AD/HD may have increasingly severe symptoms with the onset of puberty. He wrote that increased hormonal fluctuations throughout the phases of the menstrual cycle might result in increased symptomatology. With the onset of menses and monthly fluctuations in estrogen states, some women with AD/HD experience a worsening of their symptoms. The same holds true for menopausal women. Conversely, during high-estrogen states such as pregnancy, women report significant improvement.

Low-estrogen States

It has been proposed that whenever brain estrogen levels "fall below the minimum brain estrogen requirement," for whatever reason and at whatever age, brain dysfunction may ensue (Arpels, 1996). Low-estrogen states occur prior to menstruation, postpartum, and beginning at perimenopause. With menopause, there is an approximately 60 percent decrease in estrogen levels. Symptoms shared by women in low-estrogen states include depression, irritability, sleep disturbance, anxiety, panic, difficulty concentrating, and memory and cognitive dysfunction.

PMS, PMDD, and Premenstrual Magnification

Premenstrual Syndrome (PMS) is a common disorder of women that refers to physical symptoms and mild mood changes that appear predictably during the latter half of the menstrual cycle. Studies have indicted that up to 75 percent of women report some symptoms of premenstrual syndrome (Johnson, 1987). While many women report these symptoms, only about five percent of all women report symptoms that are severe enough to interfere with daily functioning (Rivera-Tovar & Frank, 1990). The diagnosis of PMS requires that the symptoms be severe enough to affect a woman's ability to function at home, in the workplace, or in her relationships with others. A thorough medical and psychiatric history and prospective daily rating of symptoms for two months should be obtained in order to make the diagnosis. Disorders such as major depression, anxiety, hypothyroidism and diabetes must also be excluded. Etiology is not fully known, but there may be a genetic component involved in PMS.

It seems that PMS worsens as a woman gets older. Symptoms can begin anytime after puberty, but most women don't seek treatment until into their thirties. What were originally manageable symptoms of PMS sometimes intensify and may become intolerable as a woman ages. Ovulation seems to be a key factor, as the disorder is not seen during pregnancy or menopause. The diagnosis of PMS is usually reserved for women whose symptoms include physical discomfort such as breast tenderness, bloating, headache, and minor mood changes. This pattern of symptoms must occur regularly at some time in the cycle after ovulation and last until menses begins. Symptoms can begin at any time, but there must be a symptom-free period during the follicular phase of the cycle. There appear to be several patterns to these symptoms. They include:

- symptoms beginning during the week before menstruation and remitting during menses;

- symptoms beginning at time of ovulation and persisting through the luteal phase;

▶ symptoms briefly occurring around ovulation with symptoms returning during 2nd week; or,

▶ symptoms beginning at ovulation and continuing through menses—leaving only a 10-day symptom-free period.

There also appears to be a subgroup of women (3% to 8%) with PMS whose symptoms are primarily related to a mood disorder. These women experience extreme mood and behavioral symptoms leading to a diagnosis of premenstrual dysphoric disorder (PMDD). These women report symptoms of irritability, tension, dysphoria, and lability of mood that seriously interfere with their functioning and relationships. They also report a higher incidence of previous mood disorders and are at risk for developing other psychiatric disorders, particularly major depression. To meet the diagnostic criteria for this disorder a woman must report five symptoms, four of which are affective in nature. The diagnosis must also be conformed by daily ratings through at least two cycles. There seems to be a genetic component, with a high concordance in twin studies. There is also a link to PMS and depression in the families of these women.

Postpubertal females with AD/HD report a high incidence of PMS symptoms involving mood disturbance. As one woman noted, "At 36, I was just diagnosed with AD/HD. I am taking Adderall and the medication is working. However, I still have severe PMS with irritability, increased impulsivity, and sleep problems."

In addition, women with a continuing mood disorder may report premenstrual magnification of symptoms or the emergence of new symptoms. A similar pattern of premenstrual increase of symptoms is reported by some women with AD/HD. Women who receive the diagnosis of premenstrual magnification may also meet the criteria for a superimposed PMS or PMDD. Premenstrual magnification most commonly occurs with mood or anxiety disorders, but has been reported by women with AD/HD.

PMS and PMDD Treatment

Symptoms of PMS or PMDD have not been found to correlate with any absolute level of estrogen in the blood (Roca, Schmidt, Bloch, & Rubinow, 1996). Women report symptoms at varying levels of estrogen, and symptoms seem to be more related to declining levels rather than absolute levels of hormone. In addition, anti-estrogen drugs such as tamoxafen and progesterone have been found to stimulate PMS symptoms in susceptible individuals (Arpels, 1996). A more recent hypothesis suggests that the problems may not be related to the level of estrogen in the blood, but to estrogen receptor sensitivity and fluctuating levels of neurotransmitters in the brain. The same receptors stimulated by estrogen are also stimulated by SSRI antidepressants. Thus PMS symptoms appear to be mediated in the central nervous system (CNS) and declining levels of estrogen in the premenstrual phase might indirectly contribute. Women with PMS appear to also have abnormalities in blood serotonin levels. Numerous studies have been remarkable consistent in demonstrating that with SSRI treatment, up to 90 percent of women with severe PMS experience almost complete relief of symptoms (Steiner et al., 1995; Yonkers et al., 1996). These findings suggest that SSRIs reduce PMS symptoms by increasing serotonin levels at the synapse.

Perimenopause and Menopausal Issues

Perimenopause is that period of several years when estrogen levels begin to drop, and menopausal symptoms start to occur, but menses has not stopped. As estrogen levels fall, beginning at perimenopause and continuing into menopause, brain volume in females begins to decline. This atrophy occurs mainly in the hippocampus and the parietal lobe, areas primarily associated with memory and cognition (Murphy, DeCarli, & McIntosh, 1996). A similar loss in brain volume is seen in males, but not until around the age of 60. This is probably because the hormone decrease with age in males occurs much later and more gradually. As a result of the continued conversion of male hormone, testosterone, to estrogen, males over 60 have approximately three times more estrogen than females. (Ferrini & Barrett-Connor, 1998). Estrogen levels may be stabilized in perimenopausal women by the use of low-dose birth control pills, with a transition to hormone replacement therapy (HRT) once periods have stopped.

Symptoms arising during these years of perimenopause/ menopause include memory problems, mood changes, and hot flashes. All of these symptoms are now thought to relate to reduced estrogen levels in the brain. Perimenopause is also a time associated with onset of depression in some women with no prior history of depression. These women report feeling sad, irritable, and worried, with energy loss, fatigue, and sleep difficulties.

Dealing with the depression and cognitive deficits associated with the decreasing levels of estrogen in perimenopause and menopause may cause women with AD/HD to become less functional as they enter this phase of their life. As these women report more impairment or increasing symptoms, physicians respond by increasing the dose of stimulant medication with little improvement noted. Instead, one needs to consider the relationship between variable or declining estrogen levels and decreased cognitive functioning, and design a more holistic approach for treatment of AD/HD in women at various stages of their lives.

Depression and Estrogen

Shepard (2001) states that while there is not an overall increase in the number of women experiencing clinical depression during perimenopause, 80 percent of women report mildly depressed mood during this time. This mild depression may be the result of decreasing neurotransmitters in those areas of the brain rich in estrogen receptors. Falling estrogen levels directly influence synaptic concentrations of specific neurotransmitters, but particularly serotonin, which plays a key role in mood regulation. In animal studies, it was found that administration of estrogen increased serotonin uptake in the frontal cortex and hypothalamus, and that the antidepressant imipramine was not effective unless estrogen was present.

Research has shown that blood serotonin levels are decreased in postmenopausal women and that hormone replacement can restore them to premenopausal levels (Gonzales & Carillo, 1993). In studies conducted on postmenopausal women, hormone replacement therapy (HRT) has proven beneficial for the treatment of depression (Zweifel & O'Brien, 1997). This has led to the speculation that antidepressant efficacy may differ in perimenopausal and postmenopausal women, and that estrogen enhances the efficacy of some antidepressants (Rodriguez & Grossburg, 1998; Schatzberg, 1999).

Recent studies confirm that the short-term administration of estrogen replacement alone relieves the symptoms of depression in perimenopausal women. In a study conducted by Peter Schmidt at NIMH, published in the August 2000 issue of the *American Journal of Obstetrics and Gynecology*, 80 percent of women with perimenopausal depression improved with estrogen patch treatment, including six of seven women with major depression and 19 of 24 women with minor depression (Schmidt et al 2000). In addition, a recent meta-analysis of 26 studies demonstrated that hormone replacement had a moderate-to-large effect on depressed mood in postmenopausal women (Zweifel et al., 1997).

Cognitive Deficits of Menopause and Estrogen

During menopause, many women report experiencing a decline in cognitive functioning, including a decrease in mental clarity and short-term memory (Frackiewicz & Cutler, 2000). Adding these symptoms to the cognitive dysfunction and language disabilities already experienced by women with AD/HD may tip them over the edge as their barely manageable life becomes unmanageable.

Several studies have now documented that women receiving hormonal therapy performed significantly better on cognitive testing. A recent meta-analysis of 17 randomized studies revealed that women with menopausal symptoms who received hormone replacement therapy improved verbal memory, vigilance, reasoning, and motor speed (LeBlanc, 2001). Estrogen was also shown to enhance both short- and long-term memory and the capacity for learning new associations. Healthy 65-year-old women who took estrogen also performed better than estrogen nonusers when matched for age, socioeconomic status, and years of formal education. Other findings suggest that estrogen helps to maintain verbal memory and enhances the capacity for new learning in women (Yaffe et al., 1998; Jacobs et al., 1998). Estrogen users performed better than nonusers on almost all neuropsychological tests, especially on those assessing conceptualization, attention, and visual practical skills (Schmidt et al., 1996).

In addition, estrogen has been shown to increase blood flow and brain activation patterns in postmenopausal women prescribed standard therapeutic doses. These changes in brain activation patterns were observed in specific brain regions associated with day-to-day memory functions (Shaywitz et al., 1999).

Thyroid Hormone, AD/HD and Depression

Thyroid hormone activity has a variety of complicated interactions with other disorders. Studies have shown that thyroid disorders can also be associated with both AD/HD symptoms and mood disorders. Thyroid hormone has been found to play a significant role in the activation of the prefrontal cortex, particularly on the shift and disengage functions of attention. Resistance to thyroid hormones has also been seen as a genetic disorder that correlated strongly with the symptoms of hyperactivity and the diagnosis of AD/HD in families (Hauser et al., 1997).

The problem with identifying hypothyroidism is that many physicians feel that they cannot make the diagnosis until levels of T3 and T4 are below normal and TSH levels are elevated. It is now known that subclinical hypothyroidism (no symptoms) is more commonly associated with psychiatric disorders and can cause significant problems in the treatment of affective and cognitive disorders. Symptoms of thyroid underactivity (and/or resistance to thyroid hormone) include weight gain, inability to lose weight, sluggish metabolism, hair loss, dry skin and hair, mental slowness, poor memory and attention, constipation, fatigue, and muscle weakness.

In addition to improving these symptoms, use of thyroid hormone augmentation or replacement can be a very useful adjunct to the treatment of depression that does not respond well to the standard antidepressants. Although most patients with depression have thyroid functioning that is in the normal range, some studies have found a pattern of T4 levels in the upper range of normal, with T3 in the lower range of normal (Maes, Metzner, & Cosyns, 1993). As thyroid augmentation has been found to be effective in the treatment of resistant depression, thyroid functioning should be routinely tested in women with depression or an anxiety disorder.

Conclusion

The key to better outcomes for women with AD/HD lies not only in better recognition of the disorder, but in the realization that, in addition to their AD/HD, these women must cope with an ever-changing hormonal environment that can have a significant impact on AD/HD and coexisting symptoms. While AD/HD symptoms respond to stimulant medication in females as well as in males, hormone levels during certain phases of the cycle may decrease effectiveness. When low-estrogen states enter the picture, a more coordinated treatment approach is needed to address superimposed or worsening symptomatology. For those women whose symptoms worsen during the monthly cycle or with menopause, estrogen administration can help stabilize mood and improve memory. Combined therapy with stimulants, an SSRI (Prozac, Zoloft), and estrogen replacement may be necessary for women with worsening of AD/HD symptoms, PMS, or PMDD. In addition, estrogen plus stimulants may be necessary to address perimenopausal depression and the cognitive dysfunctions that accompany menopause. Thyroid functioning also needs to be evaluated when response to antidepressants is limited. While these regimens haven't been tested in research settings for this particular disorder, clinical successes repeatedly validate the wisdom of trying this approach for women with AD/HD.

References

Altemus, M. (1999). *Modulation of anxiety by reproductive hormones.* Presented at the 152nd Annual Meeting of the American Psychiatric Association, Washington, DC.

Archer, J.S.M. (1999) Estrogen and mood changes via CNS activity *Menopausal Medicine, 7,* 4-8.

Arpels, J.C. (1996). The female brain hypoestrogenic continuum from the premenstrual syndrome to menopause: A hypothesis and review. *Journal of Reproductive Medicine, 41,* 633-939.

Ferrini, R.L., & Barrett-Connor, E.L. (1998). Sex hormones and age: A cross sectional study of testosterone and estradiol and their bioavailable fractions in community-dwelling men. *American Journal of Epidemiology, 147,* 750-754

Fink, G., Rosie, R., Grace, O., & Quinn, J.P. (1996) Estrogen control of central neurotransmission: Effect on mood, mental state, and memory. *Cell Molecular Biology, 16,* 325-344.

Frackiewicz, E.J., & Cutler, N.R. (2000). Women's health care during the perimenopause. *Journal of the American Pharmacologic Association, 40,* 800-811.

Gonzales, G.F., & Carillo, C. (1993). Blood serotonin levels in postmenopausal women: Effects of age and oestradiol levels. *Maturitas, 17,* 23-29.

Hauser, P., Soler, R., Brucker-Davis, F., & Weintraub, B.D. (1997). Thyroid hormones correlate with symptoms of hyperactivity but not inattention in attention-deficit hyperactivity disorder. *Psychoneurendocrinology, 22,* 107-114.

Huessy, H.R. (1990). *The pharmacotherapy of personality disorders in women.* Presented at the 143rd Annual Meeting of the American Psychiatric Association (symposia), New York.

Jacobs, D.M., Tang, M.X., Stern, Y., Sano, M., Marder, K., Bell, K.L., Schfield, P., Doonlief, G., Gurland, B., & Mayeux, R. (1998). Cognitive functioning in non-demented older women who took estrogen after menopause. *Neurology, 50,* 368-373.

Johnson, S.R. (1987). The epidemiology and social impact of premenstrual symptoms. *Clinics of Obstetrics and Gynecology, 30,* 367-376.

Justice, A.J., & deWit, H. (2000). Acute effects of estradiol pretreatment on the response to d-amphetamine in women. *Neuroendocrinology, 71,* 51-59.

Justice, A.J., & deWit, H. (1999) Acute effects of d-amphetamine during the follicular and luteal phases of the menstrual cycle in women. *Psychopharmacology, 145,* 67-75.

Kulkarni, J. (In press). Estrogen supplementation lessens schizophrenic psychosis in women. *Schizophrenia Research.*

Leibenluf, E. (1999). *Gender differences in mood and anxiety disorders: From bench to bedside.* Presented at the 152nd Annual Meeting of the American Psychiatric Association, Washington, DC.

Le Blanc, E.S., Janowsky, J., Chass, B.K.S., & Nelson, H.D. (2001). Use of HRT to improve cognitive functioning in certain patients. *Journal of the American Medical Association, 285,* 1475-1481.

Maes, M., Metzner, H., & Cosyns, P. (1993). An evaluation of basal hypothalamic-pituitary-thyroid axis function in depression: Results of a large-scaled and controlled study. *Psychoneuroendocrinology, 18,* 607-620.

Murphy, D.C., DeCarli, C., & McIntosh, A.R. (1996). Sex differences in human brain morphology and metabolism: An in-vivo quantitative magnetic resonance imaging and positron emission tomography study on the effects of aging. *Archives of Geriatric Psychiatry, 53, 585-594.*

Roca, C.A., Schmidt, P., Bloch, M., & Rubinow, D.R. (1996). Implication of endocrine studies of premenstrual syndrome. *Psychiatric Annals, 26,* 576-580.

Rodriguez, M.M., & Grossberg, G.T. (1998). Estrogen as a psychotherapeutic agent. *Clinical Geriatric Medicine, 14,* 177-189.

Rivera-Tovar, A., & Frank, E. (1990). Late luteal phase dysphoric disorder in young women. *American Journal of Psychiatry, 147,* 1634-1636.

Schatzberg, A. (1999). *The modulation of monoamine neurotransmitters by estrogen: Clinical implications.* Presented at the 152nd Annual Meeting of the American Psychiatric Association, Washington, D.C.

Schmidt, P.J., Neiman, L., Danaceau, M.A., Tobin, M.B., Roca, C.A., Murphy, J.H., & Rubinow, D.R. (2000). Estrogen replacement in perimenopause-related depression: A preliminary report. *American Journal of Obstetrics and Gynecology, 183,* 414-420.

Schmidt, R., Fazekas, F., Reinhart, B., Kapeller, P., Offenbacher, H., Eber, B., Schumacher, M., & Freidl, W. (1996). Estrogen replacement therapy in older women: A neuropsychological and brain MRI study. *Journal of the American Geriatric Society, 44,* 1307-13.

Shaywitz, S.E., & Shaywitz, B.A. (1999). Effect of estrogen in brain activation pathways in postmenopausal women during active memory tasks. *Journal of the American Medical Association, 281,* 1197-1202.

Shepherd, J.E. (2001). Effects of estrogen on cognition, mood, and degenerative brain diseases. *Journal of the American Pharmacology Association, 41,* 221-228.

Steiner, M., Steinberg, S., Stewart, D., Carter, D., Berger, C., & Reed, R. (1995). Fluoxetine in the treatment of premenstrual dysphoria. *New England Journal of Medicine, 332,* 1529-1533.

Van Hartesvelt, C., & Joyce, J.N. (1986). Effects of estrogen on the basal ganglia. *Neuroscience and Biobehavioral Reviews, 10,* 1-14.

Yaffe, K., Sawaya, G., Lieberburg, I., & Grady, D. (1998.) Estrogen therapy in postmenopausal women: Effects on cognitive function and dementia. *Journal of the American Medical Association, 279,* 688-695.

Yonkers, K.A., Halbreich, U., Freeman, E., Brown, C., & Pearlstein, T. (1996). Sertralin in the treatment of premenstrual dysphoric disorder. P*sychopharmacology Bulletin, 32,* 41-46.

Zakon, H.H. (1998). The effects of steroid hormones on electrical activity of excitable cells. *Trends in the Neurosciences, 21,* 202-207.

Zweifel, J.E., & O'Brien, W.H. (1997). A meta-analysis of the effect of hormone replacement therapy upon depressed mood. *Psychoneuroendocrinology, 22,* 189-212.

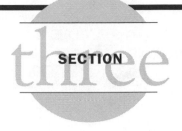

SECTION

three

NONMEDICAL TREATMENT FOR WOMEN WITH AD/HD

CHAPTER 6

Psychotherapy for Women with AD/HD

Kathleen G. Nadeau, Ph.D.

"I always knew that something was wrong. I just didn't know what it was. I always felt 'different' from other girls growing up."

"No one could understand what was the matter when I was young. Here I was, a smart girl from a nice family. I had all the advantages. But I kept screwing up. I kept disappointing my parents, and I disappointed myself."

When a woman feels that something has been wrong throughout her life . . . When she knows that she was as bright as other kids, but earned lower grades . . . Or when she earned high grades, but had to work twice as hard . . . When she felt left out by her peers and criticized by her parents . . . When her adult life seemed overwhelming and few of her dreams have come true . . . then she has to find a way to explain all of this to herself. Those explanations are often harsh and self-derogatory, aptly illustrated by the title of a book, written by two women with AD/HD, *You Mean I'm Not Lazy, Stupid, or Crazy?!* (Kelly & Ramundo, 1993).

This chapter will present a model of psychotherapy for women with AD/HD that begins by addressing this pervasive, demoralizing pattern of self-blame, helping women move from despair to understanding by reframing and accepting their difficulties as symptoms of a neurobiological disorder. Beyond developing new attitudes and understanding, however, the ultimate goal of therapy is to help women with AD/HD achieve success—success in developing better life-management tools, success in building a life-style that is compatible with their AD/HD, and success in setting and reaching goals.

The concepts discussed in this chapter are distillations of the author's clinical experience in working with many women with AD/HD over a period of years. A woman who is seeking a psychotherapist to help her learn to manage her AD/HD and related conditions should use the ideas discussed here as general guidelines. While each psychotherapist has her own approaches and techniques, psychotherapy will be more effective in working with women's AD/HD issues if it is oriented toward the practical, neurocognitive aspects of AD/HD as well as toward psychological issues.

Addressing the Neurobiological Aspects of AD/HD

Women who have AD/HD should seek a therapist whose approach always keeps in mind that AD/HD is a neurobiological condition that affects many aspects of a woman's daily functioning. Therapy should not only address psychological issues, but should also help women to develop tools to meet AD/HD-related challenges in concrete and practical ways.

Many psychotherapists, especially those trained in a more psychodynamic approach, may find such techniques alien. A psychodynamically oriented therapist may believe that practical issues should be addressed outside of psychotherapy, for

example by an ADD coach. While coaching can be a very helpful adjunct to therapy, the concrete problems faced by women
with AD/HD cannot be divorced from their psychological distress. Often, improvement in life-management skills and solutions to real-life problems can help decrease anxiety and depression. The reverse is also true. Reducing psychological distress,
and helping a woman with AD/HD to change counterproductive
attitudes can help her to be more successful in managing the multiple challenges of her daily life.

Addressing Secondary Psychological Issues

Cognitive psychotherapy is particularly well-suited to helping women focus on the psychological issues that result from
having AD/HD. With cognitive therapy, a woman with AD/HD
can learn to reframe her difficulties so that she can move away
from self-blame and demoralization toward understanding and
self-advocacy. A therapist who only uses more "traditional"
psychotherapy techniques may focus exclusively on the psychological baggage of AD/HD (depression, anxiety, poor self-
esteem)—never connecting these feelings to the AD/HD issues that have generated them.

Why Traditional Therapies Are Less Effective for Women with AD/HD

Many women who seek treatment for AD/HD have already
been engaged in more traditional psychotherapy. They have
known that "something was wrong," but neither they nor
their psychotherapist knew that their problems were related
to AD/HD. Often, such traditional psychotherapy can be
helpful in dealing with destructive early childhood experiences, trauma, or depression. However, even when such issues have been dealt with effectively, a woman with AD/
HD may be left still feeling out of control and overwhelmed
by her daily life—unable to cope with daily demands that
other women deal with more evenly. Others agree (Ratey et

al., 1991) that insight-oriented psychotherapy may be a poor match for adults with AD/HD.

When AD/HD issues are treated using neurocognitive techniques, a woman finally has the opportunity to understand the causes of problems for which she has blamed herself, and to develop effective tools to deal with them. If a woman's therapist clings to psychological interpretations of neurobiologically driven behaviors, this only reinforces her habitual self-blame. Women with AD/HD, like all women, can benefit from understanding the psychological basis of self-defeating patterns. But just as importantly, they also need to develop an awareness of patterns that are neurologically based and develop tools to manage them.

Neurocognitive Psychotherapy

The primary focus of this chapter is to introduce a structured treatment approach referred to as *Neurocognitive Psychotherapy*, that involves aspects of both cognitive behavioral therapy and cognitive rehabilitation to specifically address issues related to AD/HD. These include life-management issues, emotional issues secondary to AD/HD, and conditions that commonly coexist with AD/HD. Further, it will outline treatment issues unique to women.

Cognitive Therapy to Address Psychological Issues of AD/HD

Cognitive behavioral therapy focuses on changing attitudes and thought patterns that lead to undesired feeling states such as anxiety, depression, and self-defeating behaviors. This therapy also involves setting concrete goals for behavior change. Such an approach is ideally suited to work against the deeply ingrained self-defeating attitudes and negative self-talk engaged in by many women with AD/HD.

The Diagnosis as a Cognitive Change Agent

Rucklidge and Kaplan's research on newly diagnosed women with AD/HD suggests that the diagnosis itself has highly therapeutic effects (Rucklidge & Kaplan, 1997). Hallowell and Ratey concur, writing, "Hope begins with the diagnosis." The process of education and reframing begins immediately as "the walls of years of misunderstanding come crashing down under the force of a lucid explanation of the cause of the individual's problems . . . Everything else in the treatment evolves logically from an understanding of the diagnosis" (1994, p. 216).

Knowledge as a Cognitive Change Agent

The beginning steps of a woman's journey commence with learning about and coming to understand AD/HD. When she knows what it is and how she is specifically affected by it, she can alter her self-concept in the wake of this new-found knowledge. Hallowell and Ratey (1994) emphasize the importance of education as a first step in treatment. The better a woman with AD/HD truly understands the workings of her brain, the better equipped she is to see her challenges in a more rational, forgiving light, and the better she can formulate plans and goals that ensure a greater chance for success.

Beyond general information about AD/HD, each woman with AD/HD needs specific information about herself. Although neuropsychological testing may not be necessary to make an accurate diagnosis, such testing can be very useful in helping her to understand her own particular strengths and weaknesses. How well does her working memory function, allowing her to hang onto a thought, mid-task, when she is interrupted? How well is she equipped to resist staying in the reactive mode of living, so that she can set priorities and follow through on them? How well can she deal with the many interruptions and distractions of her day? How does she best take in and process information—visually, auditorily, or kinesthetically? How does she best express her thoughts—in verbal or written form? Where do her intellectual strengths lie? What are her abilities to self-monitor, to plan, organize, and complete tasks? In addition, it is important that a woman with AD/HD understand how she is affected by coexisting conditions such as anxiety, depression, and learning disabilities.

Reframing

Reframe—to change the frame of reference, the context or environment within which something is seen, understood, defined.
—Webster's New International Dictionary of
the English Language, 2nd Ed., unabridged

Reframing the way that one thinks about something is a classic tool of cognitive psychotherapy that is particularly useful to confront and rethink the challenges presented by AD/HD. Before she can begin to reframe her self-concept, a woman with AD/HD must challenge her negative assumptions. She may wrestle with self-doubt, asking herself, "Does having AD/HD mean that I'm defective?" Only then can she begin to build a new, more positive framework that replaces self-blame and shame with an open, growth-promoting attitude that supports her self-understanding, her sense of self-worth, and a belief in her potential.

Regret

Before a woman with AD/HD can truly focus on the future, she must come to terms with regret—regret for the opportunities lost during the many years preceding her diagnosis. She may wonder what different choices she might have made, had she understood earlier that a treatable condition was the basis of so many of her struggles. She may feel anger that her parents and teachers did not understand her problems, and were not able to help her. Sometimes her anger can become a positive force when it is directed toward advocating for her own or other children with AD/HD, to prevent them from struggling with undiagnosed AD/HD as she has.

Acceptance

A woman with AD/HD can achieve great success, but first she must come to terms with and accept her AD/HD. As Judith Viorst writes in *Necessary Losses:*

> *Accepting reality means that we've come to terms with the world's—and our own—limitations and flaws. It also means establishing achievable goals for ourselves . . . Growing up takes time and we may be a long time learning to balance our dreams and our realities.* (Viorst, 1986, p. 169).

Coming to terms with limitations and flaws can ultimately lead to greater strength. Success is more likely when it is based on a solid sense of self, and a feeling of competence that comes from real achievements instead of unrealized dreams.

Cognitive Rehabilitation Approaches in the Treatment of AD/HD

The therapeutic effects of diagnosis, understanding, reframing, and acceptance set the stage for a woman to take charge of her AD/HD by learning life-management skills, setting achievable goals, and reaching those goals. How can a therapist help a woman with AD/HD make this journey? A complex array of issues must be addressed along the way.

Goodwin and Bolton (1991) developed a three-pronged cognitive rehabilitation approach for the treatment of AD/HD in adults, focusing on:

▶ improving cognitive functions;

▶ developing compensatory strategies; and

▶ restructuring the environment.

Improvement of Cognitive Functions

In the context of treating AD/HD, the "improvement of cognitive functions" primarily involves the use of stimulant medication to enhance attention and focus. Cognitive functioning is also strongly affected by stress levels, sleep, exercise, health habits, and many other environmental factors to be discussed later. A therapist and her client with AD/HD should work together to identify and alter any habits or environmental factors that may interfere with optimal cognitive functioning. For optimal cognitive functioning, a woman may also need to carefully consider hormonal fluctuations and whether hormone regulation may need to be part of her treatment regime (see Chapter 5).

Compensatory Strategies

For those cognitive functions that are not improved by the use of stimulant medications and good daily health habits, a woman with AD/HD needs to develop techniques to compensate for these difficulties. These compensatory strategies can be *internal,* i.e., habits and behaviors developed by the individual herself, or they can be *external,* such as visual cues, programmable watches, or time management software.

1. Daily habits and strategies

The development of new habits and the consistent use of external compensations can be difficult for a woman with AD/HD to manage. If a therapist is not familiar with compensatory strategies, she may tend to relegate this critical aspect of treatment to a coach or organizer. It is essential that a therapist develop her knowledge in this area so that she can directly help her client take charge of her AD/HD effectively. Using compensatory strategies is the heart of successful treatment—*"taking charge of AD/HD."* There are many changes, both internal and external, that a woman can initiate herself, with suggestions and guidance from her therapist.

2. **Patterns of daily self-care**

Other critical compensatory strategies include patterns of daily self-care and good health habits. Although such habits are helpful for all women, they are especially important to help compensate for the chronic stress experienced by women with AD/HD.

3. **Collaborating with a coach to develop habits and strategies**

Often, the most effective way to help a woman with AD/HD develop life-management skills is for a therapist and coach/organizer to coordinate their efforts with a client (see Chapter 7). Distractibility, poor follow-through, and faulty memory sometimes combine to render weekly therapy sessions only moderately effective in developing life-management skills. When a woman with AD/HD finds that she is not able to follow through on goals set in weekly therapy sessions, it is often helpful for her therapist to collaborate with a trained AD/HD coach or professional organizer to provide more frequent structure and support.

A woman with AD/HD can be in contact with a coach for brief phone sessions during the week to reinforce strategies and behaviors that have been suggested in her therapy session. This can be especially helpful when a client with AD/HD is engaged in a complex, multistep task such as working on a dissertation, applying to college or graduate school, or engaging in a job search. Thrice weekly, and even daily contact with a coach may be needed at times to keep her moving forward, taking steps every day to move closer to her goal.

It is important to find a well-trained coach who is experienced in working with women with AD/HD, and who has a clear sense of the appropriate boundaries between coaching and psychotherapy. Brief communications between the therapist and coach are important to coordinate their efforts. A woman with AD/HD should look for a good personality match between herself and her coach, just as she should with her therapist.

4. **Using assistive technologies as compensatory strategies**
There are an increasing number of devices that have been developed to assist people with a variety of disabilities. Many of these are highly useful for women with AD/HD. A therapist who specializes in treating women with AD/HD should make an ongoing effort to familiarize herself with new technologies as they become available.

Restructuring the Environment

The third component of a cognitive rehabilitation approach involves changing various aspects of the living environment with the goal of creating an AD/HD-friendly environment. It is the task of a woman with AD/HD, with guidance from her therapist, to find or create protective factors in her adult life. These protective factors include an environment that promotes structure and predictability, a work environment that is supportive and that reasonably accommodates AD/HD traits, and the social support of friends and family who accept the negative and appreciate the positive aspects of a woman with AD/HD.

1. The physical environment

The physical environment can be made more AD/HD-friendly in many ways that can minimize AD/HD challenges, for example, choosing a low maintenance home, organizing and de-cluttering the home and office, and streamlining daily routines. A chaotic or disorganized environment can greatly exacerbate AD/HD issues; yet, creating an orderly environment is a great challenge, if not an impossibility, for many women with AD/HD. One of the most common presenting complaints of women with AD/HD is disorganization—including problems with time management, household management, and money management.

When a woman with AD/HD reports that she feels completely overwhelmed by disorganization, it can be extremely useful for the psychotherapist to collaborate with a professional organizer. A professional organizer can assist the client in a "hands-on" manner to dig out from under her chronic chaos. Then the therapist and/or coach can help the client to develop habits that can help her to maintain better organization. Many adults with AD/HD find it so difficult to remain organized that they may need to budget for occasional sessions with a professional organizer as one of their AD/HD coping mechanisms.

2. The social environment

An AD/HD-friendly social environment is one in which people are reasonably tolerant of a woman's AD/HD patterns, and focus more on what they appreciate about her than on what they find irritating or in need of change. Ideally, in an AD/HD-friendly social environment, AD/HD foibles are handled with humor and understanding. To change the social milieu, it is important to educate significant others about AD/HD. The therapist may need to play an active role in this process, involving family members in her treatment. When individuals are not receptive to learning about AD/HD, a woman with AD/HD may need to decrease her contact with them. People who are overly critical, intolerant, or disparaging will work against self-acceptance that she is trying so hard to reach. Sadly, in some cases, such "AD/HD-toxic" individuals include family members.

3. The work environment

An AD/HD-friendly work environment enhances a woman's ability to function at her best. An AD/HD-friendly job is one in which there is low stress, but optimal levels of interest and stimulation; one that provides adequate administrative support; one that provides a quiet, non-distracting workspace and a comfortable work environment; one that provides adequate structure and flexibility; one that minimizes administrative/paperwork duties; and, typically, one that entails a variety of short-term tasks rather than detailed, long-term projects. But, most importantly, one in which a woman's supervisor is flexible and supportive. Ideally, her supervisor should be willing to assign her tasks that allow her to operate in her areas of strength and to minimize job responsibilities in areas of greatest weakness.

The profession of full-time homemaker, as Sari Solden (1995) so convincingly writes, is one of the most AD/HD-unfriendly jobs a woman could consider. Homemaking involves tasks that are repetitive, often unstimulating and unstructured, and filled with interruptions. Homemaking requires attention to detail, and entails responsibility for maintaining and keeping the schedules of numerous people (family members)—a striking list of AD/HD-unfriendly job characteristics.

In general, across a range of careers, women often find themselves in support roles, where they are expected to attend to details, keep schedules for others, and process paperwork—all tasks that are AD/HD-unfriendly.

Structuring the Psychotherapy Session— a Neurocognitive Perspective

Not only does a woman with AD/HD need structure in her life, she also needs structure in the therapy session. The therapy session can be viewed as a microcosm in which the challenges of her daily life can be observed. Just as structure, compensatory strategies, and reminders are needed in her daily life, they are also needed during the therapy session.

It is rarely productive for a woman with AD/HD to ramble or free associate at length. Such rambling associations are exactly what she needs to combat in order to remain effectively focused on the issue or activity at hand.

Memory difficulties are very common for women with AD/HD (Martinez, 1997). She may have no real sense of continuity from session to session unless structure is introduced by the therapist. Audiotaping sessions can be extremely helpful, allowing her to review each session later. If taping is not done, note-taking is essential. It is helpful for her to use a small spiral notebook, easily carried with her at all times, that is dedicated to her therapy sessions. In it, she can record:

1. key issues that have been discussed;

2. key issues that occur to her during the week—so that she can remember to bring them up in the subsequent session; and

3. homework assignments that she and her therapist may establish for her to work on between sessions.

It is most helpful if her therapist has a supply of such notebooks on hand, allowing her to begin her therapeutic work in a structured fashion from the start.

A review of the prior week's homework assignments is appropriate early in each therapy session. Was the assignment accomplished? If not, why not? A brief review of medication, its effectiveness and side effects, is also helpful. It is important for the therapist to be in periodic contact with the prescribing physician to share observations regarding medication. After these routine check-in topics, she and her therapist can focus on the issues she would like to address during the current session. If both therapist and client write these topics down, the session becomes more structured. It is also often necessary for a therapist to redirect her client if she goes off on a less productive tangent, or becomes caught up in less relevant details. At the end of the session, a brief review of topics and strategies, and a new homework assignment sends a woman with AD/HD on her way with a focused approach for the week ahead.

If a woman with AD/HD routinely fails to follow through on assignments, it may be necessary to structure midweek check-ins with her therapist—by voice mail or email. The accountability factor entailed in a check-in, combined with the shorter time line of three to four days, often helps her achieve the goals that have been eluding her from one week to the next. If this increased level of structure is still not effective, then it may be appropriate to bring in a coach who can provide a higher level of structure and support between therapy sessions.

Treating Coexisting Conditions

AD/HD rarely occurs alone, without other coexisting conditions. It is critical that a woman with AD/HD find a therapist and prescribing physician who can work well together so that her AD/HD and other conditions can be effectively treated in a coordinated fashion. Depression and anxiety are very common in women with AD/HD, and can be very effectively treated in conjunction with treatment for AD/HD (see Chapters 9 and 10).

The psychotherapist and prescribing physician should remain in regular contact in order to appropriately monitor medication responses and appropriate treatment approaches. Adults with AD/HD are often poor self-observers, and may not have appropriate expectations of the benefits and limits of medication. The therapist, who has more regular and extended contact with her client than does her physician, is often in the best position to assess the effects of medication.

Co-occurring learning disabilities are also common. In adulthood, these cognitive issues might be better termed "information processing difficulties" to emphasize the wide-ranging impact that such problems can have in adulthood, extending far beyond the educational environment into many aspects of daily functioning. A complete neuropsychological evaluation can provide valuable information to the woman with AD/HD and her therapist to help guide them when career decisions are considered.

Designing a Gender-aware Treatment Approach for Women with AD/HD

Beyond consideration of gender issues in diagnosis (see Chapter 1), there are important physiological, psychological, and sociocultural factors that cause women to be impacted differently by AD/HD. It is important to find a therapist who is thoroughly familiar with how AD/HD is manifested differently in women with AD/HD, as well as the different social expectations and gender roles that can intensify the impact of AD/HD for women.

Because so few therapists have training and/or experience in treating women with AD/HD, a woman may need to advocate for herself, taking an active role in educating her therapist, bringing books and articles for her to read. A woman with AD/HD should seek a therapist who is familiar with treating adults with AD/HD, who is open to learning more about the special issues of women. Therapists and prescribing physicians who are not open to new information or new approaches should be avoided.

Sociocultural Differences

Littman (Nadeau, Littman, & Quinn, 1999) writes of the painful social experiences of girls growing up with AD/HD, including social rejection and neglect. Patterns of socialization (Gilligan, 1982) and communication (Tannen, 1991) differ between males and females. Because verbal communication, cooperation, and self-control are much more emphasized for girls, it is understandable that females with AD/HD, would feel different, wounded, more outside the social circle than would males, whose AD/HD patterns may be more consistent with gender-appropriate behavior. As a result, the well-known difficulties that many adults with AD/HD experience in social interactions—missing social cues, interrupting, becoming distracted during conversation, talking too much or too little, forgetting to return phone calls, etc.—may have a greater negative impact on women with AD/HD. Perhaps one way of describing the dilemma is that AD/HD patterns seem more discordant with female social expectations than with those of males. In treating women with AD/HD, it becomes more critical to address social skills, understanding her need for social acceptance and support. Ultimately, her goal is to reach a state of comfortable acceptance about her differentness from the stereotyped feminine ideal, and to find ways to build relationships with individuals that understand and appreciate her.

Hormonal Differences

Fluctuating hormones have a powerful and variable effect upon AD/HD symptoms in females. Beginning at puberty and continuing throughout her life, hormonal shifts must be taken into account in the effective treatment of any woman. Medication regimens that may include birth control pills, hormone replacement therapy, and the introduction of other psychotropic medications during low-estrogen states (premenstrual and postnatal) must be carefully considered, in addition to psychostimulants and other medications typically used to treat AD/HD symptomatology.

Psychological Differences

A woman with AD/HD needs a therapist who is aware of gender differences in the psychological issues that are associated with AD/HD. Research has demonstrated that low self-esteem is more common for women with AD/HD than for men. Such self-esteem issues may cause a woman to be more reluctant to make needed changes in her life. Low self-esteem may lead her to remain in a dysfunctional relationship, believing that she won't find a better partner elsewhere. Problems with self-assertion may make it much more challenging for her to advocate for herself in the workplace.

Differing Gender-based Roles

Parenting issues also pose a greater challenge for mothers with AD/HD than for fathers because women, in most families, continue to play the role of the primary parent. Furthermore, women with AD/HD may have children with AD/HD, intensifying their parenting challenges because they have difficulty with the very issues in which their children need assistance. Single parenting, faced by many women with AD/HD, presents an even greater set of challenges. A mother with AD/HD needs a therapist who can work with her on all aspects of her complex and challenging life including parenting issues (see Chapter 18).

Women's AD/HD Psychotherapy Groups

Because women's interpersonal needs and patterns of socialization differ from those of men, treatment approaches must take those needs into account. Just as women seek out one another when they struggle with child rearing issues, marital issues, and other life issues, women with AD/HD tend to seek the support of other women who can understand their AD/HD difficulties and accept their failure to live up to the idealized images of women that are so pervasive in our culture.

Social acceptance, understanding, and encouragement are powerful healing forces that can take place in a women's AD/HD psychotherapy group. In group therapy, the clinician can provide structure, guidance, and feedback that may not be present in a support group setting. In such a group, women can give each other permission to seek the structure and support that they need to function best; they can encourage one another to engage in the self-care that is necessary to reduce stress and manage anxiety; they can help one another to recognize and celebrate their strengths and to move away from their habitual hypercritical focus on areas of weakness. Often such messages are more powerful and effective when they come from other women with AD/HD, rather than from the therapist herself.

Conclusion

It is essential for a woman with AD/HD to find a therapist who possesses specialized skills and knowledge that can address all of her complex and interlocking issues. She needs a therapist who does not focus exclusively on the psychological issues associated with AD/HD, but can also help her to find concrete, practical strategies to cope with the numerous, real-life challenges that AD/HD poses in her life. Few therapists have experience or training in treating women with AD/HD, but a growing number of specialists in childhood AD/HD are beginning to treat adults as well. While women may not easily find a therapist that is highly experienced, they should look for a therapist that is open to learning how to best meet their needs.

The discovery of effective treatment strategies for women with AD/HD is only now beginning. The concepts outlined in this chapter are presented as an initial attempt to formulate a treatment approach for women with AD/HD. Treatment strategies are needed for women that can address their special challenges, such as the effects of fluctuating hormone levels upon AD/HD, the challenges of motherhood, and the intense social pressures that women face as they struggle to meet dual roles as homemakers and career women. In these very early days of discovery, women with AD/HD must take the role of pioneers, advocating for themselves, and actively educating the professionals who work with them. It is hoped that the approaches presented in this chapter will provide women with AD/HD with knowledge that can help them to find appropriate treatment— treatment that can help them take charge of their lives.

References

Gilligan, C. (1982). *In a different voice.* Cambridge, MA: Harvard University Press.

Goodwin, R.E., & Bolton, D.P. (1991). Decision-making in cognitive rehabilitation: A clinical model. *Cognitive Rehabilitation, 9,* 12-19.

Hallowell, E.M., & Ratey, J.J. (1994). *Driven to distraction.* New York: Pantheon.

Nadeau, K., Littman, E., & Quinn, P. (1999). *Understanding girls with AD/HD.* Silver Spring, MD: Advantage Books.

Prince, J., & Wilens, T. (2000). Diagnosis and treatment of adults with AD/HD. In P. Accardo, T. Blondis, B. Whitman, & M. Stein (Eds.). *Attention deficits and hyperactivity in children and adults (pp. 665-684).* New York: Marcel Dekker, Inc.

Ratey, J., Greenberg, M., & Lindem, K. (1991). Combination of treatments for attention deficit disorders in adults. *Journal of Nervous and Mental Disorder, 176,* 699-701.

Rucklidge, J.J., & Kaplan, B.J. (1997). Psychological functioning in women identified in adulthood with attention-deficit/hyperactivity disorder. *Journal of Attention Disorders, 2,* 167-176.

Solden, S. (1995). *Women with attention deficit disorder: Embracing disorganization at home and in the workplace.* Grass Valley, CA: Underwood Books..

Tannen, D. (1991). *You just don't understand.* New York: Ballantine.

Viorst, J. (1986). *Necessary losses.* New York: Simon and Schuster.

Webster's new international dictionary of the English language, 2nd edition, unabridged (1946) Springfield, MA: G. & C. Merriam Company, Publishers.

CHAPTER

Working with Coaches and Organizers

Kathleen G. Nadeau, Ph.D.

Two different but related professions have grown up in response to the increased stress of modern life—professional organizers and personal coaches. Recently, both of these professions have turned their attention toward serving the needs of adults with AD/HD. This chapter will address the interlocking and overlapping roles of therapist, coach, and organizer, as well as the types of issues and situations in which a therapist, coach, organizer, or combination of these may be most helpful.

Professional Organizing

There is considerable overlap between the work of a professional organizer and that of an AD/HD coach. Generally speaking, a professional organizer provides on-site, hands-on help. The primary focus of an organizer is to assist her client to organize her physical environment. Some organizers also teach organizing principles. Other organizers provide a minimum of hands-on help, and work more as a coach, providing structure and guidance to women as they work to organize some aspect of their environment. Because such differences exist, it is critical that a woman with AD/HD ask a professional organizer to clarify her approach before deciding to contract with her for organizing assistance.

There is no licensure or certification of professional organizers, but most reputable and experienced organizers are members of NAPO—the National Association of Professional Organizers. Organizers who specialize in working with adults with AD/HD will be the best match for a woman with AD/HD because they are familiar with typical AD/HD patterns and challenges and can approach the organizing process from an AD/HD-friendly perspective.

Judith Kolberg (Kolberg & Nadeau, 2002) describes the work of an organizer as helping a client to find organizing solutions, to purchase organizing products, to speed the process of decision-making, to motivate her, and to prevent her from feeling overwhelmed as she tackles the piles of papers, packed closets, and cluttered rooms, of her home. An organizer's non-judgmental presence can facilitate the process of de-cluttering and can help to minimize procrastination and perfectionism—two factors that often lead women with AD/HD to struggle with disorganization.

Some women with AD/HD find that it's most helpful to meet regularly with an organizer. For example, they might meet regularly on a quarterly basis after the initial organizing effort is accomplished in order to prevent her from relapsing to her earlier state of chaos. Organizing is much easier to maintain when "dig outs" occur regularly, and often women with

AD/HD need the support and structure of an organizer to accomplish these periodic attacks on disorder.

A woman with AD/HD who has lived with disorganization for years may fear that "getting organized" is a hopeless task. Even when she has a cleaning lady, her house is in chaos again a day or so after her visit. Often such a rapid return to disorder occurs because there is no official place where each belonging "lives," or at least no convenient place that she's likely to consistently use. An organizer can help a woman with AD/HD to rearrange her living space, obtain needed shelving, containers and storage units, and help her to develop AD/HD-friendly patterns that can greatly reduce her daily clutter habits. For example, if a recycling bin is not conveniently located, piles of magazines, newspapers and junk mail are likely to clutter the surfaces of the main living areas. A professional organizer can help her client develop more convenient solutions to store or discard the items that accumulate on a daily basis, contributing to the general clutter of home, auto, or office.

Coaching

The concept of coaching for adults with AD/HD was first introduced in the bestselling book, *Driven to Distraction*, by Ned Hallowell and John Ratey (1994). They described a coach as "an individual standing on the sidelines with a whistle around his or her neck barking out encouragement, directions, and reminders to the player in the game" (p. 226).

A coach typically works by phone or by email, helping a woman with AD/HD to find solutions that she can implement herself. The issues addressed in coaching are more wide-ranging than those typically addressed by an organizer. Rather than only focusing on the physical environment, a coach focuses on a broad range of life management issues, helping a woman to counteract long-standing negative patterns and create a more balanced and healthy life-style. A coach can help a woman with AD/HD clarify goals, set priorities, and build habits that can help her function better in her daily life. In addition to life-management issues, a coach can help her complete complex multistep tasks; for example, completing a long-term project, finishing a thesis or dissertation, conducting a job search, or applying to college or graduate programs.

Many women with AD/HD have long ago given up on their dreams due to repeated failures. Coaching can help a woman with AD/HD reverse this process. Cynthia Runberg (1999), a coach in Chapel Hill, North Carolina, writes:

> *Coaching is about action, about getting it done! A coach will listen to your hopes and desires, and together with you will formulate the goal. Once the goal is identified, a plan, system, or structure will be implemented into the daily routine of life to achieve the goal. Coaching provides accountability around the action you've committed to do. It's the key to progress. Creating accountability, along with the support and encouragement of a coach, will help you follow through and make progress toward your goal.*
>
> *Coaching can be a great match for women with AD/HD, empowering them to take charge of their lives instead of feeling victimized by their organizational challenges and their history of underachievement (p. 15).*

Does She Need a Psychotherapist or a Coach?

While it is clear how professional organizing differs from psychotherapy, it is less clear where psychotherapy ends and coaching begins. In fact, there are many areas of overlap between cognitive/behavioral therapy approaches and coaching. One important difference is that coaching typically takes place by telephone, while therapy typically takes place face-to-face. In fact, many clients never meet their coach face-to-face. Another important difference is that coaching is not covered by health insurance.

Both coaching and psychotherapy can involve goal-setting and concrete behavioral changes, as well as changes in attitudes that have previously interfered with reaching desired goals and objectives. However, there are important differences between therapy and coaching that should be understood and appreciated.

Readiness to Change

Coaching can work only when "the client is ready, willing and able to work in a partnership with the coach and rise to the challenge of creating a better life . . ." (Ratey, N., 1999). Often, when a woman with AD/HD enters psychotherapy, she is struggling with anxiety, low self-esteem, depression, and general demoralization. While change is the ultimate goal of both psychotherapy and coaching, immediate readiness to change is not a requirement for therapy. In fact, much of the work of psychotherapy may focus on getting ready to change—helping a woman to understand and accept herself, to reframe her self-definition in a more positive, constructive manner, and to improve relationships with the important people in her life. At that point, she may be ready to tackle the challenges of AD/HD with a coach.

Emotional/Interpersonal Issues vs. Daily Life-management

The concerns of a woman with AD/HD will be the primary determinants of whether it makes sense for her to work with a therapist, a coach, or both. If emotional issues are primary—depression, anxiety, low self-esteem, social withdrawal, parenting concerns, or relationship problems—then psychotherapy is the appropriate first step. However, if a woman has few emotional issues, but reports that her primary concerns are procrastination, poor time management, or disorganization, she may work most effectively with a coach. If she struggles with a combination of both psychological and life-management issues, as do the majority of women with AD/HD, she may find it helpful to work with a therapist who also focuses on life-management issues. As she begins to feel better in her psychological and interpersonal life, she may choose to shift to coaching. Often, there is a transition period when working with both, in tandem, can be very helpful—although this requires a greater outlay of time and money and may not be a realistic choice for many women.

Workplace Issues

Workplace issues are also a frequent concern for women with AD/HD. Depending upon her specific workplace concerns, she might choose either a therapist or a coach. A therapist might be most appropriate if she is considering a job change or career change. A therapist could help her to assess her cognitive strengths and weaknesses, and analyze her interests, values, and personality type in order to consider the most appropriate career directions. Together, they might review her past work history to identify aspects of various past jobs that have proven to be a good or bad match for her. When it comes time to take action (i.e., conduct a job search, research career alternatives, investigate retraining programs, submit graduate school applications, or explore ways to finance further training), a coach might be a better choice to help her organize and follow through on these concrete, complex multistep tasks.

When Organizers or Coaches Are Not an Option

Professional organizers are not available in all areas, and not all women with AD/HD can afford the services of a professional organizer or coach. If an organizer or coach is not an option, a "clutter buddy" can be very helpful to a woman with AD/HD. A clutter buddy can be a friend or family member, or might even be another woman with AD/HD, someone who is supportive and non-judgmental. Simply having another person present to suggest, to help, and to encourage, can be a very positive influence.

Often, a woman with AD/HD is unable to tackle her disorder because she feels overwhelmed and cannot decide where to begin. For example, she may haul everything out of her closet, making efforts to throw items into a giveaway pile. Soon, however, she becomes tired or distracted. Eventually, she puts everything back in the closet in more or less the same state of disorder.

A clutter buddy can help to divide the organizing task into bite-sized pieces and provide encouragement throughout the process. Many women with AD/HD report, with irony, that they are very good at suggesting organizing approaches to others—but are not able to stay focused and follow through on organizing tasks themselves. Women with AD/HD can provide organizing support for one another—"I'll come to your house on Tuesday afternoons, you come to mine on Thursdays, and we'll keep at this mess until things are under better control." One women's AD/HD support group in California had the creative idea to organize dig-outs, in which a group of women would arrive at one member's home to engage in a group dig-out. These organizing events became humorous, highly energizing social occasions with very positive results for everyone in the group.

Whether it's a professional organizer, a family member, a friend, or support from other women with AD/HD, hands-on help is often needed, at first, to help a woman with AD/HD gain better control over the physical disorder in her life. Later, an AD/HD coach can be helpful in teaching her ways to maintain this organization. It's important, however, that "creeping clutter" not be viewed as a sign of failure. Regular hands-on help, twice, three, or four times a year, may be an essential support for a woman with AD/HD. Physical maintenance of the home or office—cleaning, filing, sorting, and discarding—are ADD-unfriendly activities for a woman with AD/HD. A basic tenet in creating an AD/HD-friendly life is to reduce, eliminate, or delegate activities that call on abilities most impacted by AD/HD.

Setting Reachable Organizing Goals

Getting organized is about being functional, not about being perfect. When a woman with AD/HD works with an organizer or ADD coach, she should not engage in a struggle to meet unrealistic standards, or to meet standards imposed by someone else, but rather in an effort to reduce stress and to gain better control over her daily life.

References

Cantrell, P. (1999). Positively organized: A professional organizers with ADD helps you organize in an ADD-friendly fashion. *ADDvance, 2(6),* 4-7.

Hallowell, N., & Ratey, J. (1994). *Driven to distraction.* New York: Pantheon.

Kolberg, J., & Nadeau, K. (2002). *ADD-friendly ways to organize your life.* New York: Brunner-Routledge.

Ratey, N. (1999). How a coach can help make your "wishes" come true. *ADDvance, 2(5),* 26-28.

Runberg, C. (1999). Are you surviving or thriving in life? *ADDvance, 2(3),* 14-15.

CHAPTER 8

Taking Charge of AD/HD

Kathleen G. Nadeau, Ph.D.

U ltimately, a woman's goal is to take charge of her AD/HD, coming to understand herself and her strengths, as well as the challenges she faces. Although medication can be very helpful in reducing troublesome patterns associated with AD/HD, the greatest improvement comes when a woman learns how to create an AD/HD-friendly life, by developing habits and compensatory strategies that work for her. This process is often most successful when it begins in counseling or therapy with a clinician highly experienced in the practical aspects of treating AD/HD, and when the process of taking charge is supported through coaching and support groups. Gradually, a woman internalizes the messages that she has received and the strategies that she has learned so that she can move forward on her own, taking responsibility for her daily life and her future. This chapter highlights ways that a woman can take charge of her AD/HD—by changing attitudes, by making more AD/HD-friendly life choices, and by developing habits and strategies to counteract troublesome AD/HD tendencies that get in her way.

When a woman seeks treatment for her AD/HD, the therapist's role is to prepare her to take charge of herself and her life. Therapy should not only help her reframe AD/HD as a set of neurological traits—traits, some of which, under the right circumstances, can become strengths. Certainly there are AD/HD traits that typically cause stress and inconvenience, and these need to be minimized. Learning compensatory skills is an essential part of taking charge of AD/HD—skills that may be learned and practiced during counseling or coaching, but which, finally, must be used independently.

Moving from Self-blame to Self-acceptance

For a woman with AD/HD, the most painful issue is her overwhelming sense of inadequacy in fulfilling the roles that she feels are expected of her by her family and society, and that she also expects of herself. Girls are raised to apologize, to accommodate, to take the blame, and to focus on the needs of others. Sari Solden, in her book, *Women with Attention Deficit Disorder,* writes of women "coming out of the AD/HD closet" of shame and self-blame. The first challenge, then, is to stop this ingrained habit of internalization and self-blame—to move from inertia to action, from shame to self-assertion and acceptance.

It is often the diagnosis of AD/HD itself that allows a woman to take her first steps away from self-blame. The diagnosis helps women to realize that they are not "lazy, stupid or crazy," (from the title of Kate Kelly and Peggy Ramundo's book, *You Mean I'm Not Lazy, Stupid, or Crazy!?*), but rather that they have a treatable neurological condition.

However, shifting from self-blame to blaming her troubles on AD/HD, is only an intermediate step toward truly taking charge. Ultimately, a woman with AD/HD needs to stop focusing on blame and reach a comfortable, realistic self-acceptance. This self-acceptance involves a realization that she does not need to be perfect by others' standards, and an acknowledgment of her strengths and positive traits. Rather than defining herself as a woman with AD/HD, she comes to see herself as a complex human being with both strengths and weaknesses. Finally, a healthy woman with AD/HD moves away from self-condemnation and begins to celebrate her positive qualities, and appreciate her uniqueness. To paraphrase Walt Whitman, she learns to sing a song of herself, dancing to the rhythms of her own music.

Building a Support System

Both on the job and at home, women are often placed in the role of caretakers. Society traditionally expects women to *be* the support system for their families. Perhaps the greatest hurdle for a woman with AD/HD is to give herself permission to ask for and to receive support from others, to come to understand that self-care is not self-indulgent. Healthy self-preservation will ultimately benefit those who depend on her.

Support systems may be needed on both emotional and physical levels. Emotional support may come from a women's AD/HD support group. Some women seek "virtual" AD/HD support groups online, if they are not in an area where a support group is available. Often, AD/HD support can develop informally—between two women, rather than in a group. For example, women with AD/HD who are mothers of children with AD/HD may encounter one another at a parents' support group, begin to connect around their children's issues, and then, informally support one another around their own AD/HD issues as well.

Family members can be crucial sources of support. As a woman with AD/HD educates her spouse and/or children about AD/HD and how it affects her, the whole family can begin to work together to become an AD/HD-friendly family. Support can also come when a woman gives herself permission to buy or barter help in areas of functioning that are difficult for her. For example, one woman with AD/HD who was proficient at the computer, but very poor at organizing, bartered services with a professional organizer who needed help setting up her business on her computer. Coming to a comfortable acceptance of her strengths and weaknesses, her likes and dislikes, a woman with AD/HD can begin to problem-solve, acknowledging areas of life management at which she will never excel—and giving herself permission to seek help from others in those areas.

Operating in the "Green Zone"

One AD/HD coach refers to a client's areas of strength as her "green zone" and to areas of challenge as her "red zone." Green equals GO, red equals STOP—an easy way to remember an AD/HD-friendly concept. To effectively manage her AD/HD, a woman should operate in her "green zone" whenever possible, deciding to hire, delegate, barter, or reorganize her life so that her "red zone" activities are minimized and her "green zone" activities are maximized. Often the biggest hurdle for a woman with AD/HD is to give herself permission to avoid "red zone" activities, escaping from the *shoulds* of the traditional female role so that she can live in her "green zone."

Sari Solden (1995) writes of homemaking as the most ADD-unfriendly job a woman can have. Routine housecleaning and maintenance activities are typically in the "red zone" for a woman with AD/HD.

Getting out of the "red zone" may require hiring a coach or organizer to help with the reorganization of living space or to help with organizing and filing paperwork. Some women with AD/HD have a standing appointment on a quarterly basis with an organizer who can help them keep their important papers in order. Women who can't afford such services may find that they can barter services with other women.

Downsizing Dual-career Stress

Over the past generation, the struggles for women with AD/HD have intensified with the rapid rise of women in the workplace. Now, staying home to raise children is the exception rather than the rule. Most women who enter the workplace are still expected to fulfill the more traditional roles of wife and mother while also functioning efficiently and tirelessly, juggling the demands of full-time employment. These exhaustive daily demands are daunting for most women. When a woman with AD/HD encounters these dual expectations, the demands of her daily life typically exceed her ability to cope.

Each woman with AD/HD must find her own solutions when she faces impossible expectations, giving up efforts to be the "super woman" who can do it all. She may change jobs to shorten her commute, or perhaps shift to part-time or halftime employment. In addition to changing her work habits, she also needs to assess the commitments and activities of her children, streamline daily life-management tasks, and renegotiate the division of labor at home with her partner and children. Families in which the mother has AD/HD should carefully assess their budget, giving very high priority to reducing her burden of responsibilities at home. Through healthy self-knowledge and self-acceptance, women with AD/HD can learn to give themselves permission to seek the supports they need.

Single Parenting

Divorce rates are close to fifty percent in the United States, and divorce becomes even more likely when AD/HD is added to the list of marital stressors. Following divorce, it is likely the mother who remains the primary parent of her children. When a woman with AD/HD becomes a single parent, the result tends to be chronic exhaustion, emotional depletion and increasing chaos, as she struggles to juggle parenting, bill-paying, household maintenance and employment without the support of a partner.

When a woman with AD/HD becomes a single parent, her first priority must be to reduce stress and to gain support, however she can achieve it. She may need to make radical choices to maintain daily functioning. One woman with AD/HD chose to leave the metropolitan area where she had lived with her former husband, taking her two children back to the small town where she had grown up. This decision significantly lowered her cost of living and gave her immediate access to the support her parents could offer. Another woman moved from her suburban home to a large, three-bedroom apartment. In this way, she reduced the cost and complexity of managing a house, allowing her to focus her energies on her children and her job. Yet another woman with AD/HD came to the difficult, but ultimately correct decision, for her two children to live with their father during the week. The children's father had remarried, and had the support of a partner to help him meet the demanding weekday schedule, whereas she was single and had a demanding job. Her children spent weekends with her, allowing her to have extended time with them without the hectic weekday schedule of school, work, and homework.

Whatever solution a woman chooses, it needs to achieve a reduction in intolerable daily demands so that she can be successful in the areas of her life that matter most—her own well-being and that of her children.

Raising Children with AD/HD

Women with AD/HD who have a child with AD/HD face a

special challenge. Children with AD/HD can be difficult for any parent to raise. Typically, they need more structure and support, more limit-setting, and often have special educational and psychological needs. When the mother also has AD/HD, she faces the most important, most difficult task of her life—providing structure, limits, and support for her children when she has difficulty providing them for herself.

In addition to parenting challenges, she faces the ill-informed, often harsh judgment of others. "I'd never let my child behave like that!" she may hear parents of non-AD/HD children comment. From the outside looking in, it is easy for other parents to judge a woman with AD/HD when her children misbehave. But any parent of a child with AD/HD knows that he doesn't readily respond to the usual corrections and limits. Only a parent who has raised such a challenging child herself can truly understand her situation. Support groups for parents of children with AD/HD can provide a woman with AD/HD the encouragement and support that can help her succeed.

Rather than falling immediately into old patterns of self-blame—"If I weren't such an inadequate mother, my kids wouldn't have these problems."—she needs to seek the best help that she can find to raise her children effectively. Today, there are numerous excellent books on behavior management techniques for children with AD/HD. Parenting support groups, tutors, coaches, pediatricians, and child and family therapists can all help to provide a mother with AD/HD with good advice and support for her child(ren) with AD/HD.

Form or Join a Women's AD/HD Support Group

Often the biggest struggle for a woman with AD/HD is an internal one—self-imposed, unrealistic expectations, and self-blame for not meeting those expectations. Traditional female role expectations that are no longer realistic in contemporary life remain deeply ingrained in most women. Breaking out of this mold takes time and effort. A support group for women with AD/HD can be a powerful source of assistance, providing encouragement and understanding as a woman works to develop more realistic expectations and better strategies for dealing with demanding situations.

Women's AD/HD support groups, both in-person and online, have sprung up across the country. The website of the National Center for Gender Issues and AD/HD (www.ncgiadd.org) posts the names of women who are seeking support groups so that others in the same geographic area may contact them to form a group.

Whether online or in-person, the experience of meeting and interacting with other women like herself can be a heartwarming and liberating experience for a woman with AD/HD. Many women with AD/HD have spent much of their lives in hiding, afraid to be exposed as failing to live up to the standards of their non-AD/HD coworkers, neighbors, and acquaintances. Sadly, for many women with AD/HD, parents and spouses are among the most critical.

The experience of meeting other women who struggle with similar feelings and issues can be powerful, beginning a healing process, and creating a sense of belonging that has been longed for throughout a lifetime in which she has felt "different," or excluded. In a support group, these women can share "war stories," laugh together over daily disasters, and offer one another coping strategies that work.

Educate Significant Others about AD/HD

It is important that every significant other in the life of a woman with AD/HD comes to appreciate the full impact that AD/HD has upon her. Being a woman with AD/HD is hard enough without being surrounded by family members who blame her for her difficulties. A husband may feel anger and resentment over an ill-kempt house or misbehaving children, assuming that his wife "just doesn't care." Her parents may react in a judgmental fashion—questioning why their daughter's home is messy and why she may need more emotional, physical, or financial help than their non-AD/HD children.

It's best if a woman's partner and/or entire family participates in therapy so that they can understand the impact of AD/HD, and learn to problem-solve together to resolve AD/HD issues at home. A woman with AD/HD should strongly encourage her partner to attend support groups or educational meetings focused on AD/HD to listen to the stories of other families affected by AD/HD, and to more fully appreciate the challenges that a woman with AD/HD faces on a daily basis.

Once a partner comes to understand that lateness, forgetfulness, and disorder are not due to inconsideration or hostility, he or she can join in the process of constructive problem-solving. Working together with a counselor, a woman with AD/HD and her partner can develop patterns that do not overburden the non-AD/HD partner, and do not infantilize the woman with AD/HD. Responsibilities for the household and children can be redistributed to allow each person to function in their "green zone." Tasks that are in the "red zone" for both partners can be shared, or, better yet, delegated to someone else.

It's 'All in the Family'—Creating an AD/HD-friendly Household

A woman with AD/HD should work to create an AD/HD-friendly environment in her home. Chances are, if she has AD/HD, that one or more of her children have AD/HD as well. As she approaches her own AD/HD with acceptance and good humor, she is teaching her children to do the same. By creating a AD/HD safety zone at home, where AD/HD patterns are understood, the frequency of conflicts and emotional explosions can decrease, allowing her to spend her energy in more positive pursuits.

An AD/HD-friendly Family Is One That:

▶ looks for ways to simplify routines and solve problems;

▶ has a home furnished in a casual, sturdy, easy-to-maintain style;

▶ is supportive, loving, and cooperative;

▶ doesn't "sweat the details," or over-focus on mistakes;

▶ learns to be patient when people are short-tempered, and where people apologize sincerely when they "lose it" out of frustration;

▶ learns to laugh over AD/HD dilemmas—emphasizing what family members do right rather than what they do wrong;

▶ has a convenient message center, where family members can write each other notes and reminders, that is located in a place where people are sure to look;

▶ believes that it's OK to be different from each other and OK to be oneself; and

▶ makes sure to spend time enjoying each other, not just focusing on problems.

As a woman learns to take charge of her own AD/HD, she can teach her children that AD/HD is not an excuse, but a challenge that can be met with confidence and success when a family creates an AD/HD-friendly home environment.

Problem-solve to Reduce Stress

Stress is the enemy of AD/HD. One of the most critical ways that a woman with AD/HD can reduce the negative effects of her AD/HD is to conduct a stress survey of her life, and then begin a process of problem-solving to reduce sources of stress.

If her stress is financial, does she need debt-reduction counseling? Does she need help from a coach or counselor to reduce patterns of impulse spending that lead to financial stress? Does she need to make more radical decisions regarding living space and life-style in order to live within her means?

If her stress comes from over-commitment, are there activities that can be reduced or eliminated? Many women with AD/HD are chronically overcommitted, if she is a mother, her children's homework and extracurricular activities only serve to increase her over-commitment. Few commitments are so important that they justify an ongoing high stress level. Women with AD/HD often need to eliminate activities in their own and their children's daily lives, in order to create more balance.

Is her stress work-related? Does she need to change jobs? Careers? Bosses? Shorten her commute? Work for a company that is more family-friendly? Is her stress health-related? Does she get adequate sleep, exercise, nutrition?

A woman with AD/HD should examine her life, to explore the multiple sources of stress. A coach, counselor or therapist can help her make a stress analysis of her life and then begin to make decisions that can relieve that stress.

Create an AD/HD-friendly Social Network

Women with AD/HD should make extra efforts to avoid those who are overly critical and judgmental. Sometimes, judgments and criticisms come from family members. However, when she works hard to find solutions and to improve her living

situation, skeptical family members may become more supportive and receptive to learning about AD/HD. If family members
persist in critizing, she needs support from a therapist to bring
family members on-board.

Occasions for self-criticism abound. Opening any magazine
in the grocery store, a woman with AD/HD is faced with impossible ideals—of women dressed in the latest fashions, beautifully
decorated homes, lusciously prepared meals, and perfectly maintained gardens. At her child's school, she may be faced with the
perky PTA president—neatly dressed, full of energy, and always
organized. Beside the soccer field, swimming pool, or any other
gathering of parents, she is likely to hear parents bragging about
their child who has won awards, has been selected for the more
competitive team, or who earns top grades.

If surrounded by women whose standards she cannot meet,
a woman with AD/HD needs to counterbalance these demoralizing influences in her social world by seeking out others who
are warm, accepting, humorous, sympathetic, creative, and less
competitive. The rest of the world isn't perfect, but it can seem
so to a woman with AD/HD who is over-focused on her "failings" and has little opportunity for interaction with those who
understand her AD/HD and appreciate the best in her.

Self-care

Often a woman with AD/HD feels so guilty and self-blam-
ing in her struggle to meet the relentless daily grind of child
care, meal preparation, laundry, home maintenance, errands,
and workplace demands that she cannot imagine making time
for herself. And yet, it is self-care that can replenish her
energy and focus.

Neglecting herself to meet the needs and demands of
others, a woman with AD/HD often develops the habit of

stealing time for herself late at night. In a brief reprieve from daily responsibilities, she stays up to read, watch late-night TV, or surf the Internet. Depriving herself of sleep, this pattern insures that another exhausted, chaotic day will begin a few short hours later. Tired from her stolen moments the night before, she rises late, rushes to get ready for work, scolds her children through breakfast and into their school day, and leaves for work late, already feeling stressed. Such a habit only increases her AD/HD-related problems of lateness, forgetfulness, high stress levels, and disorganization.

Another destructive form of self-care is late-night food binging. Many women with AD/HD report that they console and calm themselves with carbohydrates—eating ice cream, cookies, chips, popcorn, or other snacks throughout the evening, or late at night after the rest of the family has gone to bed. The immediate pleasure and temporary sense of calm that accompanies such binges are followed by weight gain, guilt, and self-reproach.

A woman with AD/HD can only feel in charge of herself and her life when she begins to engage in *real* self-care—choosing activities that will calm and soothe her without negative consequences such as fatigue or weight gain, engaging in activities that will enhance her health and well-being, improve her ability to operate more effectively, and help her to meet the demands of each day without becoming so depleted. True self-care activities include:

Adequate Sleep

Sleep problems are very common for women with AD/HD. Women who have difficulty falling asleep should discuss this with their physician to explore the possibility of a sleep disorder. But even without a sleep disorder, a woman may struggle with chronic sleep deprivation—rarely going to bed early enough to have adequate sleep each night. The pleasure of the moment, combined with a tendency to lose track of time, defeats her best intentions night after night. If her night-owl habit is chronic, she may need to work with her counselor or therapist to develop good sleep habits.

Good Nutrition

Good nutrition often poses a challenge for a woman with AD/HD because healthy meals require planning. As a function of the rush and disorder of her daily life, she may frequently resort to fast foods or carry-out. Poor nutrition also results from the common tendency for women with AD/HD to "self-medicate" with food—typically carbohydrate-rich snack foods and desserts. A poorly balanced diet filled with starch and sugar leads to low energy, weight gain, and peaks and valleys in blood sugar level that can only increase her AD/HD difficulties.

A woman with AD/HD needs to find AD/HD-friendly solutions to her dietary problems. Complicated meal-planning is unrealistic, but better habits can be developed—such as having fresh fruit or yogurt available rather than candy bars and chips. If a woman with AD/HD finds that she turns to snack food at night to calm or soothe herself, she needs to develop healthier self-calming habits—herbal tea, meditation, or relaxation routines (see below).

Daily Stretching and Exercise

The more we understand about the human brain, the better we understand the importance of daily exercise for optimal brain functioning. Exercise is also crucial for managing feelings of restlessness or hyperactivity. A woman with AD/HD can build needed structure into healthy exercise habits by scheduling regular exercise with a friend—walking at lunch time with a coworker, or working out with a friend a couple of times a week. Ten to fifteen minutes of stretching exercises before bedtime can also help calm the mind and promote relaxation that can help her to fall asleep.

Relaxation and Meditation

Learning specific relaxation skills can be highly beneficial. A therapist or counselor can introduce a number of techniques that can be practiced, becoming more effective over time. One such technique is visual imagery. Guided by her therapist, a woman closes her eyes and imagines herself in a highly soothing, relaxing environment of her choice. This visualized environment may be actual or imaginary. As she becomes more proficient at visual imagery, she can engage in it without guidance, creating an always available break from the stress of daily life. Soothing audio tapes can be purchased to aid the visual imagery process.

Meditation is another very effective relaxation technique, although some women report being unable to "meditate" i.e., when they sit still and try to empty their minds, they find that their thoughts continue to race. For these women, a better approach to meditation is to listen to music while meditating, or even to meditate in movement, such as yoga. These approaches often seem more effective in counteracting the mental hyperactivity of AD/HD.

Beginning the morning with a calm, meditative experience can set the tone for the day— a hot cup of tea before the children get up, a few minutes alone in the garden, or fifteen minutes of yoga in a quiet room before beginning the rush of the day's activities.

Quiet Time—Daily Time-outs

Time-outs are essential daily stress reducers. A time-out is simply a quick break from being on-duty, reading for pleasure, or closing one's eyes for a few moments. A woman who is married needs to negotiate regular time-outs with her spouse—fifteen minutes before dinner, or a few moments in the morning before she's on-duty. Time-outs, however, become more challenging for a single mother to arrange. If her home is large enough to accommodate another adult, a single mother with AD/HD may want to consider offering free rent to a college or graduate student in return for help with child care and housekeeping duties, so that she can have time for self-care and stress reduction.

High stress and need for regular quiet time is not only true of women with children. A tendency to overcommit, to rush from one activity to the next, seems almost universal among women with AD/HD. Single women with AD/HD should also take care to make time for relaxation, as well, developing daily rituals to reduce stress.

Quality Time with Others

Another very important form of self-care for the woman with AD/HD is to make sure that she has daily quality time with her family and friends. It's so easy to become caught up in the daily rush that she forgets to spend time with others in a relaxed, caring way. Quality time with children can be story time just before bed, a fifteen minute walk after dinner, a ride in the car for ice cream—simple things can provide an opportunity to catch up on the day's events or simply to relax together. Quality time with friends or with a partner is just as critical—daily walks and conversation, as well as, regularly scheduled times to socialize.

Avoiding Burnout

Burnout poses a great risk for many women with AD/HD. Burnout is accompanied by an increase in AD/HD symptoms, chronic fatigue, emotional overreactions, and often a cascading chain of avoidable crises. Too often, women push themselves to their limit, only recognizing burnout after it has occurred. The key to managing burnout is learning to anticipate and avoid it, whenever possible.

One mother of two children with AD/HD recognized the importance of getting a break from the relentless demands of her two sons. Each summer, she arranged for her sons to attend sleepaway camp for a month, giving her four weeks to relax and refuel. During other parts of the summer vacation, her sons visited their grandparents at separate times. This allowed her to spend time with each son alone, a special bonding experience that each of them treasured. Recognizing her limits and seeking solutions to avoid burnout allowed her to be an effective and more patient mother during the school year.

Burnout isn't only the province of mothers. Single working women with AD/HD need to guard against a tendency toward workaholism or over-commitment to outside activities. It's important for single women with AD/HD to consciously make time to "do nothing," to relax and regenerate (See Chapter 17).

Focus on the Positive

It is so easy for a woman with AD/HD to become caught up in all the things that she has difficulty managing and never allow herself to focus on her gifts, her strengths, and the things she loves. Rather than measuring her success in terms of neatness and organization, she should celebrate her gifts — her warmth, her creativity, her humor, her sensitivity, her spirit. She should create opportunities to be her best self—even if the laundry remains unfolded! By measuring herself in terms of her own values, by operating in her "green zone" and focusing on the things she loves best, by actively looking for people who can appreciate the best in her, she can not only take charge of her AD/HD, but lead a rich and fulfilling life in the process.

References

Kelly, K. & Ramundo, P. (1993). *You mean I'm not lazy, stupid or crazy?! A self-help book for adults with attention deficit disorder.* Cincinnatti, OH: Tyrell & Jerem Press.

Solden, S. (1995). *Women with attention deficit disorder: Embracing disorganization at home and in the workplace.* Grass Valley, CA: Underwood Books.

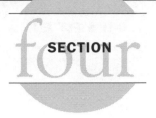

ASSOCIATED DISORDERS IN WOMEN WITH AD/HD

CHAPTER 9

An Overview of Coexisting Conditions for Women with AD/HD

Kathleen G. Nadeau, Ph.D.
and Patricia O. Quinn, M.D.

The issue of coexisting or comorbid conditions and AD/HD in women is a particularly critical concern. While there are very few clinicians who are trained to recognize and treat AD/HD in women, most clinicians are quite familiar with the range of coexisting conditions that often accompany or mimic AD/HD patterns in women. As a result, there is a strong likelihood that a woman who struggles with AD/HD will be either misdiagnosed, or that only the coexisting condition will be diagnosed while her AD/HD goes unrecognized.

A broad range of conditions commonly coexist with AD/HD in women. Tzelepis (1995) reported in a review of cases of adults with AD/HD that, at the time of diagnosis, 42 percent had another psychiatric disorder, while another 38 percent had two or more psychiatric disorders. Many women with AD/HD have received a prior diagnosis of depression, anxiety, or bipolar disorder. Because there is much overlap in the symptoms of these conditions, AD/HD is typically overlooked as a possible primary or coexisting condition.

Depression

(The following discussion of depression is excerpted and adapted from Young, J. (2002). Depression and anxiety in women with AD/IID. In P. Quinn, & K. Nadeau, (Eds.), *Gender issues and AD/HD: Research, diagnosis, & treatment.*)

There is widespread agreement that the rates of depression in females with AD/HD is higher than that in males, and that such patterns tend to increase with age, throughout adolescence and into adulthood. Given that AD/HD, the most common psychiatric diagnosis in children (Barkley, 1998b), is now recognized as a life-span disorder, and that depression is the most common psychiatric complaint in adult women (Blazer, 1995), it seems very likely that many women with AD/HD are regarded, too simplistically as being "depressed." Clinical experience supports this hypothesis. Often, women seeking an assessment for AD/HD report a prior diagnosis of depression.

Feelings of depression are so commonplace among females with AD/HD that some suggest that depression is a feature of AD/HD in females (Arnold, 1996). Littman (See Chapter 10) writes about the multiple pressures faced by females with AD/HD—societal expectations, gender roles, social pressures—that are especially difficult for women who struggle with AD/HD, and that often lead to depression.

There is much overlap between the features of depression and those of AD/HD, especially in women with predominantly inattentive type AD/HD. Women with either condition may be characterized as withdrawn, easily overwhelmed by daily events and demands, forgetful, disorganized, with low energy levels that make it difficult to rise in the morning and function with any degree of efficiency. Women with either disorder tend to engage in chronic self-doubt and self-blame, and demonstrate little optimism that their life circumstances will improve. In cases where depression exists without AD/HD, these patterns show periods of remission when depression lifts, and mood and energy level improve. Women experiencing the chronic demoralization that so often accompanies AD/HD in females, rarely report periods that are relatively symptom-free.

Especially in cases of treatment resistant depression, a clinician should consider the possibility of undiagnosed AD/HD, and consider adding stimulant medication in combination with antidepressants. Even in cases where treatment of depression is moderately successful, when a woman continues to report feeling overwhelmed, disorganized and unable to manage the tasks of daily life, AD/HD should be considered as a strong possibility. When depression and AD/HD coexist, the most effective treatment regime is a combination of antidepressants (most typically SSRIs) with psychostimulants. Some physicians prefer to prescribe Wellbutrin®, which can simultaneously address symptoms of depression and AD/HD. Generally, however, the most effective treatment for the symptoms of AD/HD are psychostimulants.

Bipolar Mood Disorder (BMD)

(The following discussion of bipolar mood disorder is excerpted and adapted from Dodson, W. (2002a). Bipolar disorder in women with AD/HD. In P. Quinn, & K. Nadeau, (Eds.), *Gender issues and AD/HD: Research, diagnosis, & treatment.*)

The differential diagnosis of AD/HD versus bipolar mood disorder (BMD) is one of the most difficult because there is considerable overlap in their primary features, including talkativeness, "racing thoughts," impulsivity, impatience, bursts of energy and restlessness, variability of mood, and impaired judgment. Because most clinicians are far more familiar with BMD, that diagnosis is highly likely, in place of an AD/HD diagnosis, for many women. One of the deciding factors often causing clinicians to lean toward a diagnosis of BMD is a family history of this disorder. It is important for clinicians to recognize the common co-occurrence of BMD and AD/HD, and not rule out AD/HD automatically if BMD is diagnosed. Biederman (1996) and Chang (2000) estimate that 20 to 24 percent of individuals with BMD also have AD/HD. Additionally, studies show that an early onset of bipolar mood disorder increases the likelihood of AD/HD (West, 1995; Faraone, 1997; Sachs, 2000).

A clinician, when attempting to make a diagnosis, should not only take a familial history of bipolar mood disorder into account, but a familial history of AD/HD as well. When these disorders co-occur, they can both be effectively treated, the most successful approach being to first address the bipolar condition, and then, to address AD/HD symptomatology, once mood lability has been stabilized.

In making a differential diagnosis, several differences in clinical features should be carefully assessed:

1. Racing thoughts, irritability, restlessness, hyperactivity, and poor judgment are seen in both. However, in AD/HD, these factors are more of a steady state. While in BMD, these manic features are episodic in nature, lasting for a period of weeks or months, followed by long periods in which such features are not seen.

2. Sleep disturbance is seen in both. However, sleep patterns should be carefully distinguished. Adults with AD/HD commonly have "delayed sleep phase syndrome" characterized by a tendency to stay up late at night, despite chronic sleep deprivation and morning fatigue. Adults with AD/HD report a "second wind" in the evening, but feel intense exhaustion when they must rise a few hours later to begin another day. Such individuals may "crash" on the weekend when they

are not required to rise in the early morning. This is contrast with BMD sleep patterns during a manic phase characterized by a markedly reduced *need* for sleep—waking energetic and refreshed after only a few hours rest. In BMD, such periods are distinct, lasting for weeks or months, followed by periods where sleep patterns are normal, or even opposite, when they enter a period of depression.

3. Rapid mood shifts seen in AD/HD are reactive—that is, they are a rapid, direct response to identifiable external events, in contrast to mood shifts in BMD that are internally triggered, unrelated to specific life events.

4. While both AD/HD and BMD are lifelong conditions, individuals with BMD will typically have periods of remission for months, even years, where mood and behaviors are normal. In contrast, those with AD/HD consistently experience racing thoughts, irritability, stress, and restlessness (among other patterns), with an increase in symptomatology at times clearly related to increased environmental stress.

Although more research is needed to study the interrelationship of bipolar mood disorder and AD/HD, clinical experience suggests that these disorders can be treated together with high rates of success.

Generalized Anxiety Disorder (GAD)

(The following discussion of generalized anxiety disorder has been excerpted and adapted from Young, J. (2002). Depression and anxiety in women with AD/HD. In P. Quinn, & K. Nadeau, (Eds.), *Gender issues and AD/HD: Research, diagnosis, & treatment.*)

Generalized anxiety disorder (GAD) is characterized by pathological worry, anxiety and muscular tension (DSM-IV-TR, 2000), with a female lifetime prevalence (5.1%) twice as high as that for males (Witchen, Zhao, Kessler, & Eaton, 1994). Symptoms of GAD are chronic and debilitating and most often, in 62 percent of cases, co-occurs with depression (Katon, Von Korff, Lin, Lipscomb, Russo, Wagner, & Polk, 1990). Many symptoms of GAD and depression overlap. These can include: dysphoria, fatigue, irritability, impatience, restlessness, impaired concentration and rapid mood swings, symptoms that are also common among those with AD/HD (Roy-Byrne & Katon, 1997).

Research into the relationship between AD/HD and anxiety disorders in adults is sparse, but overlapping symptoms suggest that AD/HD plays a role in some cases in GAD. Women with AD/HD commonly report feeling "overwhelmed" by the stresses of daily life and the demands of life-management tasks. As responsibilities increase, many women with AD/HD become increasingly stress-intolerant, reporting higher levels of stress and anxiety.

Clinical experience suggests that women with both AD/HD and anxiety are not able to tolerate stimulant medication very well, unless also taking an antidepressant with anxiolytic properties. When both disorders coexist, they must both be addressed in treatment to effectively improve a woman's level of daily functioning.

Posttraumatic Stress Disorder (PTSD)

(The following discussion of PTSD has been excerpted and adapted from Adelizzi, J. (2002). Posttraumatic stress symptoms in women with AD/HD. In P. Quinn, & K. Nadeau, (Eds.), *Gender issues and AD/HD: Research, diagnosis, & treatment.*)

Although included among the anxiety disorders, PTSD has distinct clinical features that deserve separate consideration. Clinical experience suggests that AD/HD and symptoms of posttraumatic stress may be interwoven in complex ways, and research has already suggested comorbidity between these two disorders (Famularo et al., 1992; Van der Kolk, McFarlane, & Wisareth, 1996). There is significant overlap in features of these two disorders, as concentration problems, impulsivity, and restlessness or irritability are commonly observed in individuals with AD/HD as well as PTSD (Blank, 1994).

Curiously, despite a significant overlap of symptoms, there have been few studies that have examined the relationship between AD/HD and PTSD. Famularo, Kinsherff, and Fenton (1992) write that there is evidence that the symptoms resulting in the diagnosis of AD/HD may be the result of maltreatment, and that these symptoms are a reflection of the anxiety associated with PTSD rather than manifestations of true AD/HD. Supporting this speculation, McLeer and colleagues (1994) found that sexually abused children are more likely to be diagnosed with AD/HD than with PTSD. Such a pattern is merely the flip side of the coin that leads clinicians to diagnose women with AD/HD as depressed. Clinicians tend to diagnose what is most familiar to them—AD/HD in children, depression in women.

Weinstein, Staffelbach, and Biaggio (2000) write of the importance of differential diagnosis between AD/HD and PTSD, as well as the lack of attention this has received. For example, PTSD is notably missing from the differential diagnosis list for AD/HD in the DSM-IV (APA, 1994). Furthermore, neither the Child Behavior Checklist (CBCL) (Achenbach, 1991), nor the AD/HD Rating Scale (DuPaul, Power, Anastopoulos, & Reid, 1998), two of the most widely-used AD/HD rating scales, includes questions about trauma, nor do commonly used adult rating scales include items to screen for PTSD. Further underscoring the neglect of PTSD as a differential diagnosis for AD/HD, Barkley (1990, 1998a), one of the best known researchers and writers in the field, does not mention the importance of trauma assessment in the diagnosis of AD/HD.

Jane Adelizzi has conducted a series of studies on women diagnosed with attention and learning problems who also manifest PTSD symptoms. She writes that in some cases, these women have PTSD, conforming to DSM-IV criteria, which has contributed to learning problems that mimic AD/HD. In other instances, however, women studied by Adelizzi report that the most emotionally traumatizing events in their life histories were repeated humiliations, criticisms and punishments they experienced in the classroom as a result of their learning and/or attention problems. The "PTS symptoms" resulting from this "classroom trauma" constitute an important part of their clinical presentation. Such women cannot be helped with their AD/HD issues without addressing the overlay of panic and anxiety that can be triggered, even many years later, when such women attempt to return to school to further their education. Thus, Adelizzi proposes that traumatic events causing PTSD can subsequently cause learning difficulties that are indistinguishable from AD/HD, while, conversely, AD/HD problems can lead to traumatic experiences in the classroom that result in symptoms strongly resembling those of PTSD.

While there is no clear drug treatment program for PTSD (Weinstein et al., 2000), the more successful medications appear to be monoamine-oxidase inhibitors and selective serotonin reuptake inhibitors (Maxmen & Ward, 1995), while the standard first-line medications for treating AD/HD are the psychostimulants.

Differential diagnosis becomes critical for women with both AD/HD and PTSD for two reasons. First, adverse reactions to stimulants are common among those with elevated states of anxiety (Barkley, 1998a). Second, monoamine-oxidase inhibitors, whose use is accompanied by concerns about the potential for diet- or medication-induced hypertensive crisis, may not be the treatment of choice for a group of patients vulnerable to impulsivity or forgetfulness. A clinician who screens for both conditions can then make an accurate diagnosis and choose a treatment regime optimal for this combination of disorders.

Addiction Patterns

(The following discussion has been excerpted and adapted from Richardson, W. (2002). Addictions in women with AD/HD. In P. Quinn, & K. Nadeau, (Eds.), *Gender issues and AD/HD: Research, diagnosis, & treatment.*)

Several studies have identified alcohol and other substance abuse disorders as very common among adults with AD/HD (Biederman et al., 1993; Shekim, Asarnow, Hess, Zaucha, & Wheeler, 1990; Wilens, Biederman, Spencer, & Frances, 1994). Biederman and colleagues discussed the importance of early diagnosis and treatment in the prevention of later substance abuse and addiction. And yet, the average female with AD/HD tends to be diagnosed much later than her male counterpart. As a result, women with undiagnosed AD/HD pay a high cost that sometimes that cost includes a pattern of self-medication that leads to addiction.

Conduct disorder is a well-known risk factor for substance abuse (Biederman et al., 1997). Another study of AD/HD and substance abuse suggests that comorbid antisocial personality disorder greatly increases the incidence of addiction (Biederman et al., 1995), however, the subjects of this study were predominantly male. Substance abusers with AD/HD have been found to have higher rates of anxiety and depression (Thompson, Riggs, Mikulich, & Crowley, 1996). Even when only considering adults with AD/HD without comorbid conditions, Biederman's group found that AD/HD significantly increases the risk for substance abuse.

Patterns of coexisting conditions may vary for women. One study (Biederman et al., 1994) reported lower rates of antisocial disorders among women with AD/HD, but rates of substance abuse equal to men. A more recent study (Biederman et al., 1999) found that even though the rate of conduct disorder among girls with AD/HD was one-third the rate of boys, girls with AD/HD were at *greater* risk for substance abuse. Comings (1994) found that women who are divorced, separated, or never married, (circumstances of greater social isolation) have the highest rates of heavy drinking and alcohol-related problems. Another study reported that women who have either lost or never experienced the roles of worker, mother, wife, or partner may have increased risk of abusing alcohol, again implying that lack of social connectedness may be a significant risk factor for addiction (Wilsnak & Cheloa, 1987).

When a woman has undiagnosed AD/HD, she tends to experience high levels of chronic stress, the origin of which she doesn't understand. Often these women, who may suffer from anxiety and depression as well, seek ways to reduce feelings of tension, stress, or anxiety through self-medication with alcohol or other substances of abuse. Occasional use may become habitual and eventually an addiction.

Frequently, women with AD/HD who have addictions are completely unaware that undiagnosed AD/HD is one of the complex set of problems with which they struggle. Without diagnosis and treatment for AD/HD, recovery from addictions can be difficult, if not impossible. A woman who has both addiction and AD/HD requires a comprehensive treatment plan in which both her AD/HD and addiction are treated simultaneously

(Richardson, 1997). Several studies have shown that for many adult substance abusers, when AD/HD is appropriately treated, treatment for substance abuse is more effective than prior treatment efforts (Turnquist et al., 1983; Gawin & Kleber, 1986; Schubiner et al., 1995).

Coordinated treatment for this combination of conditions is problematic at present because few professionals in the addiction treatment community have training in the diagnosis and treatment of AD/HD, while specialists in AD/HD tend to be child specialists with little training in addiction treatment. Furthermore, health care providers are reluctant to prescribe stimulant medication that has a potential for abuse to individuals with a history of addiction. Fortunately, there are a number of second-line medications for treating AD/HD that, while less effective, have little abuse potential.

Eating Disorders

(The following discussion of eating disorders has been excerpted and adapted from Fleming, J. & Levy, L. (2002). Eating disorders in women with AD/HD. In P. Quinn, & K. Nadeau, (Eds.) *Gender issues and AD/HD: Research, diagnosis, & treatment.*)

While practitioners have been aware of the impact of AD/HD on eating (Hallowell & Ratey, 1994, 1995; Nadeau, Littman, & Quinn, 1999; Richardson, 1997; Robin, 1998), there has been little systematic study of this issue. A number of authors have raised the clinical issue of problematic patterns of eating among their AD/HD clients. Richardson (1997) has discussed the use of food in the context of AD/HD and addictive behaviors. Clinical discussions have suggested that eating might help fulfill the need for high stimulation in AD/HD, decrease agitation, or satisfy a need for control (Nadeau et al., 1999; Richardson, 1997; Solden, 1995). Similarly, Robin (1998) recommends screening for AD/HD in bulimia and binge eating disorder, because of the prevalence of poor self-control and impulsivity in this population.

One recent study (Wang et al., 2001) found a strong negative correlation (r = -.84) between the density of dopamine receptors (as measured by PET scan) and Body Mass Index (BMI). Individuals with the lowest density of dopamine receptors had the highest BMIs. In other words, low density of dopamine receptors is strongly associated with being overweight. Given the substantial evidence documenting the role of dopamine in AD/HD (Faraone & Biederman, 1998; Hudziak, 2000), these results suggest that dopamine plays a role in both AD/HD and problems with obesity. In a study of adults with disordered eating patterns, over 30 percent of seriously overweight clients had significant symptoms of AD/HD that contributed to their difficulty with changing their eating behavior. This was found to be true for people with binge eating, bulimia, and for the severely obese.

How might AD/HD contribute to the development of disordered eating? Several authors (Barkley, 1997; Brown, 2000; Tannock & Schachar, 1996) have emphasized that AD/HD is characterized by problems in self-regulation. These deficiencies in self-regulation include problems with working memory, attention, primary arousal, affect regulation, and organization. Dietary regulation is a complex process (Levy, 2000; Polivy & Herman, 1993) and can be quite vulnerable to disruption. One important factor in self-regulation is an ongoing awareness of the cues for hunger and fullness (Hill & Rogers, 1998). In order to know when to eat and when to stop eating, it is necessary to be continuously aware of how one feels and of the subtle changes in these states. People with AD/HD are often characterized by a lack of self-awareness (Barkley, 1997; Fisher & Beckley, 1999; Hallowell & Ratey, 1994). Maintaining a high level of awareness of internal states, particularly when distracted by other activities, can be extremely challenging for someone with AD/HD. Illustrating such difficulties, many AD/HD/eating disordered clients in Fleming and

Levy's study reported that they often miss meals, unaware of their hunger, and only know to stop eating when they feel "stuffed."

Dietary regulation also requires a fairly high degree of organization and planning, another potential area of difficulty for those who struggle with AD/HD. Eating nutritious food at appropriate intervals requires a series of actions, including making a shopping list, buying the food, and preparing it. It is also necessary to be sensitive to the passage of time to know that it is time for refueling. A person who already feels overwhelmed by the demands of their life may not invest the personal resources to manage these dietary fundamentals. It is far easier to "make do."

Generally speaking, self-regulation requires good inhibitory control. People eat for many reasons other than physiological hunger, including boredom, excitement, anger, sadness, food availability, reward, and stress relief. Surrounded by highly desirable food, it is difficult to say "no" to the impulse to eat. Again, it is easy to understand how AD/HD might put someone at a disadvantage, since difficulties with impulse control are a central defining attribute of the disorder (Barkley, 1997; Schachar, Tannock, Marriott, & Logan, 1995).

Clinical experience has shown that the more ambiguous or unclear the rules, the more difficult it is for an individual with AD/HD to make good decisions. On a daily basis, people are bombarded with contradictory and confusing advice about how to eat properly. Furthermore, eating provides immediate gratification while the consequences of poor dietary choices are abstract and delayed. Individuals with AD/HD tend to be reactive, dominated by the moment, and, only later, regretful of their lack of foresight (Barkley, 1997; Conners & Jett, 1999; Hallowell & Ratey, 1994). On the basis of what is known about clients with AD/HD, it would seem likely that they are even more adversely affected by dieting because of their high level of impulsivity and limited abilities for self-awareness.

Women with AD/HD who struggle with disordered eating patterns need an approach that takes their AD/HD issues into account. Coaching is needed to devise a deliberate and reasonable plan for eating to replace the bad habits that arose out of AD/HD-inspired disorganization, impulsiveness, and disturbance in self-awareness. Another important issue for many women with AD/HD is the misuse of food due to boredom and a need for stimulation. These women must be helped to introduce healthier, more active pursuits into their lives to achieve their need for stimulation without resorting to overeating.

While stimulant medication can be an effective adjunct to treatment of patterns of disordered eating in someone with AD/HD, it should never be used in the absence of ongoing behavioral treatment. Stimulant medication should never be used for its side effect of appetite suppression. Adequate medication coverage is a critical issue when it comes to helping a woman with AD/HD manage her eating more effectively. For most women, the most difficult time to maintain control of eating patterns is in the evening. Here, it becomes tricky, balancing the need to maintain adequate levels of medication, while still ensuring that these medications do not interfere with sleep. Stimulant medication is used to improve executive functioning that, in turn, impacts her ability to control eating behavior.

Sleep Problems

(The following discussion of sleep disturbances has been excerpted and adapted from Dodson, W. (2002b). Sleep disorders in women with AD/HD. In P. Quinn, & K. Nadeau, (Eds.), *Gender issues and AD/HD: Research, diagnosis, & treatment.*)

Adults with AD/HD commonly report that their sleep is disturbed by mental and physical restlessness. However, as with most of the knowledge about adults with AD/HD, how AD/HD disrupts both sleeping and arousal is just beginning to be understood. In earlier attempts to define AD/HD, sleep disturbances were briefly considered a criterion for AD/HD, but were dropped because they were felt to be too nonspecific. As the focus of research has expanded to include adults with AD/HD, the causes and effects of the sleeping disturbances associated with AD/HD have become clearer. Some researchers anticipate that sleep disturbances will return as an important diagnostic criterion when the guidelines for adult AD/HD finally appear in the DSM V revision.

Thomas Brown, Ph.D., longtime researcher in AD/HD, was one of the first researchers to give serious attention to the problems of sleep in children and adolescents with AD/HD. He theorizes that sleep disturbances are fundamental to the problems of arousal and alertness in AD/HD (Brown, 1998).

The sleep disturbances associated with AD/HD generally appear later in life. In a review of 207 cases of adults with AD/HD, the mean age of onset for the sleep disturbances of AD/HD was 12.4 years (Dodson, 2002b). This phenomenon has gone unnoticed until recently because, historically, AD/HD research has heavily focused on the elementary school-aged child, prior to the typical age of onset of sleep disorders. Recently, as more attention has been turned toward adult AD/HD, sleep disturbances associated with AD/HD have begun to receive attention. In a survey of 327 adults diagnosed with AD/HD, the four most common disturbances of sleep reported are 1) initiation insomnia, 2) restless sleep, 3) difficulty awakening, and 4) intrusive sleep (Dodson, 2002b).

Among the 327 patients studied, slightly more than seventy percent of adults with AD/HD reported being unable to shut off their minds so that they could fall asleep at night. Many adults described themselves as "night owls" who feel a burst of energy when the sun goes down. Others report that they commonly feel tired throughout the day, but when they try to fall asleep, their mind clicks on, with thoughts "jumping" or "bouncing" from one concern or worry to another. Unfortunately, many of these adults describe their thoughts as "racing," often resulting in a misdiagnosis of bipolar mood disorder. In actuality, this phenomenon is the result of the physical and mental restlessness of AD/HD.

Eighty percent of adults with AD/HD studied by Dodson report falling into "the sleep of the dead" about 4 AM. Not understanding that this phenomenon is a manifestation of AD/HD, some researchers have looked for alternate explanations. Myron Brenner (1998) noted the high incidence of AD/HD individuals in the research subjects with whom he was working in his study of Delayed Sleep Phase Syndrome (DSPS), a pattern also noted by Regestein and Pavlova (1995). People with DSPS report that they can sleep a normal sleep phase— i.e., get in bed, fall asleep quickly, sleep for eight hours, undisturbed, and awake refreshed. However, this sleep phase typically occurs from 4 AM to noon. This delayed phase sleep pattern is reported by more than half of adults with AD/HD (Dodson, 2002b).

Other clinicians (Prince, 1996) emphasize the effects of hyperactivity and physical restlessness upon sleep, rather than consider the effects of mental restlessness. It is at bedtime that many adults with AD/HD feel driven, hyperaroused, and both mentally and physically restless. Indeed, the only time many women experience hyperactivity is when they are trying to fall asleep at night. Clinicians who view the source of the insomnia to be solely hyperactivity typically believe that the best course of treatment is to prescribe one of the alpha-2 agonist class of medications that were originally brought into the market as treatment for hypertension, including clonidine (Catapres) and guanfacine (Tenex). These medications cause the brain to produce less adrenalin, resulting in reduced blood pressure and decreased alertness with a side effect of sedation.

Twenty-five percent of adults with AD/HD studied (Dodson, 2002b) report either no sleep disturbance, or have the typical AD/HD-related difficulties in falling asleep, but are not helped by stimulant class medications at bedtime. For this group of adults with sleep disturbance, Thomas Brown (1998) recommends a trial of benadryl, 25-50 mg one hour before bedtime.

Learning Disabilities (LD)

(The following discussion of learning disabilities has been excerpted from Roffman, A. & Quinn, P. (2002). Learning disabilities in women with AD/HD. In P. Quinn, & K. Nadeau, (Eds.), *Gender issues and AD/HD: Research, diagnosis, & treatment.*)

The co-occurrence of learning disabilities (LD) and AD/HD has been reported to be very high. In fact, a recent study that included written language difficulties estimated the overlap at 70 percent (Mayes & Calhoun, 2000), suggesting that LD is the most common coexisting condition for those with AD/HD. Further evidence for this is found in another recent study, in which college students diagnosed with only AD/HD reported as many symptoms of learning disabilities (7.82 LD symptoms) as those students with diagnosed LD (8.78 LD symptoms) (Lewandowski, Codding, Gordon, Marcoe, Needham & Rentas, 2000).

Despite such strong evidence of overlap of symptoms and co-occurrence of LD and AD/HD, once the school years have passed, learning disabilities in adult women with AD/HD generally receive little notice. Health care professionals, typically the primary treatment providers for those with AD/HD, have little training regarding learning disabilities. Moreover, psychiatrists most often diagnose AD/HD through clinical interview and the completion of standardized AD/HD questionnaires and do not routinely recommend a neuropsychological or psychoeducational assessment to evaluate learning disabilities. This practice of overlooking coexisting LD in individuals with AD/HD occurs all too often, with significant educational and emotional impact.

A further reason why LD is often overlooked or ignored in

women with AD/HD is the mistaken belief, shared by many clinicians and physicians, that learning disabilities are only relevant when an adult is engaged in formal educational pursuits. The fact is that, just as AD/HD impacts all aspects of a woman's life, so do learning disabilities—in such basic activities as remembering directions, getting to places on time, being able to recall important names, accurately reading and recalling what's been read, completing insurance or tax forms, organizing the home environment, and even in correctly interpreting social interactions. The psychological impact of such problems is debilitating, often leaving a woman with LD so fearful of failure and so self-doubting that she limits her life options.

As its name implies, a learning disability impedes a woman's learning and often keeps her from performing at her ability level. It is important to note that, while during childhood the implications of learning problems are felt most keenly in the classroom, by adulthood they are much more broadly experienced, spilling not only into continued educational pursuits but also into friendships, marriage, parenting, work life, and day-to-day experiences in the community.

Because of the high occurrence of learning disabilities in individuals with AD/HD, it is critical that all women being diagnosed with AD/HD are also evaluated for the cognitive problems associated with LD. A thorough diagnosis will help them develop a sense of their strengths and areas of need.

Despite the everyday frustrations that result from many of the challenges associated with learning disabilities and attention deficit hyperactivity disorder, it is very possible for adults with these diagnoses to achieve a satisfying quality of life. Treatment for learning disabilities entails remediation (typically through working with an LD tutor), compensatory strategies, a career assessment that includes assessment of learning disabilities, a self-understanding that involves a clear picture of strengths and weaknesses, reframing LD/AD/HD issues in a more positive light, and strong self-advocacy skills (Roffman, 2002).

The important message for any woman with AD/HD is that she has a greater than 50 percent chance of having coexisting learning disabilities that may have been overlooked and gone undiagnosed throughout her life. With realistic understanding of her challenges, combined with a healthy appreciation of her strengths, a woman with AD/HD and LD can improve her daily functioning, enhance her job performance, and enjoy a better quality of life.

Conclusion

Awareness of coexisting conditions in women with AD/HD is critical if they are to receive appropriate, effective treatment. Careful diagnostic procedures are especially important in the assessment of women with AD/HD because clinical experience strongly suggests that the majority of women who struggle with AD/HD have received a misdiagnosis or an incomplete diagnosis of a coexisting condition. Often their AD/HD patterns are overlooked, or are interpreted as signs of a disorder with similar features. Once an accurate and complete diagnosis has been made of AD/HD and *all* coexisting conditions, then a treatment plan can be developed that appropriately addresses every condition that may contribute to the difficulties in functioning that a woman may experience. Without such a careful diagnostic process and comprehensive, coordinated treatment approach, a woman with AD/HD will not be able to gain control over her daily challenges and develop a satisfying life.

References

Achenbach, T.M. (1991). *Manual for the child behavior checklist.* Burlington: Department of Psychiatry, University of Vermont.

Adelizzi, J.U. (2002). Posttraumatic stress disorder in women with AD/HD. In P. Quinn, & K. Nadeau (Eds.), *Gender issues and AD/HD: Research, diagnosis, & treatment.* Silver Spring, MD: Advantage Books.

American Psychiatric Association. (1994). *Diagnostic and statistical manual of mental disorders (4th ed.).* Washington, DC: Author.

American Psychiatric Association. (2000). *Diagnostic and statistical manual of mental disorders (4th ed., TR).* Washington, DC: Author.

Arnold, L. E. (1996). Sex differences in AD/HD: Conference summary. *Journal of Abnormal Child Psychology, 24,* 555-569.

Barkley, R. A. (1997). *AD/HD and the nature of self-control.* New York: Guilford Press.

Barkley, R.A. (1998a). *Attention-deficit hyperactivity disorder: A handbook for diagnosis and treatment (2nd ed.).* New York: Guilford Press.

Barkley, R.A. (1998b, September). Attention-deficit hyperactivity disorder. *Scientific American,* 66-71.

Barkley, R.A. (1990). *Attention-deficit hyperactivity disorder: A handbook for diagnosis and treatment.* New York: Guilford Press.

Biederman, J., Faraone, S.V., Spencer, T., Wilens, T., Norman, D., Lapey, K., Mick, E., Lehman,. B.K., & Doyle, A. *(1993).* Patterns of psychiatric comorbidity, cognition, and psychosocial functioning in adults with attention-deficit hyperactivity disorder. *American Journal of Psychiatry, 150,* 1792-1798.

Biederman, J., Faraone, S.V., Spencer, T., et al., (1994). Gender differences in a sample of adults with attention-deficit hyperactivity disorder. *Psychiatry Research, 53,* 13-29.

Biederman, J., Wilens, T., Mick, E., Milberger, S., Spencer, T., & Faraone, S. (1995). Psychoactive substance use disorders in adults with attention-deficit hyperactivity disorder (AD/HD): Effects of AD/HD and psychiatric co-morbidity. *American Journal of Psychiatry, 152,* 1652-1658

Biederman, J., Faraone, S., Mick, E., et al. (1996). Attention-deficit hyperactivity disorder and juvenile mania: An overlooked comorbidity. *Journal of the American Academy of Child and Adolescent Psychiatry, 37,* 1091-1093.

Biederman, J., Wilens, T., Mick, E., Faraone, S.V., Weber, W., Curtis, S., Thornell, A., Pfister, K., Jetton, J.G., & Soriano, J. (1997). Is AD/HD a risk factor for psychoactive substance use disorders? Findings from a four-year prospective follow-up study. *Journal of the American Academy of Child and Adolescent Psychiatry, 36,* 21-29.

Biederman, J., Faraone, S., Mick, E., Williamson, S., Wilens, T.E., Spencer, T.J., Weber, W., Jetton, J., Krauss, I., Pert, J., & Zallen, B. (1999). Clinical correlates of AD/HD in females: Findings from a large group of girls ascertained from pediatric and psychiatric referral services. *Journal of the American Academy of Child and Adolescent Psychiatry, 38,* 966-975.

Blank, A.S. (1994). Clinical detection, diagnosis, and differential diagnosis of posttraumatic stress disorder. *Psychiatric Clinics of North America, 17,* 351-383.

Blazer, D. (1995). Mood disorders: Epidemiology. In H.I. Kaplan, & B.J. Sadock (Eds.), *Comprehensive textbook of psychiatry VI (pp.* 1079-1089). Baltimore: Williams and Wilkens.

Brenner, M. (1998) Personal communication.

Brown, T. (1998). *Problems with sleep and awakening in persons with AD/HD.* Presented at the 10th Annual CHADD International Conference, San Antonio, TX.

Brown, T. E. (2000). Emerging understandings of attention-deficit disorders and comorbidities. In T.E. Brown (Ed.), *Attention-deficit disorders and comorbidities in children, adolescents, and adults* (pp. 3-55). Washington, DC: American Psychiatric Press, Inc.

Chang, K.D., Steiner, H., & Ketter, T.A. (2000). Psychiatric phenomenology of child and adolescent bipolar offspring. *Journal of the American Academy of Child and Adolescent Psychiatry, 39,* 453-460.

Comings, D.E. (1994). Genetic factors in substance abuse based on studies of Tourette's Syndrome and AD/HD probands and relatives, II. Alcohol abuse. *Drug and Alcohol Dependence, 35,* 17-24

Conners, C. K., & Jett, J. L. (1999). *Attention-deficit hyperactivity disorder (in adults and children): The latest assessment and treatment strategies.* Kansas City, MO: Compact Clinicals.

Dodson, W. (2002a). Bipolar disorder in women with AD/HD. In P. Quinn, & K. Nadeau (Eds.), *Gender issues and AD/HD: Research, diagnosis, & treatment.* Silver Spring, MD: Advantage Books.

Dodson, W. (2002b). Sleep disorders in women with AD/HD. In P. Quinn, & K. Nadeau (Eds.), *Gender issues and AD/HD: Research, diagnosis, & treatment.* Silver Spring, MD: Advantage Books.

DuPaul, G.J., Power, T.J., Anastopoulos, A.D, & Reid, R. (1998). *AD/HD Rating Scale IV: Checklists, norms, and clinical interpretation.* New York: Guilford Press.

Famularo, R., Kinsherff, R., & Fenton, R. (1992). Psychiatric diagnoses of maltreated children: Preliminary findings. *Journal of the American Academy of Child and Adolescent Psychiatry, 31,* 863-867.

Faraone S.V., Biederman J., Mennin J., & Spencer, T. (1997). Attention-deficit hyperactivity disorder with bipolar disorder: A familial subtype? *Journal of the American Academy of Child and Adolescent Psychiatry, 36,* 1378-1387.

Faraone, S. V., & Biederman, J. (1998). Neurobiology of attention-deficit hyperactivity disorder. *Biological Psychiatry, 44,* 951-958.

Fisher, B. C., & Beckley, R. A. (1999). *Attention deficit disorder: Practical coping methods.* Boca Raton, FL: CRC Press.

Fleming, J., & Levy, L. (2002). Eating disorders in women with AD/HD. In P. Quinn, & K. Nadeau, (Eds.), *Gender issues and AD/HD: Research, diagnosis, & treatment.* Silver Spring, MD: Advantage Books.

Gawin, F., & Kleber, H. (1986). Pharmacologic treatments of cocaine abuse. *Psychiatric Clinics of North America, 9,* 573-583.

Hallowell, E. M., & Ratey, J. J. (1994). *Driven to distraction.* New York: Pantheon Books.

Hill, A. J., & Rogers, P. J. (1998). Food intake and eating behaviours in humans. In P.G. Kopelman & M. J. Stock (Eds.), *Clinical obesity* (pp. 86-111). London, England: Blackwell Science.

Hudziak, J. J. (2000). Genetics of attention-deficit/hyperactivity disorder. In T.E. Brown (Ed.), *Attention-deficit disorders and comorbidities in children, adolescents, and adults* (pp. 57-78). Washington, DC: American Psychiatric Press, Inc.

Katon, W., Von Korff, M., Lin, E., Lipscomb, P., Russo, J., Wagner, E., & Polk E. (1990). Distressed high utilizers of medical care. DSM-III-R diagnoses and treatment needs. *General Hospital Psychiatry, 12,* 355-62.

Levy, L. D. (2000). *Conquering obesity: Deceptions in the marketplace and the real story.* Toronto, Canada: Key Porter Books Limited.

Lewandowski, L., Codding, B.A., Gordon, M., Marcoe, M., Needham, L., & Rentas, J. (2000) Self-reported LD and AD/HD symptoms in college students. *AD/HD Report, 8(6),* 1-4.

Mayes, S.D., & Calhoun, S. (2000). Prevalence and degree of attention and learning problems in AD/HD and LD. *AD/HD Report, 8(2),* 14-16.

Maxmen, J.S., & Ward, N.G. (1995). P*sychotropic drugs: Fast facts.* New York: Norton.

McLeer, S.V., Callaghan, M., Henry, D., & Wallen, M.W. (1994). Psychiatric disorders in sexually abused children. *Journal of the American Academy of Child and Adolescent Psychiatry, 33,* 313-319.

Nadeau, K. G., Littman, E. B., & Quinn, P. O. (1999). *Understanding girls with AD/HD.* Silver Spring, MD: Advantage Books.

Polivy, J., & Herman, C. P. (1993). Etiology of binge eating: Psychological mechanisms. In C.G. Fairburn, & G. T. Wilson (Eds.), *Binge eating: Nature, assessment, and treatment* (pp. 173-274). New York: The Guilford Press.

Prince, J. B., Wilens, T.E., Biederman, J., Spencer, T.J., & Wozniak, J. (1996). Clonidine for sleep disturbances associated with attention-deficit hyperactivity disorder: A systematic chart review of 62 cases. *Journal of the American Academy of Child & Adolescent Psychiatry, 35,* 599-605.

Quinn, P., & Nadeau, K. (2002). *Gender issues and AD/HD: Research, diagnosis, & treatment.* Silver Spring, MD: Advantage Books.

Regestein, Q.R., & Pavlova, M. (1995). Treatment of delayed sleep phase syndrome. *General Hospital Psychiatry, 17,* 335-345.

Richardson, W. (1997). *The link between A.D.D. & addiction.* Colorado Springs, CO: Pinon Press.

Richardson, W. (2002). Addictions in women with AD/HD. In P. Quinn., & K. Nadeau (Eds.), *Gender issues and AD/HD: Research, diagnosis, & treatment.* Silver Spring, MD: Advantage Books.

Robin, A. L. (1998). *AD/HD in adolescents: Diagnosis and treatment.* New York: The Guilford Press.

Roffman, A. (2002). Learning disabilities in women with AD/HD. In P. Quinn, & K. Nadeau (Eds.), *Gender issues and AD/HD: Research, diagnosis, & treatment.* Silver Spring, MD: Advantage Books.

Roy-Byrne, P.P., & Katon, W. (1997). Generalized anxiety disorder in primary care: The precursor/modifier pathway to increased health care utilization. *Journal of Clinical Psychiatry, 58,* Suppl 3, 34-38.

Sachs G.S., Baldassano C.F., Truman C.J., & Guille C. (2000). Comorbidity of attention-deficit hyperactivity disorder with early- and late-onset bipolar disorder. *American Journal of Psychiatry, 157,* 466-468.

Schachar, R. J., Tannock, R., Marriott, M., & Logan, G. (1995). Deficient inhibitory control in attention deficit hyperactivity disorder. *Journal of Abnormal Child Psychiatry, 23,* 411-438.

Shekim, W.O., Asarnow, R.F., Hess, E., Zaucha, K., & Wheeler, N. (1990). A clinical and demographic profile of a sample of adults with attention-deficit hyperactivity disorder, residual state. *Comprehensive Psychiatry, 31,* 416-425.

Schubiner, H., Tzelepis, A., Isaacson, J.H., Warbasse, L., Zacharek, M., & Musial, J. (1995). The dual diagnosis of attention-deficit/hyperactivity disorder and substance abuse: Case reports and literature review. *Journal of Clinical Psychiatry, 56,* 146-150.

Solden, S. (1995). *Women with attention deficit disorder.* Grass Valley, CA: Underwood Books.

Tannock, R., & Schachar, R. J. (1996). Executive dysfunction as an underlying mechanism of behavior and language problems in attention-deficit hyperactivity disorder. In J.H. Beitchman, N. J. Cohen, & M. M. Konstantareas (Eds.), *Language, learning, and behavior disorders* (pp. 128-155). New York: Cambridge University Press.

Thompson, L.L., Riggs, P.D., Mikulich, S.K., & Crowley, T.J. (1996). Contribution of AD/HD symptoms to substance abuse problems and delinquency in conduct-disordered adolescents. *Journal of Abnormal Child Psychology, 24*, 325-347.

Turnquist, K., Frances, R., Rosenfeld, W., et al. (1983). Pemoline in attention deficit disorder and alcoholism: A case study. *American Journal of Psychiatry, 140,* 622-624.

Tzelepis A., Schubiner, H., & Warbasse, L., III. (1995). Differential diagnosis and psychiatric comorbidity patterns in adult ADD. In K.G. Nadeau (Ed.), *A comprehensive guide to ADD in adults* (pp. 35-57). New York: Brunner/Mazel, Inc.

Van der Kolk, B., McFarlane, A.C., & Wisareth, L. (1996). *Traumatic stress.* New York: The Guilford Press.

Wang, G. J., Volkow, N. D., Logan, J., Pappas, N. R., Wong, C. T., Zhu, W., Netusil, N., & Fowler, J. S. (2001). Brain dopamine and obesity. *Lancet, 357,* 354-357.

Weinstein, D., Staffelbach, D., & Baggio, M. (2000). AD/HD and posttraumatic stress disorder. *The AD/HD Report, 8(5),* 1-7.

West, S.A., McElroy, S.L., Strakowski, S.M., Keck, P.E., & McConville, B.J. (1995). Attention deficit hyperactivity disorder in adolescent mania. *American Journal of Psychiatry, 152,* 271-273.

Wilens, T.E., Biederman, J., Spencer, T.J., & Frances, R.J. (1994). Comorbidity of attention-deficit hyperactivity and psychoactive substance use disorders. *Hospital and Community Psychiatry, 45,* 421-435.

Wilsnack, R.W., & Cheloa, R. (1987). Women's roles and problem drinking across the lifespan. *Social Problems, 34,* 231-248.

Witchen, H.U., Zhao, S., Kessler, R.C., & Eaton, R.C. (1994). DSM-III-R generalized anxiety disorder in the National Comorbidity Study. *Archives of General Psychiatry, 51,* 355-364.

Young, J. (2002). Depression and anxiety in women with AD/HD. In P. Quinn, & K. Nadeau (Eds.), *Gender issues and AD/HD: Research, diagnosis, & treatment.* Silver Spring: Advantage Books.

CHAPTER
10

Depression in Women with AD/HD

Ellen Littman, Ph.D.

There is growing recognition that AD/HD is a disorder accompanied by many different coexisting conditions (Brown, 2000), as well as many conditions that are secondary to AD/HD. One central secondary effect of AD/HD is its impact on mood. Ratey and colleagues reported in 1992 that mood disorders were the most common diagnoses given to adults seen for treatment, prior to a diagnosis of AD/HD. Adults with AD/HD have been shown to have significantly higher rates of major depression than adults without AD/HD (36 percent vs. 7 percent) (Biederman et al., 1994). While Biederman's group found no differences in the rates of depression between men and women with AD/HD, Katz and colleagues (1998), in their study of adults with AD/HD, reported higher rates of major depression in women than in men. Mood disorders that co-occur with AD/HD include dysthymia, major depressive disorder, bipolar disorder, and cyclothymic disorder. Seasonal affective disorder (SAD), premenstrual dysphoric disorder (PMDD), and a variety of sleep disorders—all of which have been found to commonly coexist with AD/HD in women—are also characterized by depressive symptoms.

It is often overt depressive symptoms that ultimately lead a woman with undiagnosed AD/HD to seek help. With these presenting symptoms, many women report having been initially misdiagnosed with a primary depressive illness or bipolar disorder. After psychopharmacological treatment for a depressive illness, many such women found that, while their depressive symptoms improved somewhat, these medications did not address the root of their problems—their ongoing, often overwhelming struggle to manage their lives.

To date, few psychiatrists have received training in the diagnosis and treatment of AD/HD in adults, and even fewer have experience in treating women with AD/HD. As a result, it has been the tendency of the medical profession to focus on treating depressive symptoms in women without looking beyond them to consider the possibility of underlying AD/HD. While the actual relationship between AD/HD and depressive symptoms is unclear, the comorbidity of AD/HD and depression in women has been estimated to be as high as 40 percent (Biederman et al., 1994). Such a high rate of co-occurrence clearly indicates that this is an area meriting greater attention from the medical and mental health professions.

Subclinical depressive symptoms are described by Ratey and Johnson (1997) as "shadow syndromes," in contrast to a distinct mood disorder. Biederman has described depressive patterns in some women with AD/HD as "demoralization," rather than as true comorbid mood disorders. Stein and coworkers (1995) reached similar conclusions in their study comparing male and female responses to the Wender Utah Rating Scale. The "dysphoria" factor was the largest factor reported by women with AD/HD, however, the dysphoric mood described by these women was highly reactive in nature (feeling like a failure, problems making decisions, lacking mental energy) and not associated with the more vegetative symptoms of clinical depression (e.g., problems with appetite, weight, sleep, and sexual drive) described in the DSM-IV (Katz, Goldstein, & Geckle, 1998; Stein et al., 1995).

For females with AD/HD, these secondary depressive symptoms or true depressive disorders can initially appear in childhood, adolescence, or adulthood, worsening at times, remitting at others, complicating the symptom picture for diagnosis and treatment. Depression, combined with AD/HD, can result in irritability, anxiety, somatic complaints, social withdrawal, marital difficulties, academic and/or occupational difficulties, and substance abuse. If not identified and treated, the combined impact of AD/HD and coexisting depressive symptoms can lead to greater impairment and a poorer prognosis. Rucklidge and Kaplan (1997) report a significant increase in depression among women when AD/HD is added to the clinical picture. They chose to study women with and without AD/HD, *all of* whom were mothers of a child with AD/HD. In this way, they could more clearly explore how AD/HD and depression are related in women outside of the stress of parenting a child with AD/HD. One third of the women with AD/HD in their study reported current clinical levels of depressive symptoms, in contrast to only one tenth of the women without AD/HD. Two thirds of women with AD/HD reported a history of depression, twice as many as women without AD/HD.

Psychological Factors Contributing to Depression in Women with AD/HD

Replaying Old Messages

Most women with AD/HD today were raised by parents who emphasized to them the importance of behaviors that were culturally prescribed for females of that era. Their daughter's "differences" were likely found to be frustrating at best and unacceptable at worst. Many confused parents resorted to criticism, as well as controlling attempts to change the behaviors deemed unacceptable by society. Some parents may have taken extreme measures to address their daughter's behavior, perhaps engaging in physical or emotional threats, backed by punitive consequences. Most of these undiagnosed girls felt ashamed that they couldn't be what their parents desired, and believed that something was wrong with them, though not understanding what this might be. They didn't feel entitled to be angry, and only tried harder to compensate and be "normal." For many of those girls, the harsh and repetitive messages—that they were bad, stupid, wrong, lazy, or worthless—became internalized.

Women with AD/HD often look back, believing the repeated negative messages, and feeling that they deserved the treatment they received. Eventually, external blame from others becomes self-blame, leading women with AD/HD to accept and believe that they are not good enough. For these women, regardless of intellect or talent, the early negative messages have done alarming damage to their self-esteem. Many women with AD/HD experience very self-critical inner dialogues as they try to come to terms with their many difficulties in measuring up to social expectations.

Self-blame

Depressive feelings are a common reaction to the relentless struggle to compensate for AD/HD symptoms. Based on society's gender role expectations, many women with AD/HD believe that they should not feel overwhelmed in the management of their daily lives, yet they do. They tend to blame the problems on themselves rather than acknowledge the role that their neurobiological disorder plays in their daily struggles. Women tend to internalize their experiences, feeling shame and guilt, rather than to externalize their feelings by expressing irritability, anger, or aggression. Such internalization often leads to depression over time.

Low Self-esteem

On the Conners' Adult AD/HD Rating Scale (CAARS), women with AD/HD were found to score higher than men with AD/HD on the "Problems with Self-Concept" factor. This factor addresses issues of low self-esteem, self-criticism, and failure to confront challenges. Items mentioned in this factor include: not being sure of oneself, wishing one had greater confidence, getting down on oneself, acting okay on the outside but feeling unsure of oneself, finding it hard to believe in oneself in light of past failures, and a tendency to avoid new challenges (Conners et al., 1999). This factor appears to measure the low self-esteem that results from the frustration, demoralization, and sense of invalidation women with AD/HD report.

Lack of Assertiveness

In addition, women with AD/HD may lack the assertiveness skills necessary to assertively pursue the gratification of their needs without apologizing. Often, they feel they must justify their behavior, and retreat into passivity, or becoming defensive. They are uncomfortable setting limits, and often feel that they have allowed themselves to be victimized. Rucklidge and Kaplan (1997) found that the coping strategies of women with AD/HD, compared to women without AD/HD, were more emotion-oriented and less task-oriented, and therefore much less effective.

Learned Helplessness

Women with AD/HD often feel that they cannot seize control over their lives, even when they have tremendous motivation and desire to do so. The literature has demonstrated that those with histories of repeated failures, and unsuccessful attempts to rectify them, eventually blame themselves for their difficulties and become at risk for depression. According to this theory of "learned helplessness" (Abramson, Seligman, & Teasdale, 1978), as individuals continue to fail, despite efforts to succeed, they conclude that they are powerless to influence outcomes. Once they reach such a conclusion, they are no longer motivated to expend effort to solve problems.

A pattern of learned helplessness has been documented in children with AD/HD (Milich & Okazaki, 1991), and more recently reported in women with AD/HD (Rucklidge & Kaplan, 1997). Women with AD/HD often become passive, and resigned. As they often fail in their struggle to meet societal expectations, it is not surprising that many ultimately feel victimized—placing them at greater risk for emotional and physical distress.

Need for Approval

Out of a need for approval, women with AD/HD attempt to hide their inadequacies,. Feeling compelled to succeed at almost any cost, they typically sacrifice their own needs in the process (Solden, 1995). Such need for approval begins early, leading many girls with AD/HD to experience anxiety, fearing disapproval from peers, parents, and teachers (Nadeau, Littman, & Quinn, 1999).

Life Circumstances that Contribute to Depression

Relationships that Recreate the Cycle of Criticism

During a childhood focused on seeking approval from parents and other adults, many women with AD/HD grew up trained to seek validation from others. As a result, they may unconsciously recreate the patterns of harsh criticism that characterized the parent-child interaction through their choice of a marriage partner. Like the original parent-child relationship, they seek the familiar structure in which they receive explicit direction, rigid control, and negative feedback. Such negative interactions, however painful, have become linked with their experience of being cared for, providing women with a certain kind of predictability. While they may feel secure within the structure, it comes at a high cost: the old messages about their incompetence are further reinforced.

A woman with AD/HD who accepts this mindset may enter into a relationship with an unequal distribution of power. Already viewing herself as inadequate, she may believe that her significant other is entitled to judge her behavior. A critical spouse may impose harsh consequences when she is late, forgets to pick up the dry cleaning, overdraws the checking account, or has nothing prepared for dinner—scenarios that can be common for women with AD/HD.

Domestic Violence

The demoralized woman with AD/HD may live with a sense of anxiety as she tries to do things the "right" (non-AD/HD) way in order to please her companion and avoid punishment. This is the route that may lead some women with AD/HD to remain in emotionally abusive relationships, whether with a spouse, boss, or even a friend. In extreme scenarios, they may be physically abused by their significant others, all the while believing that their inadequate performance merits such treatment. Perpetually apologetic and lacking self-protection strategies, they may take the criticisms to heart. Eventually, isolated from a support system that could offer other perspectives, they may feel desperate and hopeless, doubting their own self-worth. It is likely that the incidence of women with AD/HD in abusive relationships is more common than is currently recognized. The prevalence of AD/HD among women who are victims of domestic violence is an important, but unexplored area of research.

Raising a Child with AD/HD

Several studies have shown that mothers of children with AD/HD report higher levels of depression, lower confidence in themselves as parents, and greater self-blame (Barkley, 1990; Mash & Johnston, 1983). Another study underlined a tendency of depressed mothers to over-report anxiety, depression, and behavior problems in their children, suggesting that the mother's own struggles rendered her less able to accurately assess her children (Chilcoat & Breslau, 1997). In view of these risks, treatment for the mother with AD/HD must be given an equal priority to treatment for her child with AD/HD. Only when a mother no longer struggles with depression, high stress, and low parental self-esteem can she move forward to successfully meet the challenges of raising a child with AD/HD.

Separation and Divorce

The ending of a marriage, and the prolonged stress that usually precedes separation are stressful events in the life of any woman. For a woman with AD/HD, already dealing with the chronic stress intrinsic to living with this condition, marital strife and separation may move her stress into levels beyond her ability to cope—triggering both anxiety and depression.

The loss of a spouse may also mean the loss of structure, stability and support. Although the marriage may not have been ideal, her partner may have functioned in those areas most difficult for her—for example, financial management and record-keeping.

The rejection by her partner—if the separation was not

initiated by her—may confirm her darkest fears—that she is un-lovable and that no one will be able to tolerate her AD/HD char-acteristics.

Becoming a Single Parent

Divorce rates are close to fifty percent among all marriages in the United States. Divorce and/or separation becomes even more likely when AD/HD is added to the list of marital stressors (Phelan, 2000). Following divorce, it continues to be predomi-nantly the mothers who are the primary caregivers for children, many of whom have AD/HD as well. The combination of single-parenting and AD/HD can leave these mothers in a state of chronic exhaustion, and emotional depletion, even less able to cope with daily demands.

Destructive Behavior Patterns

Whether contending with the cognitive restlessness of AD/HD or the unmotivated lethargy associated with depression, there are a multitude of ways in which women with AD/HD manage this psychological fallout. Without understanding their disor-ders and how they are impacted by them, they will continue to struggle. Without benefit of effective treatment, many of their efforts to reduce psychological distress ultimately result in even greater problems.

Self-medicating with Food

Women with AD/HD often self-medicate in an effort to deny their frustration, to escape feelings of anxiety, to slow their rac-ing thoughts, increase their energy level, assuage their irritation, or distract themselves from their distress. Food is commonly used to self-medicate, with many women abusing food to the extent that they meet the criteria for an eating disorder.

While eating may temporarily ease depression, reduce anxi-ety, and calm inner restlessness, this coping strategy always comes at a cost. Even though such consumption is usually done clandestinely, the highly visible and potentially humiliating consequence of weight gain exacerbates isolation, reinforces a sense of inadequacy, and provides an arena for self-punishing ruminations. Their attempts to reduce feelings of distress only increases their distress in the long-run.

Compulsive Shopping as a Temporary "Fix"

Many women with AD/HD shop compulsively and spend with abandon. This highly stimulating and potentially addictive activity can provide fleeting comfort and distraction from their feelings, yet at the high cost of dealing with the stress of debt, harassment by creditors, spousal recriminations, and self-blame.

Other Addictive Behaviors

Other self-medicating behaviors include smoking, hypersexuality, gambling, and workaholism. Prescription and non-prescription drug use, yet another common form of self-medication for women, is typically preferred over alcohol abuse because it is more hidden. To varying extents, these highly stimulating behaviors offer some escape from cognitive restlessness and flagging brain arousal. However, women with such addictive behaviors are not viewed kindly in our culture. While such behaviors may offer temporary relief from uncomfortable feelings, these extreme behaviors alienate others, and ultimately only increase the psychological distress they were seeking to escape.

Partner Selection as a Compensatory Strategy

Many women with low self-esteem and painful awareness of their difficulties with daily life management actively seek a life partner who functions well in these areas. While this may be a constructive coping strategy for a woman whose self-esteem is high, more often such a choice occurs when a self-esteem is high, more often such a choice occurs when a woman has little self-confidence. (See Chapter 13 for a personal account describing such a choice.) When the balance of power in a relationship is out-of-kilter, the support she sought often devolves into control and criticism, further damaging her self-esteem and contributing to depression.

Conclusion

Women with AD/HD are clearly at heightened risk for depressive disorders. Without effective treatment that addresses both depression and AD/HD, these women often resort to self-destructive coping strategies resulting in even greater dysfunction. Medications prescribed to address both AD/HD and depressive symptoms can help to augment the neurotransmitters in the brain, allowing these women to function more effectively.

Psychotherapy can help women with AD/HD better understand their strengths and weaknesses, and appreciate the ways in which AD/HD may impact their functioning. Through therapy, these women can assess the stress inherent in unrealistic role expectations, and learn to let go of the demands that don't work for them. Emotional support and psychological insight, whether in an individual or group format, can help them reframe their self-image, improve their self-esteem, and learn to practice more self-protective behavior.

With a multi-modal approach that employs some combination of these interventions, women with AD/HD who also struggle with depression can learn to value themselves. With increased self-respect, they can quit the destructive pattern of measuring themselves against standards imposed by others, and, ultimately, can create a life that honors who they *are* rather than who they are "supposed" to be.

References

Abramson, L.Y., Seligman, M.E., & Teasdale, J.D. (1978). Learned helplessness in humans: Critique and reformulation. *Journal of Abnormal Psychology, 87,* 49-74.

Barkley, R.A. (1990). *Attention deficit hyperactivity disorder: A handbook for diagnosis and treatment.* New York: Guilford.

Biederman, J., Faraone, S.V., Spencer, T., Wilens, T., Mick, E., & Lapey, K.A. (1994). Gender differences in a sample of adults with attention deficit hyperactivity disorder. *Psychiatry Research, 53,* 13-29.

Brown, T.E. (2000). Emerging understandings of attention-deficit disorders and comorbidities. In T.E. Brown (Ed.). *Attention-deficit disorders and comorbidities in children, adolescents and adults.* Washington, DC: American Psychiatric Press.

Chilcoat, H.D., & Breslau, N. (1997). Does psychiatric history bias mothers' reports? An application of a new analytic approach. *Journal of the American Academy of Child and Adolescent Psychiatry, 36,* 971-979.

Conners, C.K., Erhardt, D., Epstein, J.N., Parker, J.D.A., Sitarenios, G., & Sparrow, E. (1999). Self-ratings of AD/HD symptoms in adults I: Factor structure and normative data. *Journal of Attention Disorders, 3,* 141-151.

Cunningham, C.E., Benness, B.B., & Siegel, L.S. (1988). Family functioning, time allocation, and parental depression in the families of normal and AD/HD children. *Journal of Clinical Child Psychology, 17,* 169-177.

Katz, L.J., Goldstein, G., & Geckle, M. (1998). Neuropsychological and personality differences between men and women with AD/HD. *Journal of Attention Disorders, 2,* 239-247.

Levitan, R., Jain, U., & Katzman, M. (1999). Seasonal affective symptoms in adults with residual attention-deficit hyperactivity disorder. *Comprehensive Psychiatry, 40,* 261-267.

Mash, E.J., & Johnston, C. (1982). A comparison of the mother-child interactions of younger and older hyperactive and normal children. *Child Development, 53,* 1371-1381.

McCormick, L.H. (1995). Depression in mothers of children with attention deficit hyperactivity disorder. *Family Medicine, 27,* 176-179.

Milich, R., & Okazaki, M. (1991). An examination of learned helplessness among attention-deficit hyperactivity disordered boys. *Journal of Abnormal Child Psychology, 19,* 607-623.

Nadeau, K., Littman, E., & Quinn, P. (1999). *Understanding girls with AD/HD.* Silver Spring, MD: Advantage Books.

Phelan, T.W. (2000). *AD/HD and family stress.* Lecture presented at the Annual Conference of Children and Adults with Attention Deficit/ Hyperactivity Disorder, Chicago, IL.

Quinn, P. (1998). Women's health issues: Is SAD making you depressed? *ADDvance, 1(3),* 11, 20.

Ratey, J., & Johnson, C. (1997). *Shadow syndromes.* New York: Pantheon.

Rucklidge, J.J., & Kaplan, B.J. (1997). Psychological functioning of women identified in adulthood with attention-deficit/hyperactivity disorder. *Journal of Attention Disorders, 2,* 167-176.

Solden, S. (1995) *Women with attention deficit disorder: Embracing disorganization at home and in the workplace.* Grass Valley, CA: Underwood.

Stein, M.A., Sandoval, R., Szumowski, E., Roizen, N., Reinecke, M., Blondis, T., & Klein, A. (1995). Psychometric characteristics of the Wender Utah Rating Scale (WURS): Reliability and factor structure for men and women. *Psychopharmacology Bulletin, 31,* 423-431.

CHAPTER 11

Fibromyalgia in Women with AD/HD

Gail C. Rodin, Ph.D.
and Jerry R. Lithman, M.D.

B ecause one of the chief symptoms of fibromyalgia (FMS) is pain in "trigger points" around the body, it was long believed that FMS was a disorder of the bones and muscles. However, new evidence gathered over the past five years strongly suggests that the symptoms of FMS, including joint and muscle pain, are actually the result of dysfunction in the central nervous system (CNS). This idea has received strong support from Jay Goldstein, M.D., author of *Betrayal by the Brain* and other books about FMS. Other professionals have also become interested in a possible connection between AD/HD and FMS, including a team of German physicians led by Klaus-Henning Krause, M.D., who found that many cases of FMS respond well to treatment with stimulants and other types of medication used to treat AD/HD (Krause, Krause, Magyarosy, Ernst, & Pongratz, 1998).

As a psychiatrist (Dr. Lithman) and a neuropsychologist (Dr. Rodin), we have worked with many individuals with AD/HD, FMS, or both disorders. Our experience has led us to believe that there are links between AD/HD and FMS and that it is especially important for women with AD/HD to understand these links in order remain healthy.

The Basics—How the Brain and Body Communicate

To discuss the connections between FMS and AD/HD, it is necessary to describe how parts of the central nervous system are designed to function, as well as to explain how it controls the functioning of the body, in particular how it regulates bodily responses to stress. Medical and scientific terminology in italics will be defined directly in the text, while terms requiring longer explanations are in CAPITAL LETTERS and are defined at the end of the chapter.

The Limbic System

Our brains are actually constructed of three "brains" layered, one atop the other, wired together by a complex set of NEURAL connections. The bottom portion of the brain, and the first part to evolve, includes a set of primitive structures that control basic life processes such as breathing, heart rate, and body temperature. The top and most recently evolved part of the brain (the neocortex or simply cortex), is responsible for higher-level brain functions such as language, thought, and problem-solving. The cortex also receives external information through the senses, which it then integrates and analyzes. Between these two layers are an important set of brain structures called the limbic system that modulates the lower brain structures and is itself modulated by the cortex.

The limbic system includes brain structures necessary for emotional processing, as well as learning and memory. As the middle layer of the brain, it is positioned to mediate between the more primitive and reflexive activities of lower brain structures and the functions of the more highly evolved layer above, which is responsible for reflection, behavioral modulation, cognition and executive functions. The limbic system receives this mix of reflex and reflection, adding to it its own specialized type of knowledge that is based on emotion and experience, an important component in guiding behavior.

The limbic system is also the center for assigning emotional value or importance to information received by the brain. External information (sounds, sights, etc.) enter through the sense organs and is processed and interpreted by other brain centers before being made available to the limbic system. Internal information about the state of the body (e.g., hunger, thirst, low blood sugar, the need to urinate) in the form of chemical signals is filtered, interpreted, and acted upon by the HYPOTHALAMUS. As both external and internal information converge, it is "tagged" by the limbic system in terms of its emotional tone, significance, and importance, allowing it to prioritize incoming information. (One of the most powerful messages used by the limbic system to prioritize information is pain, which is a constant companion for people with fibromyalgia.)

The neurons in limbic brain areas have been shown to have a greater degree of PLASTICITY than do those in other parts of the brain. This heightened plasticity makes the limbic system well-suited to the encoding of new associations (learning), but also means that it is highly vulnerable to pathological processes. Many viruses, including those of the herpes family, have a special affinity for limbic regions. Some researchers believe that a viral illness can trigger FMS in susceptible individuals (Jones et al., 1985; Straus et al., 1985). Heightened plasticity means that the limbic system is especially vulnerable to the effects of STRESS.

The Hypothalamic-Pituitary-Adrenal (HPA) Axis

To understand the limbic system-stress connection, its important to understand the role of the hypothalamus. As already noted, the hypothalamus receives and interprets incoming chemical and neuronal communications from the body. It also sends information and instructions from the brain to the body. The hypothalamic nuclei are linked to the limbic system by an especially rich and complex set of neural connections designed to provide them with the wealth of information they need to carry out their primary function, that of maintaining HOMEO-STASIS. The hypothalamus uses multiple interrelated pathways to regulate body functions and keep the system as a whole functioning smoothly. These pathways ultimately act on the ENDOCRINE SYSTEM (via the PITUITARY gland) and on the AUTONOMIC NERVOUS SYSTEM (via sympathetic and parasympathetic motor neurons), both of which project widely throughout the body. In addition, the hypothalamus partici-pates in the functioning of the immune system by releasing NEUROPEPTIDES. The best understood of the hypothalamus's regulatory pathways, and the one implicated in FMS, is known as the HYPOTHALAMIC-PITUITARY-ADRENAL (HPA) AXIS.

The HPA axis functions as an interface between the central nervous system and the endocrine (hormone) system; in effect, it "translates" messages from the language of the brain into the language of the body. This is possible because the hypothalamus contains specialized neuroendocrine cells that receive input from neighboring neurons in the regular way, but can respond by secreting peptides that stimulate the pituitary gland to release HORMONES.

The hormones released by the pituitary then serve as messengers to various endocrine glands throughout the body, instructing them to produce more or less of their own specific hormones in order to support the ongoing survival needs of the individual. This is the general means by which each of us is able to adapt, on a moment-by-moment basis, to the stresses and demands that various environments and situations place on us. A number of the most important adaptations, in particular, adaptations to internal and external stressors, are brought about via the ADRENAL GLANDS, the endocrine glands which constitute the third stop on the HPA axis.

Whenever an individual is exposed to any type of stress, be it illness, injury, or emotional challenges, the brain and body react with a stress response, which is mediated primarily through the HPA axis. Parts of the stress response occur directly in the central nervous system, heightening one's levels of arousal, alertness, and vigilance, focusing our attention, and enhancing cognitive processes. Other adaptations included in the stress response are directed by the brain, but occur in the body, and are designed to allow for the delivery of energy to the CNS and to critical muscles. These include increases in heart rate, blood pressure, and respiratory rate, production of additional blood sugar, and suppression of the immune system/inflammatory response.

The body components of the stress response are produced by the HPA axis, via the following steps:

1. The hypothalamus produces two peptides: corticotropin-releasing hormone (CRH) and arginine-vasopressin (AVP).

2. CRH and AVP signal the pituitary gland to produce adrenocorticotropic hormone (ACTH).

3. ACTH travels through the bloodstream to the adrenal glands, where it:

   a) stimulates the glands' outer layer (called the adrenal cortex) to produce CORTISOL and other

GLUCOCORTICOIDS; and

b) stimulates their inner layer (the adrenal medulla) to produce EPINEPHRINE and NOREPINEPHRINE and other mineralocorticoids.

4. Glucocorticoids enter the bloodstream, allowing them to come into contact with major organ systems, and epinephrine and norepinephrine stimulate the sympathetic division of the autonomic nervous system, in order to regulate bodily functioning (e.g., increase heart rate, heighten blood vessel tone, and promote the breakdown into blood sugar of proteins stored in the liver).

5. Finally, in an all-important fifth step, the various circulating hormones and peptides come back into contact with the hypothalamus, providing it with feedback on the functioning of the HPA system. This type of closed system, called a negative feedback loop, functions like a home thermostat to turn down the system's activity level when it senses that adequate adaptation has come about.

Dysfunction of the Limbic System and HPA Axis in FMS

Many studies have shown various types of central nervous system dysfunction in people with FMS, in particular, in the limbic system and along the HPA axis (Clauw & Chroussos, 1997; Goldstein, 1993). The demonstrated abnormalities are clearly linked to major symptoms of FMS, including joint and muscle pain/weakness, sleep disturbance, cognitive dysfunction, and depression.

For example, basal levels of cortisol (those measured during normal, non-stressed periods) are lower and normal daily fluctuations in cortisol level are altered in people with FMS (Croffard et al., 1994; McCain & Tilbe, 1989). Under stressful conditions (such as exercise) the HPA axis fails to produce normal increases in cortisol level, meaning that the body is unable to mount a normal stress response (e.g., needed increases in blood flow, respiration, and energy delivery to muscles).

Alterations in the body's response to stress have also been found in the autonomic nervous system. When challenged with muscular activity or mental stress, FMS patients produce too little epinephrine and norepinephrine, needed to activate muscles (Elam, Johansson, & Wallin, 1992; Vaeroy & Morkrid, 1991; Vaeroy, Qiao, Morkrid, & Forre, 1989). They also have lower levels of neuropeptide Y, a peptide that occurs in the same locations as norepinephrine and facilitates its effects; these low levels are found both at rest and following stress.

Norepinephrine levels are also abnormally low in the central nervous systems of people with FMS (Russell, Vaeroy, Javors, & Nyberg, 1992). In the CNS, norepinephrine enhances awareness, attention, and focus. There is also evidence that SEROTONIN levels are abnormally low in people with FMS (Legangeux et al., 2001; Russell, 1995, 1996, 1998). One of the roles of serotonin is to help stimulate the HPA axis and to control its normal daily fluctuations. Serotonin is involved in decreasing pain signals in the brain, initiating sleep, fighting depression, and increasing concentration ability. One very recent study has suggested that people with FMS are more likely to have a specific variant of a gene that codes for serotonin receptors and demonstrated a strong association between this particular genotype and the severity of FMS pain symptoms (Bondy et al., 1999).

Finally, studies have shown significantly elevated (2-3 times normal) levels of substance P in the cerebrospinal fluid of people with FMS (Bradley, 1998; Russell, 1999; Russell et al., 1994). Substance P is a neurotransmitter released in the spinal cord, which plays an important role in the perception of pain and the spread of chronic pain. When too much is present, it diffuses to neighboring spinal neurons, causing them to become sensitized and leading to the perception of pain in tissues that are not themselves injured or inflamed. Further studies have demonstrated that substance P levels rise and fall in concert with pain levels in people with FMS (Larson, Giovengo, Russell, & Michalek, 2000).

Effects of Stress on the HPA Axis: The Link between Stress and FMS

The HPA axis can itself be affected and changed by stress. Like the limbic system, it has a high degree of plasticity. There is a great deal of evidence that early environmental stress can alter the activity of the hypothalamic neurons that produce CRH, and that the resulting changes in HPA axis function are detectable throughout life. The first studies to demonstrate this were done on rat pups. In one study, young rats were exposed to a highly stressful experience (being separated from their mother for 3 hours a day). The experimenters found that when these rats grew to adulthood, they exhibited an exaggerated response to stress, they produced more CRH and, as a result, more cortisol (Ladd, Owens, & Nemeroff, 1996). In another study, Plotsky and Meany (1993) subjected rat pups to a fairly mild or normal type of stress (brief daily periods of human handling). This exposure seemed to "inoculate" them against stress later in life; these rats grew to be adults who produced lower levels of CRH and cortisol than rats who had not been handled at all during infancy. Other studies have gone on to demonstrate that rats exposed to severe early stress also show later changes in the number of serotonin receptors in certain parts of the limbic system (Vasquez, Lopez, Van Hoers, Watson, & Levine, 2000).

More recent research has demonstrated the same kinds of

effects of early stress on the HPA axis in humans (Wright et al., 1993). People who have been exposed to severe or chronic stress, especially during childhood, have been shown to have hyperactivation of the HPA axis (an exaggerated stress response), as well as changes in brain structure and NEUROTRANSMITTER function that can result in heightened fear reactions, problems with learning and memory, dysthymia (chronic, low-level depression), and enhanced pain perception (Chroussos, 2000; Gunnar, 1998; McEwen, 2000). It is important to note that, in addition to demonstrating the adverse effects of stress, these studies also indicate that a person's genetic makeup determines how vulnerable he or she is likely to be to such stressful experiences.

Other researchers have shown that childhood neglect and abuse (physical and/or sexual) are associated with four specific types of later CNS abnormalities (Teicher, 2000). The first is limbic irritability, which is the tendency to display symptoms (such as unusual bodily sensations or brief alterations of consciousness) characteristic of limbic system dysfunction. The second is deficient development and differentiation of the brain's left hemisphere, which in most people is largely responsible for language and verbal learning and memory. The third abnormality involves the corpus callosum, a thick band of nerve fibers that connects the brain's left and right hemispheres, allowing them to quickly share and integrate information. Adults who were abused or neglected as children more often show a reduced density of fibers in the corpus callosum, especially in the middle section. The fourth type of brain abnormality found to be associated with early abuse is functional deficits (reduced neuronal activity and decreased blood flow) in parts of the CEREBELLUM. This abnormality is particularly interesting, since the researchers also showed that it tended to normalize when subjects were given methylphenidate (Ritalin), with higher doses bringing about greater improvement in cerebellar function.

Separate research studies have produced evidence that women with FMS have a higher rate of reported childhood sexual abuse, when compared both to healthy women and to women with other rheumatic diseases (Taylor, Trotters, & Csuka, 1995; Boisset-Pioro, Esdaile, & Fitzcharles, 1995). One of these studies also demonstrated an association between the severity (frequency) of the early abuse and the severity of FMS symptoms in adulthood (Boisset-Pioro et al., 1995).

Clinical observation and research studies also support a relationship between FMS and stress experienced during adulthood. Many people with FMS report that their illness began following either a significant acute stressor or a prolonged period of stress (Crofford, 1994; Demitrack & Crofford, 1995; Demitrack et al., 1991). Studies have also demonstrated that FMS symptoms often vary in severity with the level of stress in the patient's life and that, as a group, people with FMS report a higher level of perceived daily stress than those without the disorder (Hermann, Scholmerich, & Straub, 2000).

Finally, researchers believe they have found the first serotonin gene that is expressed differently in people with FMS, which may help explain why they are more vulnerable to the effects of stress than are people without FMS (Bondy et al., 1999; Ofenbaecher et al., 1999; Klein & Berg, 1995).

Stressors Associated with Everyday Life

As described earlier, special systems in the human brain and body in particular the HYPOTHALAMIC-PITUITARY-ADRE-NAL (HPA) AXIS—are designed to deal with external and internal STRESSORS. They set in motion a variety of physiological processes known as the STRESS RESPONSE, which allows the individual to deal with the immediate source of stress, and then return the brain and body to HOMEOSTASIS.

While we may marvel at the intricate design of this complex system, it's important to remember that it evolved to deal with the requirements of our early Homo sapiens ancestors, who lived 50,000 to 150,000 years ago in a world very different from our own. These early humans lived in small bands that traveled only as far as necessary to find sufficient food; the men crafted tools and hunted to provide meat, while the women gathered and processed edible plant materials and cared for the children. The stressors they faced were generally quite concrete and straightforward, things like hunger and thirst, predation by wild animals, and disagreements among group members, and most of their days involved the same basic activities—hunting, gathering, food preparation, child care, and basic social/sexual interactions.

Clearly, the physical and social environment in which (and for which) our brains and bodies evolved was one in which change was very much the exception rather than the rule. Present-day humans, however, have to use virtually the same brains and bodies to cope with a wide and complex world in which change is rapid and constant. A world in which an individual comes into contact with tens of thousands of other humans beings in the course of a lifetime, and in which one needs to play many social roles, the majority of which are highly demanding and often in conflict with one another. It seems likely that these fundamental differences in the demands placed on our brains and bodies today are critical to the development of "new" disorders, including FMS and its close cousin and frequent companion, chronic fatigue syndrome (CFS).

One critical factor in the emergence of such disorders is the rapidity of change that all of us must deal with. Distance and time have been reduced to a fraction of what our forebears had to contend with; in the time it took an early band of humans to cross a river, families can fly across the United States.

Only a few generations separate us from the Industrial Revolution of the late 18th century, when power-driven machines were widely introduced and people began to move from a largely rural life-style to life in urban areas and jobs in factories. Today, many own their own car, not to mention an array of electrical appliances, from curling irons to refrigerator-freezers. In our own lifetimes, the computer has shrunk from a huge, intimidating machine with blinking lights and whirling tape drives to a small, familiar appliance on our desktop or kitchen counter on which we look for information, exchange email messages, and play games.

Nearly every human invention and development has involved an increase in speed. Electricity changed long-distance communication from the handwritten letter to the phone call, and electronics added the options of fax, email, and voicemail. With the introduction of the internal combustion engine, transportation shifted from horse-drawn carriages to automobiles, and nuclear science went on to develop rockets. The printing press has given way to the word processor and the pencil to the personal computer. In short, everything around us has speeded up, requiring from us an associated increase in processing speed to keep up with our own inventions.

Some have adapted easily to the new pace of life and thrive in this world of ever-changing technology, language, and social mores. Others, however, experience the majority of these changes as highly stressful. And a significant proportion of the population—those least equipped to deal with stress and therefore most vulnerable—are not always able to cope with the modern world, and are most likely to fall victim to stress-related illnesses affecting the brain and the body.

Who falls into this last, most vulnerable group depends on a number of factors. One factor is individual genetic makeup. Numerous genes influence both our propensity to perceive events and experiences as stressful and our ability to cope with stress in an adaptive manner. In particular, genes that code for components of the brain's SEROTONIN and NOREPINEPH-RINE systems have been implicated in individual differences in stress reactivity (Adell, Garcia-Marquez, Armario, & Gelpi, 1988; Akasura, et al., 2000; Amar, Mandal, & Sanyal, 1982).

In addition, people differ in terms of early experiences that can serve to modify—either augment or inhibit—our genetically-determined stress-response tendencies. Some had a generally happy childhood, spent in intact families, surrounded by healthy, well-adjusted family members, and full of experiences of success and mastery. Others haven't been as lucky. Some may have lost one or both parents to mental or physical illness, substance abuse, or death. Others may have witnessed the verbal, physical, or sexual abuse of other family members or have been the victims of abuse; some may have repeatedly experienced failure and frustration in school, in efforts to make friends, or in trying to please their parents.

Finally, although all of us have to cope with the demands of our modern world, we differ in the specific stressors that we face and the resources we have available to help us deal with them. All three variables—genetic vulnerability, early exposure to highly stressful situations, and current stress level—are associated with the risk of developing FMS. In general, the connection is that increased stress activates the HPA axis, which in turn activates the ADRENAL GLANDS, triggering stress-related changes in the tissues and organs of the body. When these systems, which evolved to respond to brief, acute stressors (such as a charging predator), are instead persistently challenged by chronic stressors (such as childhood abuse, lack of adequate sleep, or the inability to deal effectively with the fast-paced demands of daily life), they're unable to "rest" and replenish their resources, and ultimately may begin to malfunction in ways that produce illness.

Special Stresses Associated with Being a Woman

While there are obvious differences between males and females, including differences in size, muscular development, and secondary sexual characteristics, some of the most important gender differences, are internal and not as easy to detect.

Fluctuating Hormones

One of these "hidden" differences is the far greater fluctuation in sex hormone levels that occurs in women. These include both recurrent hormonal changes associated with having a monthly menstrual cycle and fluctuations associated with reproductive transitions, such as the menarche (the beginning of menstruation in early adolescence), pregnancy and the postpartum period, perimenopause, and menopause. Given the wide variations in hormone levels that women routinely experience, it's not surprising to learn that the female brain is far more responsive to hormonal changes than its male counterpart.

Each menstrual cycle is characterized by a series of changes in the ovaries and uterus that result in ovulation (release of an ovum or egg from one of the ovaries), followed by the monthly menstrual flow if the ovum isn't fertilized. The entire process is regulated by hormones produced by the HYPOTHALAMUS and PITUITARY GLAND, which signal parts of the reproductive tract to produce the familiar female sex hormones, estrogen and progesterone. Estrogen levels rise during the first half of each menstrual cycle, falling off after ovulation, while progesterone remains at a constant, low level until ovulation, after which it increases through the third week of a typical four-week cycle, and then declines.

The hypothalamus and pituitary gland, two of the three components of the HPA axis, are both crucial to the functioning of the menstrual cycle. In order to perform its tasks, the hypothalamus in the female brain must have estrogen (and progesterone) receptors in its NEURONS, enabling it to respond to circulating hormone levels.

However, the hypothalamus isn't the only region of the female brain with a high density of estrogen receptors. Other brain areas highly responsive to estrogen levels include:

▶ The amygdala and hippocampus (LIMBIC areas crucial to emotional functioning, as well as learning and memory);

▶ Lower brain areas responsible for the synthesis of he MONOAMINE NEUROTRANSMITTERS (DOPAMINE, norepinephrine, and serotonin);

▶ The basal forebrain (an area that includes both limbic structures and the BASAL GANGLIA, which are implicated in AD/HD); and

▶ Frontal, prefrontal, and cingulate CORTEX (areas known to play a role in AD/HD, depression, and obsessive-compulsive disorder (OCD).

All of these brain areas rich in estrogen receptors are affected by women's monthly fluctuations in sex hormone levels. When estrogen levels are high (especially during the middle of the menstrual cycle when ovulation occurs), neurotransmitter receptors in these brain areas are sensitized and work more efficiently; in addition, more dopamine and serotonin receptors are produced and these form more synapses (connections between neurons). These changes typically result in euthymia (good mood) and increased cognitive efficiency, especially in the areas of language, verbal memory, and fine motor skills.

In contrast, lowered estrogen levels (especially just prior to menstruation) are associated with less efficient functioning of the monoamine (dopamine, norepinephrine, and serotonin) receptors in these areas of the female brain, as well as decreased receptor and synapse density. The result is a greater likelihood of dysthymia (depressed or irritable mood) and reduced cognitive efficiency, as well as possible PREMENSTRUAL SYNDROME (PMS).

Similar effects are seen with the changes in estrogen and progesterone levels that occur with various reproductive transitions across the female life cycle. Increased density and sensitivity of monoamine receptors, with associated high levels of emotional and cognitive functioning, occur during high-estrogen states, most notably during pregnancy. And low-estrogen states, such as the postpartum period, perimenopause, and menopause, bring about decreases in the number and density of such receptors, with associated difficulties with mood and cognitive functions.

How are hormonal fluctuations and associated transmitter changes related to FMS? The clear benefits of estrogen for emotional and cognitive functioning have led researchers to call it "nature's psychoprotectant." But for a sizable percentage of women, having higher levels of this beneficial substance proves to be a two-edged sword. While the brain functions well during peak periods of estrogen, every month it must cope with the withdrawal of this function-enhancing hormone—meaning that for a sizable portion of each month during their reproductive years, many women struggle to compensate for the relative cognitive deficits brought about by this withdrawal.

While conclusive studies have yet to be carried out, our clinical experience strongly suggests that in some women this repeated buildup and withdrawal of estrogen (along with associated changes in progesterone levels) constitutes a significant stress on the central nervous system. Like other chronic stressors, it can lead to dysfunction in some or all components of the HPA axis, which may ultimately result in the development of FMS.

Gender Differences in Response to Stress

For fifty years or more, numerous studies have demonstrated that stress produces a "fight-or-flight" response, mediated by the body's release of norepinephrine, ADRENALINE, and COR-TISOL. However, it now appears that this response to stress is actually characteristic only of men, for whom the chemical release is also accompanied by increases in testosterone level (Taylor et al., 2000).

In contrast, the stress response in women triggers an accompanying release of the hormone OXYTOCIN, which is boosted by estrogen (Taylor et al., 2000). Oxytocin is also released during childbirth and breastfeeding and is known to regulate mood, decrease anxiety and depression, and promote affiliation. While testosterone fuels the "fight-or-flight" response in men, the release of the "friendlier" hormone oxytocin in women produces a different type of response to stress. The study's authors have dubbed it the "tend-and-befriend" response, as it encompasses a tendency when under stress to protect one's children and/or to form social bonds with others.

The typical female stress response is more likely than its male counterpart to contribute to the survival of the group as a whole while it facilitates an individual woman's ability to cope with a stressor. However, it differs in an important way from the prototypical male response in that it's likely to be far less effective in terms of bringing about an end to the stressful situation. While men are hormonally programmed to fight off stressors or remove themselves from the sources of stress, the female stress response is much more likely to keep a woman "in the line of fire." This increases the likelihood that the experience of stress will become prolonged, if not chronic. And, as we've stated, it's chronic stress that's most likely to trigger the dysfunction associated with FMS, as well as a variety of other brain and body ailments.

Stress Related to Gender Role Expectations

Finally, cultural realities may also contribute to a higher "stress quotient" for women than for men. Despite the significant societal changes brought about by the women's movement, women continue to be overrepresented in jobs with lower status and lower pay and, whatever their occupation, are generally paid less for the same work than their male counterparts. Whether or not they work outside the home, women are more often responsible for the majority of childcare responsibilities, and for those who are single parents (by choice or by fiat) the burden is even greater. In addition, the burden of caring for sick and aging parents more often falls to women than to men. Overall, it appears that women must more often juggle a dizzying array of responsibilities that includes work, tending to the needs of family members, homemaking chores, and community activities—just the recipe for chronic stress!

Special Stresses Associated with Having AD/HD

Women with AD/HD are likely to have more stress-related illnesses such as FMS than their counterparts without AD/HD for several reasons. First, growing up with AD/HD—particularly undiagnosed AD/HD—is likely to expose one to a greater amount of chronic stress. Second, a host of acute stressors have been shown to be associated with living as an adult with AD/HD. And finally, there is growing evidence that one of the core deficits in AD/HD is an impaired ability to deal with stress in an adaptive manner. Below, each of these predisposing factors is considered.

The Stress of Growing Up with AD/HD

Early exposure to chronic stress has been found to have a lifelong influence on the functioning of the HPA axis. Certainly, many children with AD/HD are likely to experience some of the following significant childhood stressors:

▶ criticism and negative reactions from parents, teachers, and other adults;

▶ repeated punishment for misbehavior;

▶ increased risk of abuse;

▶ poor academic performance;

▶ difficulty making friends; social ostracism;

▶ repeated experiences of frustration and failure;

▶ feeling misunderstood or unfairly treated;

▶ feelings of helplessness at being unable to control one's own behavior; and

▶ feelings of guilt, shame, and remorse.

Many girls with AD/HD, struggling with academic, behavioral, and/or social difficulties, come to feel like failures and eventually develop dysthymia, a chronic state of low-level depression that can be accompanied by feelings of hopelessness or apathy. Nothing their parents, friends, or teachers say can undo their profound sense of inadequacy. Depending on her temperament, the girl with AD/HD may eventually give up trying, avoiding academic challenges and perhaps becoming involved with undesirable friends and activities. Alternatively, she may redouble her efforts, pushing herself to the limits until she succumbs to exhaustion and physical breakdown. Many bright girls with AD/HD eventually "hit the wall" as academic expectations inexorably rise to a level that exceeds their ability to compensate.

The Stress Associated with Being an Adult with AD/HD

As adults, people with AD/HD are also more likely to experience many types of stressful life experiences. Some of these stressors are linked to AD/HD-related impulsivity, others to difficulties with focus and persistence:

▶ difficulties with organization and time management;

▶ social difficulties;

▶ lower educational attainment;

▶ problems on the job; more frequent job changes;

▶ financial difficulties;

▶ more frequent moves;

▶ higher risk of traffic accidents;

▶ unplanned pregnancies;

▶ marital discord and divorce;

▶ increased risk of depression, anxiety, and other neuropsychiatric disorders; and

▶ raising children with AD/HD.

While all of the above are significant stressors, it's the last—the challenges of raising one or more children with AD/HD while trying to cope with AD/HD oneself—that often proves to be the "straw that breaks the camel's back," exhausting the AD/HD woman's ability to effectively compensate and cope. Supporting this idea is a recent study that demonstrates that there are in fact unique stressors associated with parenting an AD/HD child, especially for mothers (Kaplan, Crawford, Fisher, & Dewey, 1998).

A group of 248 parents (mostly mothers) indicated how much they agreed with statements such as, "There are lots of bad feelings in the family," "We don't get along well together," and "We are not able to make decisions on how to solve problems," reflecting their degree of satisfaction with their family life. More than half of the parents studied had children who were experiencing academic difficulties, some due primarily to AD/HD, others primarily to a reading disability (dyslexia), and others with both AD/HD and a reading disability. Not surprisingly, the researchers found that parents of children with academic problems were less satisfied with family life than those whose children were meeting expectations. However, the dissatisfaction was significantly higher in the parents of AD/HD children than in those whose children had reading disabilities.

AD/HD Affects the Ability to Cope with Stress

Paul Wender, M.D., one of the first physicians to recognize and write about AD/HD in adults, has discussed the fact that many adults with AD/HD appear particularly susceptible to the effects of stress. In his book, *Attention-Deficit Hyperactivity Disorder in Adults,* Dr. Wender writes,

Many AD/HD adults relate that they are over-reactive to the ordinary stresses of daily life, that they lack resilience and are unable to persevere. They respond excessively or inappropriately to ordinary demands, particularly if unanticipated. They describe themselves as easily confused, "discombobulated," "stressed out," and "hassled." These anxious feelings often induce a vicious cycle: the AD/HD adult under stress becomes more impulsive, more disorganized and less competent, generates further difficulties, and becomes increasingly overwhelmed and demoralized (pp. 29-30).

It's important to keep in mind that everyone—AD/HD or not—is affected by stress in a fairly predictable manner. Mild levels of stress generally improve learning and memory, e.g., students often find that they can't concentrate on course reading until they start feeling a little anxious about an upcoming exam. Higher levels of stress, however, adversely affect cognitive functions and thus interfere with learning and memory, e.g., in the hours just prior to the exam, many students are too anxious to process anything they read and may even fail to notice that they've walked directly in front of an oncoming car.

The problem for the person with AD/HD is that her brain and body may be much more sensitive to stressors, so that what the majority of her classmates experience as "mildly stressful" may feel overwhelming to her. To extend the above example, even a week before the exam the AD/HD student may feel highly stressed just thinking about the upcoming exam and find that words seem to swim on the page when she tries to sit down and study. Procrastination becomes an understandable response when situations seem overwhelmingly stressful.

The Path from Stress (via AD/HD) to FMS

Numerous studies demonstrate that inappropriate distribution of the neurotransmitters dopamine and norepinephrine—too much to the limbic system, not enough to the frontal lobes—underlies the symptoms of AD/HD (Grace, 2001; Solanto, 2000). The frontal lobes have insufficient "fuel" to carry out important attentional and executive functions, while the limbic system, bombarded by excess neurotransmitters, is put into overdrive. As described earlier, the job of the limbic system is to evaluate input coming from both the external environment and the internal milieu, compare it with previous experience, and tag it with appropriate emotional coloration. This integrated and enriched information is then routed to the frontal lobes to be acted on, as well as to the endocrine, immune and autonomic nervous systems (via the hypothalamus) to ensure that the necessary "support services" (such as energy and strength) are available for the anticipated behavioral response.

This process doesn't always go smoothly in the AD/HD brain, however. Because of the lopsided distribution of neurotransmitters, the messages primarily travel "downstream" (to the body systems), readying the person for a series of goal-directed activities. But guidance as to what to do, which should come from the frontal lobes, may not be forthcoming, due to their underactivation. As a result, the task stays undone and the limbic system re-sends its messages for action and support. While the sluggish frontal lobes are likely to experience this "second request" as if it were brand new, the already stimulated hypothalamus and its downstream systems may go into hyperdrive.

As this pattern is repeated time and again (perhaps exacerbated by hormonally-mediated fluctuations in mood and cognition), the owner of the AD/HD brain feels increasingly emotionally stressed. Additionally, various brain and body systems may begin to change in more permanent ways, e.g., serotonin levels may fall and SUBSTANCE P levels rise, triggering increased perception of pain. The pain then serves as additional input to the limbic system, which should recognize its importance and route instructions to resolve it. But the systems it needs to activate to do so—the HPA axis and its extensions—have "burned out" from their chronic, ineffective efforts to deal with stress and are unable to respond appropriately. The immune system also gives way under this barrage, paving the way for opportunistic infections and maladaptive responses to external or internal agents (called, respectively, acquired sensitivities and autoimmune disorders). Thus, stress breeds additional stressors, which further challenge systems already weakened by chronic stress, until the cycle eventually breaks down into FMS or other overt states of illness.

Dealing with the Stressors that Can Lead to FMS (or Already Have)

It is important that women with AD/HD, who are at heightened risk for developing FMS, learn ways that they can counter these risks and improve their odds of staying healthy. The following are eight recommendations for women who are concerned about developing FMS, as well as for those who may already have it:

1. **Get accurate diagnoses.** A high-quality diagnostic evaluation is essential. No disorder can be properly treated and no stressful situation effectively modified until it has been appropriately identified. A woman who hasn't received a definitive diagnosis of AD/HD should consult with a clinician who is knowledgeable about AD/HD and the host of other disorders that often co-occur with AD/HD. Each woman, as well as the health professionals she works with, needs to know with certainty what disorder(s) she has and how they interfere with her functioning, in order to develop an effective treatment plan (see Chapter 9 for a discussion of other coexisting conditions). Understanding the nature and severity of stressors in her life—both current and in the past—should also be part of a good AD/HD evaluation, and will help set the stage for dealing effectively with those stressors.

   Similarly, a woman who thinks that she may have FMS should get a thorough physical exam from a physician with knowledge and experience in dealing with this disorder. Many other conditions may produce symptoms similar to those of FMS (thyroid problems, iron-deficiency anemia, sleep apnea, chronic viral infections, and other autoimmune disorders, to name just a few). In determining whether a woman has FMS, her physician will need to rule out these and other disorders, or treat them if they're found. In particular, if the thyroid gland is operating at low- or mid-normal levels (T3, T4, TSH and free thyroid levels), the physician should raise these levels three fourths of the way into the accepted "normal" range. (TSH will drop, but this is not a real value to follow when using exogenous sources of thyroid hormone.)

2. **Take AD/HD medication(s) as prescribed.** Medication prescribed for AD/HD and related conditions such as depression or anxiety, should be taken as prescribed every day, every dose. Medication is the only treatment for AD/HD that corrects the underlying anomalies in neurotransmitter distribution that can lead to FMS, but the neurotransmitters are only normalized when medications are taken as directed. Women who have difficulty remembering to take all prescribed doses should work with their therapist or AD/HD coach to develop an effective reminder system—setting an alarm watch or establishing a link between taking medication and an external cue (e.g., putting pills next to a toothbrush or in a lunch bag). A woman whose mood, attention, or other cognitive functions vary with her menstrual cycle should keep notes on these variations for a month or two and then talk with her prescribing physician about the possibility of tailoring her medication regimen to provide optimal effectiveness throughout her cycle.

3. **Work to maintain a healthy life-style.** Women with AD/HD and FMS should strive to get regular and adequate sleep, eat healthy, well-balanced meals, and stick with a reasonable program of regular exercise. A daily multivitamin—with iron to supplement that lost through menstruation—can also help maintain good health. Smoking should be avoided and alcohol intake should be kept at a healthy level; weight, blood pressure, and cholesterol levels should be regularly monitored. While these recommendations are important for everyone,

they're especially critical for people with AD/HD, who may have more difficulty finding the time for things like sleep, exercise, or doctor appointments.

4. **Learn effective stress-management techniques.** A woman with AD/HD and FMS should carefully assess her stress level. If stress levels are high, it may be helpful to work with a therapist or counselor on stress reduction. Using structured problem-solving techniques, a good therapist can help her identify stressors she can eliminate or reduce and which she can learn to deal with more effectively.

Of course, not all stressful events can be eliminated or controlled; to better cope with these, it is important to learn how to control the ways in which the brain and body respond to stress. Meditation, guided imagery, yoga, and biofeedback training can all be effective. Stress-management classes using these and other techniques are offered by many health clubs and wellness centers and through workplace Employee Assistance Programs (EAP's), as well as by psychologists and other mental health professionals. The best time to learn these skills is before stress levels have become overwhelming, when practicing them can function almost like a vaccination against the harmful effects of stress. But women already facing high stress levels can benefit from these methods as well.

5. **Establish a working relationship with a gynecologist.** Again, while it's important for all women to have a partnership with their gynecologist, it's especially important for the woman with AD/HD, who may be at increased risk for hormonally-mediated illnesses. Each woman with AD/HD needs a knowledgeable

gynecologist who will work cooperatively with her to manage hormone-related health issues such as menstrual irregularities, PMS, changes associated with pregnancy and the postpartum period, and the effects of perimenopause and menopause. A gynecologist can also monitor and manage changes in other hormone systems (e.g., thyroid, growth hormone, insulin) that interact with estrogen and progesterone.

6. **Find a physician who understands FMS.** Because FMS is a complex disorder and its etiology is not yet fully understood, some doctors persist in viewing it as a psychiatric or psychosomatic disorder, or as simply a physical manifestation of anxiety or depression. When faced with a physician having these attitudes, a woman with AD/HD and FMS should educate him/her or find a new doctor. Scores of research studies have documented that FMS is a bona fide medical disorder and have described the physiological abnormalities associated with it. In efforts to educate her physician, a woman can share a copy of this chapter along with an article or two from a reputable website on FMS and related disorders (www.nih.gov/niams/healthinfo/fibrofs.htm, www.immunesupport.com, or www.teleport.com/~nfra/).

7. **Form a treatment team.** Because of its complexity and stubborn persistence, FMS usually requires treatment from multiple health professionals. To optimize the effectiveness of treatment, a woman needs to insist that all her physicians and other health-care providers (therapist, accupuncturist, nutritionist, physical therapist, massage therapist, etc.) work together and are aware of one another's interventions. She should ask the most knowledgeable of her providers

to be the "quarterback" or team leader, responsible for getting team members' questions answered and information shared. One simple way a woman can begin facilitating communication among providers is to be sure each one copies all other providers every time she is seen or a change is made in her medication or treatment regimen.

8. **Explore a variety of pharmacotherapy options.** Psychostimulants such as Ritalin®, Dexedrine®, Adderall®, and Concerta™ remain the "gold standard" for treatment of AD/HD. By bringing about needed changes in the distribution of neurotransmitters, they may also be helpful in addressing the stress cycle that can lead to FMS.

Once FMS has developed, additional medications are usually necessary. Next in line are medications that reduce pain and inflammation in affected tissues. The most effective of these are opioid derivatives, which work by affecting endorphins, neuropeptide hormones that bind to opiate receptors in the brain to reduce the sensation of pain. To avoid these medications is a grave mistake, as numerous studies have demonstrated their high degree of effectiveness and low likelihood of abuse among patients with pain syndromes. GLUCOCORTICOIDS (such as cortisone) and MINERALO-CORTICOSTEROIDS are another important group of medications in the FMS armamentarium, as can be some nonprescription herbal preparations and supplements such as ENADA® (an oxidizing COENZYME), Co-Q 10 (another coenzyme), and DHEA (a steroid compound).

Because limbic system dysfunction underlies FMS, the use of anticonvulsants can also be quite helpful. Klonopin® can help in a highly specific way with kindling and anxiety disorders, and Neurontin® appears to be helpful with pain in

FMS patients. To help with good sleep hygiene, medications like trazodone and low-dose tricyclic antidepressants can be beneficial.

Conclusion

While we still have much to learn about both AD/HD and FMS, it's becoming increasingly clear that these disorders are related and that effective treatment of either requires aggressive treatment of both. We believe that a cornerstone for the prevention and treatment of FMS is the recognition of underlying AD/HD and initiation of its treatment with medication (usually a psychostimulant) that effects the necessary redistribution of monoamine neurotransmitters. This, along with the appropriate treatment of secondary pain syndromes and life-style modifications, can bring about healing and resetting of the underlying homeostatic pathways.

Definitions of Terms

ADRENAL GLAND—Two small ENDOCRINE gland which sit atop the kidneys and are the final link in the HPA AXIS. Each adrenal gland consists of an outer layer (adrenal cortex) and an inner layer (adrenal medulla) (see text for their functions) ADRENALINE—A hormone neurotransmitter produced by the ADRENAL GLANDS as part of the STRESS RESPONSE, which causes increased heart rate and other metabolic effects needed to respond to STRESSORS. (Also called epinephrine.)

AUTONOMIC NERVOUS SYSTEM—One of two major divisions of the peripheral nervous system (the other is the somatic nervous system, which is responsible for controlling voluntary muscle movements). The autonomic nervous system regulates "smooth" muscle, the type over which we don't have voluntary control (e.g., in the walls of blood vessels or lining the GI system). One division of the autonomic system, called the sympathetic division, is responsible for regulating processes that occur when the body needs to draw on its energy reserves (e.g., increasing heart rate and blood sugar level, increasing blood flow to the voluntary muscles). The other division, the parasympathetic, handles the reverse side, that is, it controls processes that help the body take in and store energy for later use (e.g., secretion of saliva and digestive juices, increased blood flow to the stomach and intestines).

BASAL GANGLIA— A collection of large nuclei (aggregations of neuronal cell bodies) including the putamen, caudate nucleus, and globus pallidus, which sit below the brain's frontal lobes, with one set in each hemisphere. Among the important functions of the basal ganglia are the execution of planned sequences of movements and shifting of attention.

CENTRAL NERVOUS SYSTEM—The human nervous system is divided into two major components. The central nervous system includes the brain and the spinal cord, while the peripheral nervous system contains all the remaining nerves throughout the body.

CEREBELLUM—A small structure at the back of the brain, attached to the brain stem, that looks like a miniature version of the brain (cerebellum is Latin for "little brain"). The cerebellum has long been recognized as playing an important role in balance, posture, and the coordination of complex voluntary muscular movements. More recently, it has also been shown to be involved in attention and complex cognitive processes.

COENZYME One component of an active enzyme system, usually containing a vitamin or mineral. Enzymes modify and increase biochemical reactions in the body without being consumed in the process.

CORTEX—The outermost layer of the brain, made up of neuronal cell bodies. Cerebral cortex is largely responsible for higher brain functions, including sensation, voluntary muscle movement, thought, reasoning, and memory.

CORTISOL—One of the steroid hormones (collectively called GLUCOCORTICOIDS) produced by the ADRENAL GLANDS; regulates carbohydrate metabolism and maintains blood pressure. (Also called hydrocortisone.)

DOPAMINE—Yet another MONOAMINE NEUROTRANSMITTER found in both the central nervous system and various body systems. In the brain, dopamine is important to the initiation of voluntary movements as well as cognitive processes, especially attention and executive functions.

ENDOCRINE SYSTEM—A body system made up of glands, including the thyroid, ADRENAL, PITUITARY, pancreas, etc., which secrete HORMONES directly into the bloodstream.

EPINEPHRINE & NOREPINEPHRINE—two chemically similar NEUROTRANSMITTERS. Epinephrine (also called adrenalin) is produced by the ADRENAL medula and stimulates the sympathetic division of the AUTONOMIC NERVOUS SYSTEM. Norepinephrine (also called noradrenalin), while also produced by the adrenal medulla, is found mainly in the CENTRAL NERVOUS SYSTEM, where it fuels brain systems critical for arousal, attention and emotional reactions.

GLUCOCORTICOIDS—Steroid-like compounds produced by the ADRENAL GLANDS that have an antiinflammatory effect on body tissues. The best known glucocorticoid is CORTISOL.

HOMEOSTASIS—A steady state or state of equilibrium, in which all body systems are working and interacting efficiently. When homeostasis is interrupted (e.g., by response to a stressor), the body attempts to restore it by adjusting one or more physiological processes.

HORMONES—A substance produced by one type of body tissue and conveyed by the bloodstream to another type of tissue to affect its activity level. Hormones are divided into two types, PEPTIDES (chain of amino acids) and steroids (fat-soluble molecules small enough to pass directly into body cells).

HYPOTHALAMIC-PITUITARY-ADRENAL AXIS (HPA AXIS)—A major component of the body's STRESS RESPONSE SYSTEM. The HYPOTHALAMUS receives input from both the body and the environment and determines how best to respond (adapt) to it; it then chemically signals the nearby PITUITARY gland, which in turn sends chemical messages to the ADRENAL GLANDS. These glands then secrete substances that appropriately activate parts of the ENDOCRINE SYSTEM and of the sympathetic division of the AUTONOMIC NERVOUS SYSTEM.

HYPOTHALAMUS—A brain structure adjacent to the LIMBIC SYSTEM that consists of numerous small nuclei (collections of neuronal cell bodies); one of its major functions is to work with the PITUITARY gland and ADRENAL glands to regulate bodily states in response to STRESS.

LIMBIC—Pertaining to the limbic system, a group of deep brain structures including the hippocampus and amygdala, associated with olfaction (sense of smell), learning and memory, emotion, and motivation.

MINERALOCORTICOSTEROIDS—Steroid hormones secreted by the ADRENAL GLANDS that regulate the body's balance of water and electrolytes (ions such as sodium and chloride required by cells to regulate their electric charge and the entry/exit of water). (Also called mineralocorticoids.)

MONOAMINE NEUROTRANSMITTERS—Neurotransmitters are chemical substances that transmit nerve impulses from one neuron to another across the intervening synapse (interneural space). The three monoamine neurotransmitters are DOPAMINE, NOREPINEPHRINE, and SEROTONIN.

NEURAL—Pertaining to neurons, the nerve cells which make up the nervous system. Each individual neuron uses an electrical impulse to transmit information along its length, then releases one of a number of special chemicals, called NEUROTRANSMITTERS, that signal the next neuron in line to "pass it on."

NEURONS—The nerve cells which make up the nervous system. Each individual neuron uses an electrical impulse to transmit information along its length, then releases one of a number of special chemicals, called NEUROTRANSMITTERS, that signal the next neuron in line to 'pass it on.'

NEUROPEPTIDES (or PEPTIDES)—One of two classes of HORMONES produced by neurons (including some in the HYPOTHALAMUS) and by glands of the ENDOCRINE SYSTEM. Peptides may themselves function as NEUROTRANSMITTERS, or they may act as modulators of the effectiveness of other neurotransmitter substances (such as NOREPINEPHRINE and SEROTONIN). Examples of peptides mentioned in this article include corticotropin-releasing hormone (CRH) and arginine-vasopressin (AVP) (both of which are secreted by the hypothalamus and serve as neurotransmitters), and neuropeptide Y (which modulates the actions of the neurotransmitters EPINEPHRINE and NOREPINEPHRINE).

NOREPINEPHRINE—Another of the MONOAMINE NEUROTRANSMITTERS, which fuels brain systems critical for arousal, attention, and emotional reactions. (Also known as noradrenaline.)

OXYTOCIN—A hormone released by the PITUITARY gland that stimulates uterine contractions, facilitates the release of breast milk, and plays a role in the STRESS RESPONSE, especially in women.

PITUITARY—A small, oval, ENDOCRINE-activating center richly connected to the HYPOTHALAMUS; part of the HPA AXIS that responds to STRESS. Because pituitary secretions control the other endocrine glands of the body, it is sometimes referred to as the master gland.

PLASTICITY—The ability of body systems to change in form and function as a result of experience and previous function. In the CENTRAL NERVOUS SYSTEM, the changes occur via the formation of new connections between NEURONS, which support the learning and retention of new information, associations, and behaviors.

PREMENSTRUAL SYNDROME (PMS)—A group of symptoms, including abdominal bloating, breast tenderness, headache, fatigue, irritability, and depression, that occur in many women from 2 to 14 days before the onset of menstruation.

SEROTONIN—One of the MONOAMINE NEUROTRANSMITTERS found in both the central nervous system and various body systems. In the brain, serotonin is important in regulation of sleep and mood, concentration, and pain control; it also helps to stimulate and regulate the HPA AXIS.

STRESS—A stimulus or disturbance (metabolic, physiologic, traumatic, inflammatory, infectious, or psychological/emotional) that interferes with the body's HOMEOSTASIS and leads to activation of stereotypical stress-adaptation mechanisms, including the HPA AXIS and sympathetic division of the AUTONOMIC NERVOUS SYSTEM. Technically, the triggering stimuli are known as stressors, while the body's reaction to them is called the stress response. Examples of stressors include illness, injury, frightening events, anxiety-producing experiences, and worry.

STRESS RESPONSE—The body's reaction to a STRESSOR. (See HYPOTHALAMIC-PITUITARY-ADRENAL AXIS.)

STRESSOR—An internal or external stimulus that triggers the body's STRESS RESPONSE. Examples of stressors include illness, injury, frightening events, anxiety-producing experiences, and worry.

SUBSTANCE P—A neurotransmitter involved in the transmission of pain impulses from the body to the brain.

References

Adell, A., Garcia-Marquez, C., Armario, A., & Gelpi, E. (1988). Chronic stress increases serotonin and noradrenaline in rat brain and sensitizes their responses to a further acute stress. *Journal of Neurochemistry, 50,* 1678-1681.

Akasura, M., Nagashima, H., Fujii, S., Sasuga, Y., Misonoh, A., Hasegawa, H., & Osada, K. (2000). Influences of chronic stress on central nervous system. *Nihon Shinkei Seishin Yakurigaku Zasshi, 20,* 97-105.

Amar, A., Mandal, S., & Sanyal, A. K. (1982). Effect of brain monoamines on the secretion of adrenocorticotrophic hormone. *Acta Endocrinologica (Copenhagen), 101,* 180-186.

Boisset-Pioro, M. H., Esdaile, J. M., & Fitzcharles, M. A. (1995). Sexual and physical abuse in women with fibromyalgia syndrome. *Arthritis and Rheumatism, 38,* 235-241.

Bondy, B., Spaeth, M., Offenbaecher, M., Glatzeder, K., Stratz, T., Schwarz, M., de Jonge, S., Kruger, M., Engel, R. R., Farber, L., Pongratz, D. E., & Ackenheil, M. (1999). The T102C polymorphism of the 5-HT2A-receptor gene in fibromyalgia. *Neurobiology of Disease, 6,* 433-439.

Bradley, L. A. (1998). *Abnormal pain perception and functional brain activity in women with fibromyalgia.* Invited presentation, Gender and Pain, National Institutes of Health, Bethesda, MD, April 7-8.

Chrousos, G. P. (2000). *Neuroendocrinology of stress: Developmental aspects.* Invited presentation, The Intersection of Stress, Drug Abuse, and Development, National Institute on Drug Abuse, Bethesda, MD, January 20.

Clauw, D. J., & Chrousos, G. P. (1997). Chronic pain and fatigue syndromes: Overlapping clinical and neuroendocrine features and potential pathogenic mechanisms. *Neuroimmunomodulation, 4,* 134-153.

Crofford, L. J. (1994). Neuroendocrine aspects of fibromyalgia. *Journal of Musculoskeletal Pain, 2,* 125-132.

Demitrack, M. A., & Crofford, L. J. (1995). Hypothalamic-pituitary-adrenal axis dysregulation in fibromyalgia and chronic fatigue syndrome: An overview and hypothesis. *Journal of Musculoskeletal Pain, 3,* 67-73.

Demitrack, M. A., Dale, J. K., Straus, S. E., Laue, L., Listwak, S. J., Kruesi, M. J., Chrousos, G. P., & Gold, P. W. (1991). Evidence for impaired activation of the hypothalamic-pituitary-adrenal axis in patients with chronic fatigue syndrome. *Journal of Clinical Endocrinology and Metabolism, 73,* 1224-1234.

Elam, M., Johansson, G., & Wallin, B. G. (1992). Do patients with primary fibromyalgia have an altered muscle sympathetic nerve activity? *Pain, 48,* 371-375.

Goldstein, J. A. (1993). *Chronic fatigue syndromes: The limbic hypothesis.* Binghamton, NY: Haworth Medical Press.

Goldstein, J. A. (1996). *Betrayal by the brain: The neurologic basis of chronic fatigue syndrome, fibromyalgia syndrome, and related neural network disorders.* Binghamton, NY: Haworth Medical Press.

Grace, A. A. (2001). Psychostimulant actions on dopamine and limbic system function: Relevance to the pathophysiology and treatment of ADHD. In M. V. Solanto, A. F. T. Arnsten, & F. X. Castellanos (Eds.), *Stimulant drugs and ADHD: Basic and clinical neuroscience.* New York: Oxford University Press.

Gunnar, M. R. (1998). Quality of early care and buffering of neuroendocrine stress reactions: Potential effects on the developing human brain. *Preventive Medicine, 27,* 208-211.

Jones, J. F., Ray, C. G., Minnich, L. L., Hicks, M. J., Kibler, R., & Lucas, D. O. (1985). Evidence for active Epstein-Barr virus infection in patients with persistent, unexplained illnesses: Elevated anti-early antigen antibodies. *Annals of Internal Medicine, 102,* 1-7.

Kaplan, B. J., Crawford, S. G., Fisher, G. C., & Dewey, D. M. (1998). Family dysfunction is more strongly associated with ADHD than with general school problems. *Journal of Attention Disorders, 2,* 209-216.

Klein, R., & Berg, P. A. (1995). High incidence of antibodies to 5-hydroxytryptamine, gangliosides and phospholipids in patients with chronic fatigue and fibromyalgia syndrome and their relatives: Evidence for a clinical entity of both disorders. *European Journal of Medical Research, 1,* 21-26.

Krause, K.H., Krause, J., Magyarosy, I., Ernst, E., & Pongratz, D. (1998). Fibromyalgia syndrome and attention deficit hyperactivity disorder: Is there a comorbidity and are there consequences for the therapy of fibromyalgia syndrome? *Journal of Musculoskeletal Pain, 6,* 111-116.

Ladd, C. O., Owens, M. J., & Nemeroff, C. B. (1996). Persistent changes in corticotropin-releasing factor neuronal systems induced by maternal deprivation. *Endocrinology, 137,* 1212-1218.

Larson, A. A., Giovengo, S. L., Russell, I. J., & Michalek, J. E. (2000). Changes in the concentrations of amino acids in the cerebrospinal fluid that correlate with pain in patients with fibromyalgia: Implications for nitric oxide pathways. *Pain, 87,* 201-211.

Legangneux, E., Mora, J. J., Spreux-Varoquaux, O., Thorin, I., Herrou, M. Alvado, G., & Gomeni, C. (2001). Cerebrospinal fluid biogenic amine metabolites, plasma-rich platelet serotonin and [3H] imipramine reuptake in the primary fibromyalgia syndrome. *Rheumatology (Oxford), 40,* 290-296.

McCain, G. A., & Tilbe, K. S. (1989). Diurnal hormone variation in fibromyalgia syndrome: A comparison with rheumatoid arthritis. *Journal of Rheumatology, 16,* 154-157.

McEwen, B. S. (2000). Effects of adverse experiences for brain structure and function. *Biological Psychiatry, 48,* 721-731.

Offenbaecher, M., Bondy, B., de Jonge, S., Glatzeder, K., Kruger, M., Schoeps, P., & Ackenheil, M. (1999). Possible association of fibromyalgia with a polymorphism in the serotonin transporter gene regulatory region. *Arthritis and Rheumatism, 42,* 2482-2488.

Plotsky, P. M., & Meaney, M. J. (1993). Early, postnatal experience alters hypothalamic corticotropin-releasing factor (CRF) mRNA, median eminence CRF content and stress-induced release in adult rats. *Brain Research–Molecular Brain Research, 18,* 195-200.

Qiao, Z. G., Vaeroy, H., & Morkrid, L. (1991). Electrodermal and microcirculatory activity in patients with fibromyalgia during baseline, acoustic stimulation and cold pressor tests. *Journal of Rheumatology, 18,* 1383-1389.

Russell, I. J. (1995). Neurohormonal abnormal laboratory findings related to pain and fatigue in fibromyalgia. *Journal of Musculoskeletal Pain, 3,* 59-65.

Russell, I. J. (1996). Neurochemical pathogenesis of fibromyalgia syndrome. *Journal of Musculoskeletal Pain, 4,* 61-92.

Russell, I. J. (1998). Advances in fibromyalgia: Possible role for central neurochemicals. *American Journal of Medical Science, 315,* 377-384.

Russell, I. J., Orr, M. D., Littman, B., Vipraio, G. A., Alboukrek, D., Michalek, J. E., Lopez, Y., & MacKillip, F. (1994). Elevated cerebrospinal fluid levels of substance P in patients with the fibromyalgia syndrome. *Arthritis and Rheumatism, 37,* 1593-1601.

Russell, I. J., Vaeroy, H., Javors, M., & Nyberg, F. (1992). Cerebrospinal fluid biogenic amine metabolites in fibromyalgia/fibrositis syndrome and rheumatoid arthritis. *Arthritis and Rheumatism, 35,* 1538-1539.

Solanto, M. V. (2000). *Dopamine dysregulation in AD/HD: Integrating clinical and basic science research.* Online Proceedings of the 6th Internet World Congress for Biomedical Sciences (INABIS). Available from URL: http://www.uclm.es/inabis2000/symposia/files/125/index.htm.

Straus, S. E., Tosato, G., Armstrong, G., Lawley, T., Preble, O. T., Henle, W., Davey, R., Pearson, G., Epstein, J., Brus, I., et al. (1985). Persisting illness and fatigue in adults with evidence of Epstein-Barr virus infection. *Annals of Internal Medicine, 102,* 7-16.

Taylor, M. L., Trotter, D. R., & Csuka, M. E. (1995). The prevalence of sexual abuse in women with fibromyalgia. *Arthritis and Rheumatism, 38,* 229-234.

Taylor, S. E., Klein, L. C., Lewis, B. P., Gruenewald, T. L., Gurung, R. A., & Updegraff, J. A. (2000). Biobehavioral responses to stress in females: Tend-and-befriend, not fight-or-flight. *Psychological Review, 107,* 411-429.

Teicher, M. H. (2000). Wounds that time won't heal: The neurobiology of child abuse. *Cerebrum: The Dana Forum on Brain Science, 2,* 50-67.

Vaeroy, H., Qiao, Z-G., Morkrid, L., & Forre, O. (1989). Altered sympathetic nervous system response in patients with fibromyalgia (fibrositis syndrome). *Journal of Rheumatology, 16,* 1460-1465.

Vazquez, D. M., Lopez, J. F., Van Hoers, H., Watson, S. J., & Levine, S. (2000). Maternal deprivation regulates serotonin 1A and 2A receptors in the infant rat. *Brain Research, 855,* 76-82.

Wender, P. H. (1995). *Attention-deficit hyperactivity disorder in adults.* New York: Oxford University Press.

Wright, L. B., Treiber, F. A., Davis, H., Strong, W. B., Levy, M., Van Huss, E., & Batchelor, C. (1993). Relationship between family environment and children's hemodynamic responses to stress: A longitudinal evaluation. *Behavioral Medicine, 19,* 115-121.

SECTION

five

SUPPORT FROM THE ENVIRONMENT

CHAPTER 12

Self-acceptance for Women with AD/HD

Lynn Weiss, Ph.D.

W hen Gwen was twenty-three years old, she had a vision. It didn't seem strange to her that she had a picture in her mind. She had always seen pictures, kind of like watching a perpetual stage play. Pictures were how she thought. To be sure, she didn't think about what happened in her mind as "thinking." Actually, she didn't *think about it* at all. She blithely assumed that all people *saw* as she saw in her mind's eye.

Nonetheless, if asked, she might have said she had an active imagination. And it was this imagination that kept her hopeful that somehow she would find a better world than the one in which she lived.

Years later, she remembered that vision vividly—the vision that came to her at age twenty-three. That day, she saw herself as an old woman sitting on the edge of her bed, smiling and swinging her feet. Her old self was nearing the end of her life.

The young woman wondered what that older self would see when she looked back through her aged eyes at the life path she had traveled. Would she see that she had followed a practical, safe, acceptable route, one that others understood and applauded? Or would she see that she'd followed one that was made of the dreams in her heart and mind? Would she rather have risked failing to accomplish her dreams than not to have tried?

"Maybe," she pondered, "I'd better follow the route I've been told is the way go." But thinking this made her belly ache. Her throat tightened, and she wanted to cry.

As she looked directly at the old woman on the bed, she felt torn within herself. She did not have the courage in her twenties that would come to her later. But, as she viewed the old woman with the smile and the swinging feet, she somehow knew what she *had* to do. She really did not have a choice, not if she wanted to live pain-free in her gut and her heart. She had to honor her desires—and that frightened her. What if she made a mistake?

Actually, the groundwork for her choice had been laid earlier, by the time she was five years old. But at twenty-three, she'd forgotten about her childhood. Darkness and despair clouded her memory. She simply didn't recall until much later that the little girl also saw the truth about herself with clarity. In her imagination, the child *knew* that truth about herself. But she simply wasn't strong enough to maintain her connection to that belief.

Little Gwen had had a heart that was filled with joy. Within, she knew feelings of wonderfulness. Her mind pictures portrayed colorful swirls of Fantasia-like designs, flying animals and talking plants. Colors took on a life of their own in her spontaneous imagination, each speaking their tones of red, yellow, magenta, blue, green and purple. And all these shown in the warm sunlight of gold surrounded by billowy clouds against azure skies. Rainbows danced overhead and flowers and grasses bent in synchronized waves to the rhythm of gentle breezes.

Gwen reveled in the flight paths made by butterflies. She identified with the birds' calls. She spoke with the nature fairies of wind, fire, fog and rain.

And, best of all, Gwen knew, too, that she could make music with the birds, dance with the rainbows and paint the pictures in her mind using her color-rich palette. She believed that anyone viewing and hearing her productions would experience warmth in their hearts as she did.

But then something happened that threw a blanket of gray over the truth she understood at such a young age. To her surprise, others did not rejoice with her. They didn't seem to see what she saw. And they spoke a language that separated her from them.

In retrospect, she realized that was the time when she packed her dreams away for safekeeping. She didn't really mean to, but it happened. It began when she started school. She learned that there was a *right* way to do her work, draw her pictures and remember her lessons. She was supposed to sit upright and not move so that she could learn to read. She was expected to divide her work up into equal segments, doing one-fourth of her work on each of four days so that she would be done with her project on the fifth day. She discovered that others put more value on learning to call something by name than on being able to demonstrate its use or purpose.

Gwen learned that she was supposed to think about things in words rather than using the wonderful pictures in her mind. She even was taught there was *a right way* to design her pictures and that she must memorize a set of words to describe what she did naturally. Her stories no longer flowed as she tried to learn a framework for grammar and words. The flow and sounds of words were not enough. The grand ideas of her stories and writing were pressed into dry, windowless boxes that stripped them of their meaning. Her wonder-filled imagination was imprisoned, becoming emaciated and spiritless.

She did what she was told to do, abandoning *her way*. As she did, the grayness smothered her more and more, turning her world darker and darker.

Where was the path her curiosity wished to follow? She could no longer see it. She even forgot there was one.

If she hadn't been such a good little girl, well-liked by grown-ups, she would have asked, "Why can't I explore, learning while I ask a million, zillion questions?" Or she would have complained, garnering adult disapproval as she proclaimed, "It's not fair!" She might even have simply refused to do the work at all.

But, instead, she not only tried, she forced herself to work and work and work. Her childhood vanished and she became the model child. Adults liked her. The gray-turned-black cloud completely surrounded her, separating her from her True Self—the Self with which she was born; the Self that carried her talents and intelligence; the Self that the world sorely needed.

Gwen's story, though, isn't really a sad story. It's only one that took time to unfold. She had to reconnect with her True Path, the one from which she had become separated. She had to find the ways that were her ways to accomplish her goals. She had to grow out of her dependence on others for approval so that she could use the guidance system that was within her—one that had always been there. She had to realize that each person is unique, excluding the possibility that there is a right way to be or one right way to do anything. She had to learn there is only individuality.

Though guilt chased her and disappointment dogged her, she continually reached out to opportunities that came her way, opportunities that made her feelings quicken and her lips smile. To be sure, she also did what she was *supposed to do* for many years to come, but at the same time she made room to also follow her rainbows.

Over the years, unexpected surprises often came her way. These opportunities were ones that she had not imagined. They were not the predetermined, acceptable routes that many of her peers followed. Yet she seemed to recognize them as *right* for her when they presented themselves. They were often creative in nature—providing her with an opportunity to develop a new program, learn a new expressive skill or take what was old and reconstruct it into something new. They rarely followed the path most traveled.

When Gwen followed these unexpected opportunities, she often achieved at a much higher level than she did when she adopted the ways most accepted by others. The gray cloud dissipated. Her energy soared, and her happiness increased.

It wasn't until many years later that she connected her improved productivity and heartfelt joy with the way in which she undertook her goals. Eventually though, she could not deny that there was a direct connection between the way in which she accomplished her tasks and the quality of her life in general and her productions specifically. Part of her eventual empowerment came as she clearly recognized a basic law of her Universe. "Do what fits in a way that fits, and you will be successful and fulfilled."

By middle age, she'd taken control of her life—at least to the degree to which any human being can. And either her gray cloud was absent or she knew how to shed it when she inadvertently strayed from the path that innately belonged to her.

Now, as an elder, she sees clearly, understanding that her way is perfect for her as the way of others is perfect for them when they honor what fits them. And, indeed, the rainbows dance, the flowers sing, the fairies rejoice and her heart is full.

Gwen is not an unusual or outrageously gifted person. She is simply a *real* person—one who has strengths and weaknesses, talents and liabilities, dreams and fears. So why has her life worked out so well for her? Can others hope for similar outcomes? Of course!

When I first met Gwen, she was labeled with a diagnosis called *Attention Deficit Disorder*. She fought bouts of depression and had mood swings, was impulsive, reactive, and bounced around like a rubber ball. She didn't work up to her potential and had difficulty with follow-through. She wasn't able to keep track of details. She considered herself disorganized. She believed that she had a poor memory. And she often felt miserably inadequate, as if there was something innately wrong with her.

At first, when she obtained a diagnosis, she felt relieved. "Whew," she thought, "Now I know what's *wrong* with me."

Finally, she had a tangible reason for not having succeeded like other people. The identification of AD/HD explained why she'd always fallen short in school, unable to make the highest grades even though she worked hard and felt smart inside herself. The best schools hadn't admitted her and the best companies hadn't hired her. Yet, despite her experiences, she'd always felt very, very special.

She could never quite come to the conclusion that she was deluding herself. But she worried, "Maybe I'm not as special and good as I think I am."

No one else seemed to mirror her sense of herself. Few external awards or indicators validated her inner feeling of excellence. So, she tried even harder to modify her belief about herself. But she couldn't convince herself that she was not special or talented.

Torn between others' perceptions and her own inner self-vision, Gwen's feelings vacillated between the deep depression that is a part of grieving and the passionate joy of sensing the wonder within herself, her potential, as yet unrealized.

As we worked together, Gwen began to understand that she spent an enormous amount of time doing things that she didn't like and wasn't particularly good at. She thought she *should* be good at them. When she wasn't, she felt bad inside. "See, I'm really not adequate," she said over and over to herself.

The things that she did well, she figured, were of little count. They were so easy for her to do. Surely everyone could do them. Since she hadn't been acknowledged for her talents, she figured that anything she could do wasn't of much value.

What never occurred to Gwen was that many of the people who won awards and gained recognition were also doing what they did well. And they didn't even attempt to do the things that she did well. Mostly they didn't need to. For Gwen lives in a culture that doesn't see imagination, creativity, vision, or the ability to talk to the fairies and dance with the grasses as a part of valued achievement.

It turned out that one of her greatest talents was her sensitivity to read other people and situations; to know what others are thinking or are about to do. She could see within others and instantly knew what they needed or what was off-kilter physically or emotionally. But her ability to instantly read what others were feeling and respond with supportive input was rejected, because this was not considered the acceptable ways to attain insight into people and their problems. *Proof* had to be obtained through laborious attention to detail. The facts had to be presented in a stereotypical form with agreed-upon labels.

Unable to provide the kind of proof required, she discounted her skills, just as everyone else discounted them. When those in the mainstream couldn't see what Gwen saw, they failed to realize that it was their inability to access the information in the way Gwen did that created the problem. Those in the mainstream were unable to imagine that someone could instantly know another's thoughts, feelings and physical status, much less make accurate assessments. It was not that Gwen's way didn't work. It was just that they couldn't understand her way.

When I and a few others began to recognize Gwen's abilities, things began to change for Gwen. They began to see that

Gwen's intuitive assessments of others were correct. Gwen no longer felt alone on her quest for recognition once others validated her abilities. She realized she had been right about herself all along. Her self-belief blossomed and her power grew once the crack appeared in her fears about her skills. The resurrection of her childhood potential became only a matter of time.

Gwen's AD/HD *problems* turned out to be non-problems when she began to give herself permission to do things in ways that fit her. This meant, too, that she had to begin to seek goals that fit her, instead of seeking the goals that well-meaning others chose for her—the goals they labeled "sensible." She also had to pursue her goals in ways that worked for her, which often took her off the path most tread. She had to learn to listen to feelings rather than make decisions based on what someone else considered logical. She had to realize that her system of logic was simply different from the more commonly held style of logic.

One of the most difficult aspects of Gwen's escape from her gray cloud was to go beyond the diagnosis of AD/HD—the very diagnosis that initially came as a relief. She had to realize that there really wasn't anything innately wrong with her. There never had been. She was the victim of mismanagement. She was the victim of a misconception.

To be sure, when she, like millions of others, is expected to perform in ways that don't fit her, she becomes *functionally* disabled. Would you try to teach a fish to fly? Would you expect a cactus to grow in a swamp? There's nothing wrong with the fish or the cactus. They simply can't do something that is completely against their nature. And there was nothing wrong with Gwen, either.

Not only was Gwen initially cheated from having an opportunity to learn and perform in ways that fit her, she was further hurt by the very act of being forced to learn and perform in ways that did not fit. Rather like having one's feet bound because the culture believes that small feet are more beautiful, she was forced to learn in ways that didn't fit because the culture thinks there is a preferred was to be taught and tested. The result: crippled feet, crippled minds and crippled psyches.

For a time, Gwen wanted to hang onto her diagnosis. After all, the diagnosis meant she could get accommodations to help her accomplish some of her goals. All she had to do in order to be taught in a way that fit her needs was to say, "I am *handicapped.*"

She felt trapped.

She felt she needed this accommodation to be given the opportunity that would, in turn, grant her the power to do the job she was capable of doing. And she needed this power if she hoped to make changes in the way people's individuality was viewed in the future. But she also wanted to make changes to a system that sees one type of brain construction as superior to another. If she did not give in to the *pathologizing* of her particular way of working, she would be kept from doing the very things she had the skills and ability to do.

As she grew in strength and self-belief, the more and more she disliked having to be called names in order to be given opportunities. It reminded her of what it would be like for women to have to concede to being disordered in order to be given the opportunity to do a job that had previously been the domain of men. It smacked of the belief that people of color were truly less adequate than whites and, therefore need extra help. She felt this kind of thinking was humiliating.

Gwen finally became free when she found what fit her and sought ways to accomplish her goals—ways that were often creative in nature—so that she did not have to choose between being denied opportunities or saying she was *disabled.* She finally reconnected with the part of her self that saw herself as perfectly adequate, perfectly acceptable and most definitely not damaged.

Eventually, she came to truly believe in herself. She found the paths that surely led to the best outcomes—outcomes that reflected her potential.

With success in hand, she no longer saw herself as disabled. Sure, she has what is called an AD/HD-style of brain construction. That's why she is as good as she is at what she does well. And the world is a better place because of the way in which she is constructed. She offers what others with differing brainstyles cannot offer. And she has found that by teaming with others in an environment of mutual respect, everyone's style becomes valuable. Jobs get done in a way that accomplishes more than any one person can hope to achieve alone.

Gwen no longer worries about making mistakes as she did when she was young. She has come to realize that, because of her brainstyle, she learns from every step she takes. If one step feels off-track for her, she quickly recognizes it and adjusts her reactions. Then she reconnects to her goal path; often using the very experience that might be called an error. The out-of-line step ultimately enriches the journey as well as the end product.

She now knows that honoring the desires of her heart *is* the means by which she uses the skills of her internal guidance system. When she does this, she achieves success in whatever she seeks. As she honors *her* way, she cannot but be who she was always intended to be, her own unique person.

Gwen is a beautiful woman, as all women are, as all people are. Gwen's AD/HD is her greatest gift. It is so because she has come to believe it is so. Now, no one can tell her differently. That's why she is a success. For what she believes about herself is what is so. As she believes, so she creates.

CHAPTER 13

Understanding for Women with AD/HD

Gayle Voigt

Having AD/HD in a non-AD/HD world is not always easy—akin to being a saltwater fish trying to survive in a freshwater tank. No matter where we live, work, or play, we are constantly surrounded by people with little experience of AD/HD, whose perceptions of us are often grounded in misunderstanding. The greatest challenge for me as a woman with AD/HD is to convey to the important people in my life—parents, siblings, teachers, spouses, coworkers, and friends—the challenges, strengths, weaknesses, and needs inherent in having AD/HD. As their understanding grows, my navigation through life is greatly enhanced.

I sometimes wonder how different my life might have been if I'd known as a child that I had AD/HD. Would my teachers and parents have provided extra support and helped me with organization and planning? Would I have set goals and pursued a higher education? What if I'd known I had AD/HD before I got married? Perhaps my husband would have turned and run for his life before pledging his love and devotion to the impulsive, fun-loving, unambitious young woman I was. On the other hand, maybe it would have been me who shied away from lifelong commitment to a man who had no need to complicate his life with danger, adventure, and risk. Needless to say, my AD/HD has created some unique challenges, both in marriage and in life.

In contrast to me, my husband's course was always stable, well-planned, and goal-oriented. He knew what he wanted in every arena of life, and when I arrived on the scene, he had little trouble fitting me into the picture. Eager-to-please, yet confused and insecure, I looked for someone to tell me who I was, and what I should be, a role my husband-to-be assumed with little delay.

Once I had received my assignment, I set about to accomplish it. I was to be a wife, and, in due course, a mother. I was determined to be the very best of both. First came the wedding, next came family four children in all—while my husband pursued his educational and professional goals, progressing through his stages like clockwork. But, despite appearances, all was not well for me, though I didn't dare admit it. Deep down, there was an awareness of problems that I never allowed to rise to the surface.

The years were busy ones, raising the children, meeting the constant needs of a family—housekeeping, entertaining, educating, managing (sort of)—spending all of my energy to keep up the act. All the while, I longed to quit, to take off the mask and get down off the stage, but it seemed too much was at stake. I was still unaware of my AD/HD and its forces at work in my life. Inside, I secretly carried a tremendous guilt for the resentment I felt toward my husband and children. Outwardly, I looked like the perfect wife and mother, yet I knew I was a fraud—an imposter who would be discovered sooner or later. I worried constantly about keeping up the act, and often wondered whether any other woman had ever attempted such a feat.

In proportion to the inner unhappiness that plagued me was a need for external commotion to keep me stimulated, distracted, and outwardly focused. Fortunately, this was abundantly available in our house, as I had bestowed my AD/HD genes on all four of our children. By the time I learned about AD/HD and received my diagnosis, I felt like a bird in a cage, the circumstances of my life crisscrossing around me, holding me captive. There I was, already a housewife and mother of four, as the realization hit that these are two of the most AD/HD-unfriendly jobs a woman could have.

If I'd thought I'd been busy and stressed before, the post-diagnosis years proved even more challenging. The children were, by then, in school. With all the organization and scheduling necessary to run an active family, I was barely keeping my head above water. But at least, after my diagnosis, "the act" was over. I was no longer pretending to be superwoman, and began giving myself permission to be less than perfect, particularly in those jobs that drew heavily on my weaknesses, such as housework. Indeed, I could not have kept up the act if I'd tried. It was simply too draining, both emotionally and physically.

Having children with AD/HD presented more challenges than I would have liked, but I think my biggest stressor was a gnawing sense of underachievement, and lack of personal fulfillment. Don't misunderstand me. I would not have missed the joy of sharing my life with someone, nor of being a mother, even if I'd known earlier all that I know now. What *would* be different is that I would have believed in myself and my abilities. I would have set goals and pursued an education, delaying marriage and family until I'd established an identity and felt satisfied within myself. Instead, my need to appear normal and to hide my disability was an all-consuming force that had driven my early choices.

As AD/HD becomes more readily identified in women, I hope that more girls will be appropriately diagnosed before reaching young adulthood. This is the time in life that a woman makes momentous decisions that impact her future, even the rest of her life—setting goals, pursuing educational tracks or vocational training, and choosing life partners. This latter task involves more than simply falling in love if the union is to survive the lumps and bumps inherent in all marriages, but particularly those of AD/HD stock. I'm certain my marriage would have been less rocky had my husband and I known about and understood my AD/HD. Throughout my life, I have often found myself wishing . . .

I Wish They Understood My Need for Change

While others can get comfortable in ruts, I long for the stimulation of changing routines, variable surroundings, different activities, and flexible schedules. I love spontaneity—to be truly in touch with life and be responsive to the various faces and moods it presents. Detours are always welcome on the path of routine, and I never know what new or exciting possibilities I might encounter to expand my horizons.

Take this summer, for example. I decided not to register for summer classes as I have done in previous years. As May merged into June, I sensed a nagging fear that being home all summer would bore me to death. However, I needn't have feared. On an impulse, I packed myself and my son off to a family camp for five days and had loads of fun. Then, no sooner had I arrived home than I learned of a seminar in California of interest to me, and set about making reservations. Finding no vacancies at the local hotels, I packed my tent and spent five more wonderful days camping while attending the seminar. This experience opened other doors of opportunity to me.

A week later, I was jetting back to northern California to volunteer at a life-style center for ten days. Enriched by the experience, my AD/HD brain began overflowing with ideas. The rest of the summer was spent planning and implementing seminars in my hometown, interspersed with family events and vacation. So, what might have been an uneventful summer turned into one of the most memorable of my life, but only because my AD/HD antennae were continually scanning for interesting possibilities. Of course, when college begins in the fall, my spontaneity will be somewhat curtailed, but I'll always make room for the unexpected, and have need for the unplanned happenings that crop up in daily life.

My husband frequently laments my spontaneity, labeling it "lack of planning." He doesn't seem to understand that, for me, my unplanned spontaneity is not a problem to be solved, but the expression of a need. It's part of having AD/HD, and cannot be adequately explained outside that context. I realize the abrupt changes that steer my course through life also affect those around me, and I try to appreciate the hardships others might encounter because of it. There are many sidetracks that I choose not to follow—regardless of their pull and attraction for me—simply because it would be irresponsible and selfish to do so.

I Wish They Understood My Need for Excitement and Stimulation

Without stimulation, provided by the unknown or by risk, the consequences for me would likely be inactivity, depression, and poor self-image. My need for stimulation is probably the most crucial aspect of AD/HD that needs to be understood by those around me. If they understood my need for stimulation, they would support and encourage my search instead of thwarting my efforts to find stimulating activities.

Chaos serves my need for stimulation. A frenzied search for some misplaced document, the crazy schedule I set, the ambitious goals I scramble to meet—keep me feeling alive, although these patterns may leave an onlooker reeling. It is important that those around me realize that the alternative to chaos is likely to be depression and paralysis.

It's as if I've been born with a stimulation thermostat that's set rather high. Whenever it drops below the mark, I descend into depression and listlessness unless I find something to trigger a new surge of energy. I approach life with intensity, and find myself drawn to "the edge." This is the place that affords me the best view of life. It is the line between safety and danger—success and failure. Why would anyone wish to court failure? Perhaps it's because of the excitement that comes from taking risks. My risk-taking sometimes assumes the form of overloading myself, committing to too many tasks. The more I have to do, the more stimulating my pursuit of accomplishment. But it's not only the stimulation of activity that motivates me, it's also the danger of failing.

My procrastination is prompted by the stimulation I feel when I risk failure. Many people procrastinate for as many different reasons, but I find myself deliberately doing so until the pressure becomes so great that it stimulates me to get a job done. If I give myself plenty of time for a project, I work inefficiently, and succumb easily to distractions. But when the pressure is on, the stimulation can be tremendous, depending, of course, on how important I perceive the job to be.

Stimulation comes in many forms—danger, procrastination, change, or exhilaration—providing the current that keeps my life humming. Exhilaration is often pursued by those with AD/HD through sports or recreational endeavors, such as skydiving, windsurfing, mountain-biking, scuba-diving, or other activities that divert attention from the mundane and ordinary. Pursuing such activities, however, can be difficult to justify. Others see it as just "having fun," something to be reserved as an occasional reward for hard work. For me, this kind of stimulation is an intense need. If relationships are to be nurtured and strengthened, it is essential that my family and friends understand. When I can access stimulation from sports or recreation, there is a greatly decreased chance that I will seek more stress-producing or self-destructive avenues for meeting those needs.

Unfortunately, many women are trapped in jobs and life situations that offer little stimulation. Under such circumstances, it doesn't take long for their spark to be extinguished. Risk-taking and novelty-seeking are integral characteristics of AD/HD for those at the more hyperactive end of the AD/HD continuum. It is this stimulation-seeking phenomenon that makes the job of emergency medical technician, fire fighter, law enforcement officer, pilot, or navy diver so attractive to men with AD/HD. Women with hyperactive traits have these same needs, although they have less opportunity to have a career that meets them. I run best on adrenalin, not on invariant routine. While structure and routine can help keep me functional, there must be an outlet for stimulation if I am to function at my best. Instead of becoming frustrated with my need for stimulation, I wish those around me understood this as a basic need, related to my AD/HD.

I Wish They Understood My Need for Time Alone

Although my approach to life is intense, I also need time alone. While I seek the stimulation of "the edge," I expend a lot of nervous energy there, and need to back off and recharge. These cycles of energy and rest are such an integral part of my AD/HD, yet so often I find myself working against these natural "tides"—trying to fit myself into the non-AD/HD mold that others would like to fashion for me. Instead of operating according to my natural cycles, I find myself running in circles to maintain my home and family in a manner expected by those around me.

I Wish They Understood My Need for Down-time

My hectic, often chaotic life-style leaves little room for rest. I begin my day with high energy, thinking about all the possibilities I can pack into it; however, I have learned that my energy has definite limits. When I reach that limit, I need rest. What seems so hard for my family to understand is that I benefit most when this time is spent alone. Being an "at-home" mom, especially when my children were young, made it difficult for me to find time for myself. I wish I had had the understanding and help of a close friend or relative to give me some time alone.

For a woman whose work is never done, considerable guilt can be generated by time spent doing nothing. I have to continually remind myself, as well as my family, that rest is as important as work, and necessary for maintaining balance in my life. Frequently, my rest time is sabotaged through misunderstanding or ignorance of my needs. To have my family's approval to take time out for myself is important, and their cooperation is appreciated immensely.

I Wish They Understood My Organizational Deficits

Organization is not a strength for a woman with AD/HD. I wish others could understand the many ways that my disorganization impacts me. Being disorganized is not my choice. It seems I was born with the need for a personal organizer by my side throughout life. I have spent tremendous resources on systems and gadgets to aid with organization, only to find I lack the momentum to make them work long enough to get relief. Making lists, for instance, seems a logical way to compensate for disorganization, but reading the list items at the critical time, or even having the list with me when I need it is not so easy. I write on my hand; I tie pens and note pads in strategic places; I set timers; I buy filing systems, wall pockets, shelves, and organizers; I wear aprons with massive front pockets; but all to little avail. I still forget to put out the recycling, to pick up the dry-cleaning, to pay the phone bill, or to fill the gas tank.

Years ago, as a young woman, I felt driven in pursuit of a husband who possessed organizational abilities to compensate for my own deficits. Without understanding why, I chose a man based on his abilities to balance the checkbook, pay bills on time, file taxes, keep track of appointments, maintain appliances in working order, and generally keep my life functional. While this seemed a worthy goal, it was unrealistic to expect all my problems with planning and organization to be solved in this way. The reality was that my husband and I assumed different and separate roles, and while his life was organized, I was left scrambling to manage in my own realm.

Because my husband valued organization, he became increasingly frustrated with my disorganized style. This had the potential to create personal and marital stress. There had to be honest dialogue in order to understand how to constructively create an AD/HD-friendly environment. When those around me are accepting of my poor planning and time-management skills, a burden is lifted from my shoulders, as I continue to manage my daily life as best I can.

Nothing ever happens on time in my house; in fact, time is an abstraction I've never been able to master. I constantly marvel at how time just disappears, leaving me to continually play "catchup." I am often plagued by the futile wish that time would stand still long enough for me to "get a grip." Every new day seems to start while I'm still entrenched somewhere in the previous one—scrambling to complete yesterday's work.

It's not always fun living in the disorganized world of AD/HD. I need the support of family and friends who understand that I can't simply "snap out of it" and organize my life. Possessing internal organizational deficits, I rely heavily on external assistance from those around me. Time management is an ongoing challenge for me, and a great deal of frustration is generated by my well-intentioned, yet clumsy attempts to develop skills in this area.

I Wish They Understood the Difficulties
I Face in the Home

It's easy for me to envy women who have jobs outside the home, although in reality, these women usually carry a double load. Even in this enlightened age of women's rights, women still carry the major share of work inside the home. This presents a problem for those of us who struggle with tasks that require organization, planning, and consistency. Few could argue that housekeeping presents one of the greatest challenges to women with AD/HD, yet keeping a well-ordered home is still commonly held as the measure of a woman's worth. Certainly our self-esteem is tied, no matter how loosely, to our success or failure in the home.

Understanding the core symptoms of AD/HD reveals clues as to why some women might not be well-suited to domestic responsibilities. Disorganization, stimulation-seeking, intolerance of tedium, and distractibility place the AD/HD woman at a distinct disadvantage when undertaking her work in the home. Within this environment, distractibility is tremendous. Unable to filter out surrounding stimuli and focus on one task at a time, I'm left running in circles, accomplishing very little of what I set out to do. Housework is definitely not my forte!

There is something banal and tedious in doing a job that must be done over and over again. I can't achieve satisfaction from running on the treadmill of housekeeping, and there are too many chances for distraction in the course of such work. The highly repetitive nature of the job, as well as its limited opportunities for creativity, makes housework difficult to start, much less to complete in an efficient manner. Most domestic duties require a certain degree of organization and systematic action, making the methodical nature of the work under-stimulating, and quite outside the comfort zone of women with AD/HD.

Neither is housework suited to my stimulation-seeking tendencies and my intolerance of boredom. It can feel downright imprisoning to be working every day in a task that goes against one's natural abilities and strengths. Few women with AD/HD achieve success as a homemaker without paying a high price, feeling significant stress and accomplishing little, a surefire recipe for demoralization.

I Wish Others Understood My Search for Personal Fulfillment

For many years prior to my AD/HD diagnosis, I had become well-entrenched in a pattern of behavior, striving to attain an image that I believed was expected or desired of me. While my outward presentation approached the prescribed ideal, I felt little personal fulfillment. Not understanding that I was affected by AD/HD, I had little faith in my own abilities. My low self-esteem led me to seek the approval of others—conforming to what my family, my husband, and society in general expected of me.

With the enlightenment that came from my diagnosis of AD/HD, it became painfully obvious to me what had been wrong throughout my life. The personal liberation I felt after diagnosis was dampened by grieving over lost opportunities, and limited by others who expected me to maintain the image of the perfect housewife and mother that I had worked so hard to attain. Once I understood what I had struggled against all my life, what I wanted most was the freedom to be myself—the person I am, not the one I had tried to become. It seems a small thing to ask, to be oneself. But I felt denied this possibility. Family and friends expected the "old" me and couldn't understand the "new" me that was struggling to emerge.

Before my diagnosis of AD/HD, I lacked the insight to make the best choices for myself. My belief in my own abilities took a beating over the years as I struggled to maintain outward appearances, gallantly trying to hide my frustrations, fears, and failures. After the diagnosis, once I realized there was a name for my discomfort, my initial relief could hardly be contained. I felt renewed and energized as I began to emerge from the constraints that had bound me for so long. But I found myself on slippery ground as social and psychological forces of past, present, and future converged upon me. I wanted those close to me to understand and celebrate this new journey, as I sought to reclaim my self-esteem, and to establish myself on solid ground.

In my quest for personal discovery, I have had to learn to avoid my weaknesses and build on my strengths. Becoming educated in self-knowledge involved examining my history in order to know my own heart, and holding true to my convictions throughout the enlightenment process. But metamorphosis does not occur in a vacuum. To embrace my AD/HD and value myself as a unique woman, I must transform self-expectations and self-perceptions, as well as receive a corresponding response from others. I sometimes daydream about how great it would be if I could suddenly be transported to a different place, surrounded by different people, where I could make a fresh start. I would wear my AD/HD badge proudly, and just be myself. I would build my life with people who liked me the way I am, and would seek work that enhanced my creativity and productivity.

It's not so easy to make changes within a long established environment. An AD/HD diagnosis is like being handed the keys to unlock your cage. To establish a new life of freedom means not only change from within, but also that others must relate to and interact with you differently. For instance, once I understood myself in the light of AD/HD, I was no longer willing to strive to maintain near perfection in housekeeping to the exclusion of everything else. I wanted to have time to explore my talents and discover my skills. Yet, as my housekeeping standards deteriorated, I found subtle forces working against me to push me back into conformity, back into my old patterns. Of course, an easy solution to the housekeeping problem was available in the form of a maid service, but it was not as easy to solve the problem of entrenched expectations, and unyielding attitudes of others. I perceived attitudes of condemnation when my actions deviated from previously proscribed patterns. Personal fulfillment remained an elusive hope without the willingness of others to be flexible and supportive in relation to my personal growth.

I Wish Others Could Accept Me, Replete with Ups and Downs

It is rarely possible to have AD/HD and not experience the highs and lows that often accompany it. It is a law of nature that the higher one bounces the further one has to fall. The need for stimulation may lead a woman to take risks and encroach on extremes, but her thrill is often short-lived, followed by a period of dejection, depression, or despair. This pattern repeats itself ad infinitum, and in all probability serves as an auto-stimulation mechanism to keep her existence from becoming boring.

I find that when an activity is captivating I put my whole heart and soul into it. Inevitably, when nothing seems enticing, I hit bottom. It is a constant challenge to keep an even keel. When I embark on an assignment that interests me I can produce my very best; however, the prospect of facing jobs such as housework or paperwork sets my emotional barometer plunging, where it remains until some captivating new activity presents itself.

The impulsive nature of some women with AD/HD plays a factor in the ups and downs of our lives. We're stuck on a roller-coaster ride. While we seek the fun and stimulation of the ride, we often find ourselves trapped and unable to get off when we need to rest. Many times I throw myself enthusiastically into some impulsive venture, then plunge from the heights as I find myself unable to muster sustained attention once the novelty wears off.

When this happens my self-esteem takes a beating as I face up to my failures over and over again. It seems I don't easily learn from experience.

Impulses can be the spark that ignites action in the woman with AD/HD, since impulsive actions are often laced with risk and excitement. If I could take the time to think through each situation before acting on impulse, I would often feel no interest in pursuing the course. But then my life would become rather flat, devoid of the spark I rely on to motivate me. Because I am highly critical of myself when impulse leads me into trouble, facing the criticism of others is both unnecessary and embarrassing. Having someone to laugh with me at my mistakes instead of lecturing me on my faults would be a great relief.

Another factor in my roller coaster ride is my tendency to overload myself with commitments. Whether it's difficulty saying no, miscalculating my time, misjudging my ability, or just seeking activity to focus me, I find my typical day is just too full. In high moments, I feel energetic, capable, and optimistic of accomplishing much, but I forget that as energy runs low, productivity rapidly follows suit. Having a day that is too full of commitments and activities also subtracts from my sleep, making me tired and inefficient, and prompting me to feel down. It is only natural to feel let down when goals aren't accomplished and plans fail. It all relates back to deficits in organization and planning. Over time, I am gradually learning ways to regulate my ups and downs, but only to the extent that stimulation is not completely extinguished.

I Wish Others Understood How Much I Need Encouragement and Support

Life can be unkind to those of us who are inherently distractible, impulsive, disorganized, perhaps dyslexic, and often forgetful. It seems that just getting through each day is hard work, and the exhaustion felt at the end of it seems hardly justified by the little that was accomplished. The encouragement of others, whether family, friends, or co-workers, is of inestimable worth, helping me to navigate the rocky path of AD/HD.

I frequently forget appointments, miss deadlines, lose keys and other necessary items, and the lament often escapes my lips, "I'd lose my own head if it wasn't screwed on!" While it is possible to learn compensations to overcome the difficulties caused by memory impairment, it can still be a source of negative messages that erode a woman's sense of self worth. "I'm such a klutz," or "I can't believe I forgot that again," or "No wonder I can't get a decent job," becomes the subconscious self-talk that women begin to believe about themselves. Often being late leads to feelings of incompetence, or simply exasperation. When others recognize the source of our difficulties, they are more likely to lend support and encouragement, than if they are ignorant of AD/HD. Hearing positive messages from those around me could help me laugh at the mistakes and believe in myself.

Not only does time pose a challenge to women with AD/HD, often direction does too. I remember writing in bold letters the words "left" and "right" on my respective gym shoes in high school. While this was considered a joke among my peers, I now feel safe to admit that it was a necessary strategy to overcome confusion whenever someone referred to these directions. Reading maps and reversing directions also pose significant difficulties for me. I find myself twisting maps sideways and upside-down to match the road I'm traveling on. I regularly get lost and sometimes don't even attempt some activities in order to avoid the effects of this deficit. Perhaps it's tied to my dyslexia, but I also have difficulty reversing directions, so that I might find my way to some place, but am at a loss to get home again. I remember pulling over to the side of the road to consult a map years ago, and hearing my three-year-old son in the back seat utter with total exasperation, "Are you lost again, Mom?" It is easy for others to denigrate and criticize a woman for these traits, yet sensitivity and understanding would prove a far more compassionate approach.

I Wish Others Could Know How Grateful I Am for Their Love

I've not been a perfect mother—I guess no one ever is. It has not been easy raising four children, all having AD/IID. For a long time, I was plagued by the guilt that my children's greatest disability was having a mother with AD/HD. Without organizational abilities of their own, they looked to me to set structure, routine, consistency, and follow-through, and I felt a great burden since I lacked these skills. Not only that, but children who have AD/HD are at risk for all kinds of dysfunctional responses to life, including depression, anxiety, school failure, substance abuse, risk-taking, criminal behavior, and suicide. And we had our share of trouble. At times I felt ready to despair, but I kept fighting—for it often seemed life was a battle—and eventually the rewards began to pay off.

However, I could not have survived effectively without the understanding and support of others. The AD/HD support group, CHADD, has been an invaluable source of information and encouragement, and I feel that the friends I made there are more like family than friends. CHADD is the only place where I can "tell it like it is," a place where I know I am fully understood.

While my husband and extended family have had difficulty understanding my AD/HD, nevertheless, their efforts to provide support have been greatly appreciated. I write this at a friend's beach house. While I'm sitting here feeling overwhelmed at the thought of packing and cleaning before we leave today, my husband is mobilizing the children and giving instructions for the job to be carried out in a systematic and efficient manner. He seems to know when I need him to step in and take charge, and for this I am grateful. My friends show that they're true friends by loving me in spite of my deficiencies and failures. They may not understand the struggles I encounter in daily life, but they're always there for me, ready to lend their help and support in any way they can. And finally, I've accessed strength through spiritual growth, and can truly say with the Psalmist of the Bible, "God is my refuge and strength, a very present help in trouble . . ."

After such a long discussion of my struggles, I would be remiss not to mention that certain strengths accompany AD/HD as well. Creativity abounds among those with AD/HD, and it even seems that organizational deficits are conducive to creativity. Women with AD/HD are adept at discovering new ways of doing things, recognizing the obscure, inventing new methods. As we come to understand ourselves better, as more women experience the same "enlightenment" that my diagnosis brought about, and as more people come to understand us, perhaps we can begin to focus on and celebrate those qualities that bring us joy and sustenance.

Above all else, I'd like to be valued—not just in spite of my AD/HD—but because of it. I want my family and friends to celebrate with me the unique gifts I possess, to share my tears and my joys, and to love me for who I am—not for what they think I should be. With understanding comes infinite possibility . . .

Deprogramming
Women with AD/HD

Thom Hartmann

Modern women with AD/HD face many of the challenges confronted by men with AD/HD, but to all these they have two added layers of difficulty. Subtle, yet pervasive and powerful, these two layers are composed of *cultural barriers* and *cultural programming/expectations*. These work together to wound women—particularly those who were born as neurological Hunters instead of Martha Stewart Farmers—and frustrate their attempts to find success and emotional balance.

Cultural Barriers

Franklin Delano Roosevelt pointed out that "those who forget history are doomed to repeat it." Yet, most modern men and women never learned in our schools the cultural history of the role of women. Lest we repeat that history (there are those who are strongly suggesting we should), it's healing to quickly review it.

While we find equality between women and men in most indigenous cultures (their *roles* may be very different, but their relative *power* within the family and community is in balance), this has very much not been the case since the eruption of our modern civilization in Sumeria around 7,000 years ago. Even though logic would indicate that a creator of new life would have a womb, monotheism brought with it the notion that if there was to be only one god, this god must have a penis. According to his priests and scribes, this male god explicitly directed the quarantine or slaughter of all peoples who worshipped goddesses, a process that continues to this day in much of the world.

The men of these early agricultural and pastoral Younger Cultures vilified women as the source of first sin, banned worship in the natural world, and listed only males (with very few exceptions) in their historical and religious literature. They produced histories, myths, and fables that taught women their (inferior) role, and instituted laws (often punishable by death) insuring that their new view of women was adopted. They tortured and murdered millions of women in Europe over several centuries as they brutally crushed all traces of Europe's Older Culture's natured-based, female-centered religions, medicine, and rituals— and continue to do so in much of the world today. Midwifery and herbology were renamed witchcraft, women who respected and interacted with nature were called consorts of a devil, and girls were officially banned from formal education. The echoes of this cultural departure from millennia of matriarchy or cooperative Older Culture were again heard in the opinions and beliefs of the male-dominated European psychology profession as it was birthed in 1690 by England's John Locke ("An Essay Concerning Human Understanding") and Germany's Christian Thomasius in 1692 ("Further Elucidation by Different Examples of the Recent Proposals for a New Science for Discerning the Nature of Other Men's Mind").

When Paul created the Pauline Church to compete with (and eventually replace) Peter's Jerusalem Church, he told his church in Ephesus that wives must submit to the authority of their husbands. This single phrase was enshrined in British law about a thousand years ago, and became a cornerstone of American colonial law in the 1700s.

Among the earliest laws passed by the Colonies were those putting power over women into the hands of men. A married woman was not allowed to make out a will, because she was not allowed to own land or legally control anything else worthy of willing to another person. Any property she brought into the marriage became her husband's at the moment of marriage, and would only revert to her if he died and she did not remarry. But even then, she'd only get one-third of her husband's property, and what third that was and how she could use it were determined by a court-appointed male executor, who would supervise for the rest of her life (or until she remarried) how she used the third of her husband's estate she "inherited." When a widow died, the executor would either take the property for himself or else decide to whom it would pass. The woman had no say in the matter because she had no right to sign a will. Women could not sue in a court of law, except by the weak procedures allowed to the mentally ill and children, supervised by men. If the man of a family household died, the executor would decide who would raise the wife's children, and in what religion. She had no right to make those decisions and no say in such matters. If the woman was poor, it was a virtual certainty that her children would be taken from her. It was impossible in the new United States of America for a married woman to have legal responsibility for her children, control of her own property, own slaves, buy or sell land, or even obtain an ordinary license.

While women got the right to own property in the mid-1800s, to vote in 1920, and laws against discrimination were passed in 1962 and 1964, it was only in 1973 that the U.S. Supreme Court (in *Roe v. Wade*) overturned the 1873 *Bradwell v. State* Supreme Court decision that "the Law of the Creator" defined the "paramount destiny and mission" of women as limited to "the noble and benign offices of wife and mother."

Today, in this 21st century, we still live in a world where "women's work" is very much a defined reality. Nurses, waitresses, teachers, secretaries, child-care workers, and maids—-from hospitals to hotels to big business to our nation's schools, the patriarchal idea of women's roles is still very much with us. The archetypal spectrum runs from deified to cursed, from Madonna to prostitute, but at almost every level the role is still very much one subordinate to and in service of men. And the nature and quality of a woman's service to men demands, in almost all cases, a very non-AD/HD type of focus.

"You've come a long way, baby," and other slogans of our time promulgate the myth that men and women are operating on a level playing field. It's a useful myth for those who want to keep their secretaries and avoid further rebellion by women, and it's a particularly useful archetype for corporate marketers who want to put their hooks deep into women's psyches, but it's false. (While this may come as a revelation to some men, I imagine most women reading this are well aware of this fact.)

Born in 1951, I spent a bit more than the first decade of my life in an America where women and minorities were routinely and legally oppressed. It shaped my world view, as well as that of my contemporaries of both genders. None of us escaped unaffected; and neither have our children. The consequence of the reality that women have only recently achieved the legal protections and prerogatives that men have enjoyed for 6,000 years is substantial and far-reaching, and we see it clearly on at least three different levels.

First, many women say that they experience a deep sense of disempowerment in modern culture. Louise Hartmann tells the story of how, when she ran an advertising agency in Atlanta in the 1990s, men would often call her "Honey" or "Sweetie" and use an adult-talking-to-child tonality to establish who was in charge of the discussion. "I learned to ignore it," she said, "because, if I confronted it, I'd become a 'bitch.' When men have power, they're called alpha dogs or leaders; when women take power they're called bitches." In April, 2001, I was in a meeting with author and social activist Marianne Williamson when word came that the Supreme Court had just ruled that police could arrest, strip search, and imprison people for "crimes" for which there were no jail penalties (such as jaywalking, littering, or not wearing seatbelts). Commenting that the ruling effectively eviscerated the Fourth Amendment's protections against unreasonable search and seizure, Marianne said, "Now white men can get a taste of what black people and women have been experiencing for centuries in this country."

Second, many women share a sense of "outsiderness" that comes from a long lineage of exclusion, control, and domination by men. While for some this also creates a sense of solidarity (witness women's groups and the various feminist movements), it's the solidarity of the oppressed. Women, who are and always have been an absolute majority in our culture, are still treated as a minority by both the males in charge and, to a large extent, by themselves.

Third, when women come into contact with the largely male-dominated medical, educational, and pharmaceutical industries, they are often treated with condescension, categorization, or— even worse—invisibility. Being patted on the head and told to go home and take your pills is bad enough; being told that you "just have a female problem" or that you're a "ditsy blonde" is wounding.

Compounding this for women with AD/HD is the fact (in my humble opinion) that what they're expressing in either their acting-out or their daydreaming is a fundamental and visceral human need to experience their own aliveness. Just as for men, when women are confined in highly structured schools or Farmer-type workplaces, their need for aliveness is unmet. Men, however, are encouraged to meet this need by reaching out and interacting with the world around them; women are told to sit down, shut up, and "be a lady." If aliveness can't be found in the physical world, people will find it in their internal world—we call this "inattentive AD/HD."

Cultural Programming/Expectations

To a large extent, the special wounding of women with AD/HD begins in school. In the first three decades of the twentieth century, European and American public education went through a startling change. Legislators and educators looked at the systems of the industrial revolution, at the wild success of Henry Ford and others using assembly-line techniques, and said to themselves, "We should make our schools more efficient, too!" In addition, there was pressure on educators to produce more students who were "factory-ready," pre-trained to handle boring, repetitive tasks. Factories produced a standardized product, and needed a standardized sort of laborer; thus, education should become standardized to turn out these "industry-ready" workers. (Of course, for the upper class children who would become the rulers of the next generation, a separate school system was already in place. It was called private school or prep school, and operates as such to this day.)

The task of producing standardized worker-citizens was first defined in 1909 by president Woodrow Wilson, who said: "Let us go back and distinguish between the two things that we want to do [in our schools]; for we want to do two things in modern society. We want one class of persons to have a liberal education, and we want another class of persons, a very much larger class, of necessity, in every society, to forego the privileges of a liberal education and fit themselves to perform specific difficult manual tasks. You cannot train them for both in the time that you have at your disposal."

During the 1920s—an extraordinary period of change in American and European education—our schools were transformed from places of mentorship, tutelage, and participation into "education factories" where a standardized child was put on a multi-year conveyor belt and moved along the assembly line of the school through standardized grades so she could graduate as a standardized citizen and worker. It all worked quite neatly and elegantly, producing an explosion in the number of children who were thus "educated."

But when designing this assembly-line educational system, nobody considered what to do with the neurologically non-standard child. As a result, such children were given punishment, humiliation, segregation, and labeling.

Children who could learn very well in other settings —who had successfully learned to walk, speak an entire language, and interact with others in just the first few years of their lives—were now told they were slowing down the system, gumming up the works, that they must be "learning disabled." With this simple phrase, which came into vogue in the 1970s, responsibility for success in education was neatly and elegantly lifted from the shoulders of college trained adults (teachers) and placed squarely onto the backs and shoulders of seven- and ten-year-olds. *They* are the problem, this label says: *they* have the defect; *they* came to school with a non-standardized brain. The proof was that there is an abundance of children who were standard at entry, perfectly capable of moving through the school-factories, scoring well on standardized tests and graduating as standardized people. If they could do it, then those who couldn't must be the problem, not the system itself. The message the non-standard children hear is, "Why can't you be like the rest of them? Just try harder!"

Some, of course, would succeed. They'd figure out ways around and through the system, or even use internal brute-force techniques or drugs to retrain their own body's and brain's wiring to function similar to the standardized way, "just like the others." Others, however, would bear the scars of their failure for their entire lives. The wounded ones adopted their teacher's story that they, the children, are the ones with the deficit or disorder, the broken brains or dysfunctional abilities. They lived out this story, generalizing it in their lives. It became their secret excuse and public explanation, their self-story and identity. The teacher said it, it must be true: I'm not as good as the others. Even if it was never said out loud, they know they didn't do as well as others seem to. They become "impaired." And their impairment becomes the centerpiece of their lives. They raise their hands as if in an AA meeting and say, "I'm Susan, and I have AD/HD."

Add to the school wounding done to neurologically non-standard girls the expectations of our culture (that started long before women were allowed to attend school) that women were created to serve men and can only find their fulfillment in that role, and you cut right to the bone.

I remember well the shock I experienced the first time I read the story of Cinderella to one of our daughters; I later told my wife, Louise, that I felt like I'd just participated in a cultural experiment or brainwashing session.

Cinderella was the good girl and the pretty young woman. She was compliant, uncomplaining, hard-working (as a maid!) in the service of authority, and spent a lot of time in a dream world. Her stepsisters were women who knew what they wanted and were on a mission to get it. Thus, they were characterized as ugly and undesirable. The object of all this competition was the appropriate and inevitable goal of every woman, according to the Cinderella story, a man to submit herself to. But not just any man—this was a man of wealth and power, which allowed everybody to overlook the fact that he was so self-obsessed that after dancing with Cinderella for several hours, he still couldn't remember what her face looked like.

The messages of the story are frighteningly clear, and to find out if they've been picked up by the females of our culture, just spend ten minutes in a shopping mall and watch the teenage girls as they primp and preen and compete for the attention of the boys.

Add to this the fact that modern girls and women are more often the targets of market-directed advertising than boys and men, and thus are more likely to take to heart the message of modern advertisers. And what a powerful message that is! Corporations *need* consumers with low self-esteem, and work hard to create them. To sell nonessential items, companies must "manufacture needs and wants," a process that first strips away one's self-esteem, then offers to sell back tattered remnants of self-esteem if one buys and uses the company's products. Whether it's bleached teeth or hairless legs, breast size or hair color, height-increasing shoes or wrinkle-free skin, girls and women are explicitly told that they're unfeminine, unworthy, and undesirable (by males) if they don't modify their bodies with corporate products. While self-esteem-destroying messages are also directed at boys by corporate advertisers, the level of intensity is octaves lower and they rarely focus so much on body image or appearance.

In this regard, our culture is now organized as a self-fulfilling feedback loop. Women are defined as powerless beauty objects for the pleasure of men, and so fairy tales communicate this to little girls, who then grow up to carry the story that their role is to be powerless beauty objects for the pleasure of men. When women try to break out of that loop, national talk show hosts and bigots refer to them as "FemiNazis;" less articulate men call them "bitches."

In the morning-after of the 21st century, Cinderella is still present and accounted for, but midnight is now past and she's in a world of pain, especially if she wasn't born with a neurology that would make it easy for her to be a maid, secretary, or, to quote Jerry Falwell on the appropriate role of women, "called by God to be mothers [and] to nurture…"

Healing the Wounds

It's axiomatic that healing begins with recognition of the situation. Both men and women heal as they're exposed to the raw realities of the history of women's rights in America, as they realize the dangers in the growing political movement to roll back women's recently-won gains, and as they come to recognize the institutions and beliefs that fuel the entire process. They recover part of their identity and power when they realize that spirituality and religion are separate things, and that it's absolutely possible to have deep and meaningful spiritual experiences in any church, mosque, or synagogue while still understanding the dysfunctions inherent in human-made institutions (particularly ones created and run by men).

But just knowing the history is only the beginning. In order to truly heal, people must move beyond this past and see before them a clear, shining image of themselves and a world in which they can be powerful and dynamic forces for change and success. We know what we're against. Let's now create what we're *for*.

The Iroquois were very clear that we don't inherit the Earth from our ancestors, but instead, borrow it from our grandchildren. Therefore, they had an absolute injunction built into their system of governance that stipulated that every decision taken must be made in the context of its impact on the seventh future generation. Imagine how a similar policy would transform our political and corporate processes.

But the Iroquois also knew that there was one group among

them that was more concerned with the seventh generation than others: women. Therefore, in four of the five nations of the original Iroquois Confederacy, only women could vote on matters of long-range importance. When Ben Franklin invited 42 members of the Iroquois Confederacy to attend the Albany Plan of Union in 1754 (an early attempt to write a U.S. Constitution), he said in a speech to the Albany Congress:

"It would be a strange thing . . . if six nations of ignorant savages should be capable of forming such a union and be able to execute it in such a manner that it has subsisted for ages and appears indissoluble, and yet that a like union should be impractical for ten or a dozen English colonies."

(Franklin later agreed with Jefferson and Madison that the Iroquois way of voting was backward and should be changed so that only men could vote in the new U.S.A.)

But the evidence of archeology and anthropology clearly indicate that egalitarian cultures are our greatest and most long-lasting history. There have been (and continue to be around the world, largely among indigenous peoples) thousands of cultures based on egalitarian principles, where women play a real and important role in the politics and structure of the community, and where individual women can rise as far as they can dream. Since this is more the absolute norm for tribal peoples, and such people make up the majority of your and my ancestors, regardless of our race or national origin, egalitarianism is encoded in us, at the core of our humanness, built into our genetic code. We are most directly wired for cooperation rather than domination.

So let's work together to create a world where men and women peacefully coexist without either dominating the other, where women are respected and supported in all of their endeavors whether at home or in the world, and where we can safely raise our AD/HD and non-AD/HD girls with pride and respect.

Let's transform our schools back into places of stimulation, interest, and a passion for learning. Let's work to create opportunity and cooperation, a bright future for our children, and a world that works for all.

There may still be time . . .

LIFE STAGES
FOR WOMEN
WITH AD/HD

CHAPTER 15

Transition to Independence for Young Women with AD/HD

Kathleen G. Nadeau, Ph.D.

Young women with AD/HD must cope with a broad array of changes and challenges in their lives as they transition from dependence upon parents to independence. The challenges may seem even greater if a young woman is newly diagnosed with AD/HD, and is only beginning to understand how AD/HD affects her and what she must do to take charge of her increasingly independent life.

Entry into adulthood is accompanied by greater demands for judgment, organization, self-control, and long-range planning skills. The very psychological traits that one normally associates with maturity—ability to delay immediate gratification in order to achieve long-term benefit, ability to act based on reason rather than on immediate emotional impulse, and the ability to make plans and to carry through on those plans—are all traits that are among the most challenging for individuals with AD/HD.

Sam Goldstein and Michael Goldstein (1998) write that

successful treatment of AD/HD in children requires both symptom relief as well as protective factors that enhance their resilience, allowing them to recover from stress and leading them toward a successful transition into adulthood. These critical protective factors include an appropriate, supportive school setting, the support of friends, and, perhaps most important, family support. For young women with AD/HD, all of these factors remain relevant as they enter adulthood. In addition, protective factors relating to the workplace become critical.

Young women with AD/HD can ease the transition to independent adult life, by seeking or creating the same sorts of protective factors that support children with AD/HD:

1. an environment that promotes structure and predictability;
2. a work or school environment that is supportive and that reasonably accommodates AD/HD traits; and
3. the social support of friends and family who are accepting of the negative and appreciative of the positive in them.

Decreasing Structure and Support

If the young woman with AD/HD has been fortunate, she has had parents who worked to provide her with an AD/HD-friendly environment as she was growing up—an environment that is structured and predictable, with regular routines that support the completion of the daily activities necessary for a healthy, productive life. Such predictability may have eroded as she entered her teens and struggled to assert her independence. As she becomes a young adult, routines may have become lax, even if she is still living in the family home.

As she moves into the world of adult independence, her task is to find ways to create for herself the structure and support that she needs. This chapter will focus on the choices, challenges, and risk factors faced by a young woman with AD/HD as she makes a transition from home to independent living.

Risk Factors

Parents, quite naturally, are concerned, sometimes over-focused on the risks their daughter with AD/HD faces as she makes her first moves toward an independent, self-sufficient adult life. These risk factors are real, and should not be underestimated. However, there are many steps that parents and their daughters can take to reduce such risks.

❱ Pregnancy

Studies suggest that young women with AD/HD run a greater risk of an unplanned pregnancy (Arnold, 1996). A young woman with AD/HD may be more sexually impulsive than her non-AD/HD peers, and is also less likely to maintain consistent, effective birth control methods. Whether or not she decides to continue an unplanned pregnancy, she faces emotional stresses. If she terminates the pregnancy, she often risks intense feelings of guilt and remorse that may last years, if not a lifetime. If she gives birth, but decides to give up her baby for adoption, she again faces the possibility of lifelong feelings of guilt and regret. If she decides to keep her baby, she is typically very ill-equipped for motherhood, leading to increased risk factors for both herself and her child.

❱ Sexually Transmitted Diseases

In this era of AIDS, few are unaware of the dangers of sexually transmitted diseases, however, many young adults naively believe that sexually transmitted diseases are only a problem for "other" people. Combining such misguided beliefs with the impulsivity that so often accompanies AD/HD can sometimes lead to tragic consequences.

◗ **Dysfunctional Romantic Relationships**
A young woman with AD/HD who is passive and dependent may choose a boyfriend who is protective and "in command," only to find her self-esteem eroded by his assumption that she can't take care of herself. At the other extreme, young women with more hyperactive/impulsive AD/HD patterns may choose an "exciting" boyfriend who increases her dysfunctional tendencies through drug usage or through a chaotic, irresponsible life-style.

◗ **Impulse/Rebellion/Shame**
Research suggests that young women who have been rebellious or sexually impulsive as teens or young adults struggle with prolonged feelings of shame as they mature, sometimes to the extent that they make great effort to hide certain aspects of their past from friends and family (Johnson & Bishop, 1993).

◗ **Low Self-esteem Leading to Low Expectations**
Low self-esteem often leads to very low self-expectations, a pervasive risk factor for women with AD/HD. Studies have shown that the consequences of such negative self-appraisal are pervasive and destructive (Rucklidge & Kaplan, 1997), affecting many life choices.

◗ **Poor Life-management Skills**
The life lessons learned by a young woman with AD/HD may be expensive lessons indeed. For example, the potential consequences of repeated speeding tickets and "fender benders" can be enormous if she becomes an "assigned risk" and must pay thousands of dollars per year for automobile insurance. The impact of unpaid bills can be large if she develops a poor credit rating.

The impact of poor time management can compound if she loses her job due to chronic lateness.

▶ **Self-medication/Substance Abuse**

Self-medication is common among young women with undiagnosed or untreated AD/HD. Biederman and colleagues (1999) found that 14 percent of teenage girls diagnosed with AD/HD have a substance abuse disorder, and that girls with AD/HD were even more likely than boys with AD/HD to smoke cigarettes. Binge eating and compulsive overeating is a common method of self-calming for young women with AD/HD, as is cigarette smoking and overuse of caffeine-containing drinks to increase focus and concentration. Alcohol is often abused, as is marijuana, in attempts to self-calm or reduce anxiety.

▶ **Financial Chaos**

Difficulty managing finances is common for many young adults, but a young woman with AD/HD may experience extra challenges due to impulsivity, difficulty tracking expenditures, and problems with bill-paying. She risks acquiring thousands of dollars of charge card debt that may take her years to pay off. Out-of-control spending may ruin her credit rating, causing future problems when she applies for an automobile or home loan.

Protective Factors

Although the risks faced by young women with AD/HD are very real, there are many factors that can significantly reduce these risks, including a supportive family, supportive friends, and a supportive school environment. Once a young woman with AD/HD leaves school, a supportive work environment becomes another critical factor.

Family Support

Family support continues to be a critical component, even after a young woman has left home. However, parental roles must shift in order to allow her to appropriately develop independent living skills. Parents and daughters need to work toward developing a different relationship with one another—one that allows independent decision-making, and ultimately, an independent, self-sufficient life. While this can be a difficult task in any family, it can become especially difficult when the young woman in question has AD/HD. As an adult with AD/HD she may need guidance and support throughout her life in certain areas, but will feel more in charge of her life if this support comes from people other than her parents. Parents must walk a tightrope, balancing between their daughter's need for support and her need to learn self-reliance.

As a young woman with AD/HD, she may lag behind her peers in her capacity to take charge of her own life and make her own decisions. Often, when a young woman with AD/HD continues to need guidance and structure from adults, someone other than her parents may better provide this guidance as she works toward independence. An older adult—a relative, teacher, coach, therapist, or counselor can provide much needed guidance about the potential consequences of impulsive or ill-considered actions, while "lectures" from parents may fall on deaf ears.

Supportive Friends

A young woman with AD/HD will function best when she has the support of friends who understand and accept her AD/HD, and who encourage her to make good choices. Ideally, she will find other young women who are also working hard to build a future for themselves. A close bond with a best friend or roommate can provide a solid base as she faces the multiple challenges of young adulthood.

The choice of boyfriend is often pivotal in young adulthood, affecting a young woman's ability to function well as she leaves the shelter of her parents' home and tries to establish herself independently. Often, young women with AD/HD are drawn to young men with similar tendencies. She may feel more comfortable with a boyfriend who shares her struggles, rather than one who seems to "have it all together." But, unless her boyfriend is also working hard to take charge of his life, a destructive pattern may develop in which they pull each other down. To be successful, a young woman with AD/HD must take her needs and goals seriously, and look for a partner who helps her grow in confidence and independence.

Supportive School and Workplace Settings

A wise choice of educational program, following high school can often mean the difference between failure and success. A young woman with AD/HD will need supports and accommodations to function at her best academically. She may make better choices with professional guidance from someone who is familiar with various programs and with the needs of students with AD/HD.

Workplace choices are more complicated. While many colleges and universities have developed excellent programs for students with AD/HD, this is not true of the workplace. Few employers understand the needs of their employees with AD/HD, and, despite the Americans with Disabilities Act, the protections provided for adults with AD/HD in the workplace are limited. Good career counseling and job placement are important, but hard to find. The reader may want to refer to *ADD in the Workplace* (Nadeau, 1997), *ADD on the Job* (Weiss, 1996), or *Finding a Career That Works for You* (Fellman, 2000) for more detailed information on how to choose or change a work environment so that functions as a protective factor rather than a risk factor for AD/HD.

Risks of Over-protection

Parents often worry about risks their daughter with AD/HD may face if their guidance is withdrawn, but are less aware of the risks of overprotection. Parents may fear the consequences of an ill-prepared departure from home, perhaps into the arms of a highly undesirable boyfriend, or into a disordered, unstable life-style. At times, however, such protective impulses can lead to a pattern of prolonged dependence and immaturity. A young adult woman with AD/HD benefits most from parenting that gives her a feeling of emotional security, but at the same time promotes competence and confidence. She needs help in learning real-world skills. Even as she receives family support, it is essential that her parents communicate their expectations that independence and self-reliance are the expected outcomes.

Making AD/HD-friendly Life Choices

One of the great advantages of seeking treatment as a young adult is that the most important defining life choices still lie ahead. With the benefit of therapy, life choices can become informed choices, helping to build an AD/HD-friendly life. Typically, a young woman has not yet chosen her life partner, has not become a parent, and has not made great commitments of time or money toward any single career or profession. Understanding herself—her strengths, weaknesses, interests, and passions—within the framework of AD/HD, can help her make choices that can have a positive impact upon her AD/HD.

Constricted Choices during High School Years

The high school experience is often demoralizing for teenage girls with AD/HD. As they are bombarded with increasing academic demands from multiple sources, their native intelligence is often no longer enough to support them. Reading and writing assignments lengthen in high school. Girls can no longer get by just by paying occasional attention in class and hurriedly scribbling

homework assignments. During high school years, there is relatively little choice available to them. They must conform to the
standard curriculum and are required to sit and listen passively
for many hours each day, taking classes that may hold little interest for them.

Expanding Opportunities

As she leaves the narrow confines of high school, a young
woman with AD/HD can choose from a much broader array of
options: attending community college, obtaining vocational training, going away to college, going to work, traveling abroad in
student exchange programs, taking the opportunity to travel and
work in other parts of the country, living at home while preparing for independence, or moving into a group house or apartment with other young adults, to name but a few. She also can
make varied choices in friends, no longer confined to the narrow
social hierarchy of her high school.

Making Informed Choices

Young adult years can be a time of tremendous opportunity
for a young woman with AD/HD because her possibilities suddenly expand. For the first time, she can make choices that suit
her interests and preferences. A young woman who is aware of
her AD/HD has the chance to make much more informed life
choices by understanding her own strengths and weaknesses. If
she goes to college, she can take advantage of the many supports
and accommodations that weren't available until the past few
years. If she enters the work force, she can use her self-understanding to make a better job choice.

A young woman's choice of educational attainment, of career, of whether and whom she will marry, of where she will
live, and whether she will have children are all ahead of her.
These transition years are an ideal time to enter counseling or
psychotherapy with a professional who can help her learn more

about herself and her AD/HD so that she can make life choices that will help her function at her best.

Whether she is headed to college or the work force, this is an excellent time to undergo ability and interest testing before she has invested valuable time, money, and energy pursuing an unsuitable career. Both personality testing and interest testing can be very useful in charting a career direction. Her choice needs to be made with careful consideration of how AD/HD affects her life, as well as a clear understanding of her cognitive strengths and weaknesses (Nadeau, 1997; Fellman, 2000).

Creating an AD/HD-friendly Lifestyle

One of the most powerful approaches to reduce the negative impact AD/HD is to create an AD/HD-friendly lifestyle. In making important life choices—where to live, with whom to live, whom she will choose for a romantic partner, where she will work, what sort of work she will do—a young woman should take her AD/HD into account, so that her choices will reduce rather than increase her stress levels, will allow her to operate from her strengths, and will provide her with acceptance and emotional support from the people most significant to her.

Assessing Readiness for Independence

As young women with AD/HD approach the end of their high school years, two major decisions loom: whether to stay home or move out, and whether to go to college or to work. Both of these decisions are critical because they will set the stage for her transition to adult independence. False steps aren't fatal, but overestimating how much independence a young woman can handle often leads to failure and lowered self-confidence that makes the next step more difficult. This can be a very useful time for psychotherapy, where these decisions can be considered more dispassionately. An eighteen-year-old young woman may have her heart set on a particular course of action—for example, getting her own apartment or going away to college simply because her best friend or boyfriend is making this choice. Psychotherapy can provide a place for her to step back and consider whether she is truly ready for this level of independence, without the reaction she may feel toward "overprotective" parents.

Is College the Right Choice?

One of the first big choices facing a young woman with AD/HD is whether to go to college after high school. This decision is often fraught with anxiety for the parents, as well as for their daughter. Many parents feel that a college education is a necessity in today's economy. They may fear that, if their daughter doesn't attend college right away, she will lose the opportunity. A thorough, up-to-date psychoeducational evaluation may help with this decision-making process. Consultation with a college-placement professional who specializes in the needs of students with attentional and learning problems is also very useful. Often, students and their parents are not aware of the best choices of schools for students with AD/HD. Success in college is much more likely if a student receives careful guidance in choosing a college, in choosing a course of study, and in requesting and receiving appropriate supports and accommodations. For young women who do not feel ready to leave home, one option that may work well is to attend a local community college for a couple of years and then transfer to a four-year college.

Going to Work

A young woman with AD/HD may choose to work after high school rather than go on to college. Despite current conventional wisdom, college is not for everyone. Many young women with AD/HD may feel pressured to go to college, despite their misgivings, only to drop out after a few semesters. This scenario is very expensive for parents and demoralizing for a young woman who must now cope with feelings of failure and parental disappointment. Going to work immediately after high school can be a very valuable experience, allowing a young woman to focus on learning important life-management skills without added academic pressures. Through working, she can learn to budget her money, better manage her time, and learn appropriate workplace behaviors.

Many older adults with AD/HD report that, although they were not ready for college at age 18 or 20, they have gone back to school with success when they were more mature. Often, once a woman with AD/HD has identified a career interest, she has a stronger motivation to succeed in earning a college degree.

Choosing a Career, Not a Job

Whether she goes to college or directly joins the work force, it is critical that a young woman with AD/HD make a job choice that is a good match for her skills, interests, and personality type. Many young women only think in negative terms—attempting to avoid areas of weakness. Instead, with the guidance of an experienced clinician, she can focus on her strengths, choosing a career that is a good match for her, something that she can enjoy and excel at, rather than settling for a job that she merely tolerates (see Chapter 19).

Moving Away from Home

Each young woman must decide, based on her particular circumstances, whether she's ready to leave her parents' home. Ideally, this is a decision made jointly with her parents. Some young women feel ready to leave home at 18, while many others postpone their departure. Young adults with AD/HD often mature more slowly than their peers.

In making her decision, she needs to consider what supports she will need to succeed. If her decision is to go away to college, her success will be depend upon making a good choice of schools. College campuses vary tremendously in size and in the level of support available to students who are away from home for the first time.

If she moves into an apartment and takes a job, other issues must be carefully considered. Will she need financial assistance from her parents for a while? Are her parents willing and able to provide such assistance? Both parents and young women with AD/HD should be aware that it is not unusual for a young woman with AD/HD to return to the nest once or twice before her wings are truly prepared to keep her aloft. Learning the many skills required to live independently takes time.

Developing Life-management Skills

Today, many options are available to young women, and much greater independence is expected of them now than in the past. In addition, life has become more complex. Young adults need to learn about money management, handling charge cards, balancing check books, purchasing automobiles, car and health insurance, interest rates, record-keeping for tax returns, financial investing, and modern technology, to name only a few. Developing such skills should begin in high school, and continue during the college years or the early years of employment.

Not only is contemporary life very complex, but young women with AD/HD often experience difficulty in managing the "simple" tasks of daily life—meals, laundry, home maintenance, and personal health habits (sleep, exercise, health care).

Timeliness often poses great difficulty, and difficulties with time management often have greater consequences once a young woman is in the workplace. Though she may have been admonished for lateness in high school, most likely there was no neagative response for being late to class in college. Entering the world of work can be a rude awakening, where even fifteen minutes of tardiness can create a very negative impression.

Support from Professionals

Typically, when a young woman with AD/HD is still at home, she lives her life with "training wheels"—with parents and other adults available on either side of her to keep her from toppling over. As she leaves home to start her adult life, she may need continued help in order to ride successfully. AD/HD coaching is particularly well-suited to helping a young woman with AD/HD gradually "take off the training wheels" without crashing (see Chapter 7 on coaching). But riding without falling is not enough; she also needs to choose the direction in which she will ride. Psychotherapy can provide the structure and guidance needed to chart her course (see Chapter 6).

Coaching

Consequences of poor decisions tend to add up, whether it's on her driving record, her financial record, or her work record. A series of poor choices can quickly lead to dire consequences. AD/HD coaching is often an ideal support that can help her avoid painful and costly life lessons. Coaching can help a young woman with AD/HD learn daily life-maintenance activities such as meal planning, laundry, cleaning and ordering her living space, time management, priority setting, and money management. She may also need coaching to develop and maintain daily self-care activities—regular exercise, adequate sleep, and good nutrition. When parents are no longer around to provide structure and support, often these very basic activities are performed erratically, if at all.

Regular contact with a coach, by phone, by email, or in-person, can help her to set concrete goals, stay on track, and follow through as she learns the skills necessary to manage her life and her AD/HD patterns.

Psychotherapy

Psychotherapy is often the best choice when a young woman with AD/HD faces more than just the "practical" issues of life-management. Psychotherapy with a professional who is highly experienced in the issues of young women with AD/HD can help her as she struggles with issues of self-esteem, as she works to change her relationship with her parents, and as she struggles with the consequences of poor choices and learns to make better ones.

The following case history is presented to illustrate some common tendencies in young women with AD/HD that, in "Carrie's" case, have become exaggerated. The dysfunctional patterns in Carrie's family had been long-established before Carrie entered psychotherapy.

Case History of a Young Woman with AD/HD

Carrie was a highly intelligent young woman, a college graduate, who was experiencing great difficulty in launching her life as an independent adult. Her intelligence had carried her far academically, but very strong AD/HD patterns had led to daily problems with time management, self-discipline, organization, and the performance of daily life-management tasks. When she entered psychotherapy to treat her AD/HD, she was living at home with her parents, working only sporadically, and spending her days in a highly unstructured fashion.

Reflective of her emotional immaturity and relative comfort in depending upon her parents, it was Carrie's mother, not Carrie, who sought the initial consultation. Carrie reported that she had been diagnosed with AD/HD, hyperactive/impulsive subtype, during high school.

Her academic performance in high school had been good, despite her AD/HD, due to a highly structured lifestyle. She had competed in long-distance running, which gave her vigorous daily exercise, reducing her hyperactivity. Carrie attended a highly structured private school with small class size and very involved teachers. Carrie's brother, four years older than she, was already away at college during her high school years, so she received her mother's undivided attention, and lived in a calm, non-distracting home environment. Those structures at school and at home had kept Carrie on track.

In college, Carrie survived through a combination of high intelligence and personal charm. She related, humorously, that she had never turned a paper in on time, but, nevertheless had never had her grade lowered by turning in assignemts late. Her disorganization and procrastination, combined with a strong tendency toward perfectionism, led her to work on her papers for countless hours, far into the night, and sometimes for days after the deadline had passed. Interested in writing, she took a variety of courses in college, changed her major repeatedly, finally graduating with a degree in communications after five years as an undergraduate.

Following college, with very unclear goals, Carrie entered graduate school, more as a means to continue her student lifestyle than to prepare for a career. After two semesters, Carrie dropped out of her master's program. She returned home, and, since then, had worked in a variety of underpaid, short-term jobs, while she continued her collegiate lifestyle of late-night socializing.

When Carrie entered psychotherapy, she had been living at home for three years. Although 25 years old, her attitude and lifestyle were more like that of a 19-year-old. She had lost several jobs due to lateness, impulsively entered into romantic relationships that were ill-considered, and had made no concrete plans for the future.

Although living at home during high school had provided her with structure that helped her to succeed (protective factors), living at home after college seemed to promote and foster a very nonproductive, prolonged adolescent state (overprotective factors). Carrie's parents, not Carrie herself, voiced concern over her loss of jobs, her lack of planning for the future, and her unstructured, unproductive lifestyle.

Due to her parents' overprotection, Carrie never suffered the consequences of her immature behavior. It seemed clear that, unless her parents were actively involved in her treatment, Carrie would be unlikely to make changes. Her mother also seemed to enjoy having Carrie at home, and was very protective of her. Her father, however, expressed anger and frustration over Carrie's dependence and irresponsibility. The therapist's task was to engage both Carrie and her parents in a dialogue about the need to structure her environment, to impose consequences for irresponsible behavior, and to set realistic short-term and midterm goals for Carrie to work toward. Her father's angry responses did not motivate Carrie to change. Rather than make changes that would prevent her father's outbursts, she simply learned to avoid her father.

The therapist encouraged Carrie's parents to insist that she find a job as soon as possible. Carrie's goal in therapy would be to build structure into each day, including a consistent bedtime and rising time—a rising time that would assure arriving at work on time. Carrie and her parents agreed that Carrie would give them 50 percent of her paycheck as payment for room and board. This money would be set aside toward the goal of moving out, getting her own place to live, and leading a financially self-sufficient life within six months.

If Carrie failed to find and keep a job for six months, their agreement was that Carrie would be given a set amount of money (from her almost depleted education fund) with which she was expected to immediately find a place to live and move out—tough love with a soft landing pad. The sum would be enough for Carrie to live on for several weeks and would force her to actively seek employment to support herself.

The key to the success of this plan was that Carrie's mother was finally "on board," realizing that her behavior had enabled Carrie's prolonged dependence and irresponsibility. Carrie had lived in a world that, for years, had tolerated and accommodated her chronic lateness and inconsistent follow-through—first in college, and later at home.

As Carrie came to realize that her parents were no longer willing to tolerate her over-dependence, she began to take her task more seriously—to learn the skills and habits necessary for

independent living as a young adult. Her parents were coun-
seled that she might need repeated attempts to fly from the
nest before she was successfully launched. Her parents, how-
ever, needed to consistently communicate their expectation of
self-sufficiency.

After handing over half of her paycheck for several months,
Carrie decided that it would be more enjoyable to find an apart-
ment to share with a friend who had returned to the area. She
and her therapist planned to continue their work together as
she entered this next phase of her life—learning to make her
own decisions and be responsible for her own actions. Life
would be her teacher and circumstances her motivator as she
began the hard work of taking charge of her AD/HD.

The months to come would be filled with challenges for
both Carrie and her parents as they all worked to develop a
different relationship with one another. Carrie's mother learned
not to jump in to rescue Carrie or to excuse her behavior.
Carrie's father, feeling that he and his wife finally had the
same agenda, was able to become less angry and critical. Car-
rie was able to come to her father for advice without fearing
the barbed comments that had accompanied his advice in the
past. Carrie was finally engaged in therapy for herself—want-
ing to learn the skills she needed to manage her life. She had
far to go, but she was on her way.

A more traditional therapist might have involved the parents little, if at all. A more traditional therapist might have
focused the therapy on talking about feeling of depression and
anxiety, rather than on taking actions that would reduce these
feelings. Therapy that is effective in helping young women
with AD/HD typically focuses on the simple, concrete notion
that success breeds success. The therapist worked with Carrie
and her parents to find concrete ways to achieve small degrees
of success that would make later successes more likely.

Conclusion

While young women with AD/HD face many risks and challenges, there are also many positive aspects of this phase in the life of a young woman with AD/HD. With adequate protective factors in place, with encouragement from parents to develop self-sufficiency, and with education and guidance about ways to create an AD/HD-friendly life, this can be an exciting and fulfilling time—a time to explore newly available options, develop strengths, and make positive choices that can set her life on a track toward success and fulfillment.

References

Arnold, L.E. (1996). Sex differences in AD/HD: Conference summary. *Journal of Abnormal Child Psychology, 24,* 555-568.

Biederman, J., Faraone, S. V., Mick, E., Williamson, S., Wilens, T. E., Spencer, T. J., Weber, W., Jetton, J., Kraus, I., Pert, J., & Zallen, B. (1999). Clinical correlates of ADHD in females: Findings from a large group of girls ascertained from pediatric and psychiatric referral sources. *Journal of the American Academy of Child and Adolescent Psychiatry, 38,* 966-975.

Fellman, W. R. (2000). *Finding a career that works for you.* Plantation, Florida: Specialty Press, Inc.

Goldstein, S., & Goldstein, M. (1998). *Managing attention-deficit hyperactivity disorder in children: A guide for practitioners.* New York: John Wiley.

Johnson, J., & Bishop, K. (1993). The impulsive woman as client: Treating the legacy of shame. In W. McCown, J. Johnson, & M. Shure (Eds.), *The impulsive client: Theory, research, and treatment* (pp. 361-386). Washington, DC: American Psychological Association Press.

Nadeau, K. (1997). *ADD in the workplace: Choices, changes, and challenges.* New York: Brunner/Mazel.

Rucklidge, J. J., & Kaplan, B. J. (1997). Psychological functioning in women identified in adulthood with attention-deficit/hyperactivity disorder. *Journal of Attention Disorders, 2,* 167-176.

Weiss, L. (1996). *ADD on the job: Making your ADD work for you.* Dallas: Taylor Publishing.

CHAPTER 16

The College Experience

Belinda Guthrie, M.A.

W omen with AD/HD attending colleges and universities across the nation form a student body diverse in terms of identity, race, ethnicity, age, socioeconomic status, sexuality, educational background, individual interests, and personal goals. In a recent study among freshmen with disabilities, two in five students (41%) reported having a learning disability and/or attention deficit disorder (Henderson, 1999).[1] Forty-two percent of students with learning or attention disorders enrolling in two- and four-year academic programs are women. The decision to go to college for women with attention deficit hyperactivity disorder (AD/HD) is just as exciting, confusing, and liberating as it is for every young woman choosing to pursue a degree. This excitement, however, can be tempered for women with AD/HD by concerns about whether they will succeed in college and

[1]The American Council on Education defines a learning disability as a disorder in one or more of the basic psychological processes involved in understanding or using language, spoken or written, which manifests itself in an imperfect ability to listen, think speak, read, write, spell, or do mathematical calculations. This term, for statistical purposes, includes such conditions as Attention Deficit Disorder and Attention Deficit Hyperactivity Disorder.

live up to their potential, and whether professors and peers will somehow view them as less capable because of their diagnosis. Women with AD/HD experience the same personal and cognitive growth as their non-disabled peers, however, they also face additional challenges that can either foster or undermine their goal of higher education.

The question is not whether women with AD/HD are going to college. The question is whether women with AD/HD are merely *surviving* rather than *thriving* in college, and what factors make the difference. While there is no universal experience for women with AD/HD in college, these women enter higher education facing some common roadblocks that require each student to identify her own unique approach to learning, identify strengths and interests, and develop strategies for achieving academic success. The case history that follows provides a critical lens to examine factors which contribute to student success at the postsecondary level for women with AD/HD. This case history also provides a canvas for exploring the college experience as it relates to self-esteem, internal motivation, and personal growth of women with AD/HD.

"Olivia"   diagnosed with AD/HD at age 20

Olivia is a 23-year-old student enrolled at a highly selective four-year college. She is currently only three classes and a senior thesis away from completing her bachelor's degree—the end of a journey, which Olivia recalls as being very difficult, but instrumental to her development as a young woman. Olivia remembers her first year as one of "merely surviving." Professors viewed her as bright and capable, but undisciplined, and irresponsible. Messages such as "You need to take more responsibility," and "You're one of the brightest students in the class, I don't understand why you won't get your work in on time," seemed to echo voices from her childhood. Olivia recalls working hard and staying up all night to finish papers, but still found herself falling further and further behind in her classes. She knew of other students who seemed to have similar problems, but most of her friends were getting it done. Olivia was definitely not "getting it done."

Olivia believed that her failure was due to lack of responsibility, laziness, and not being smart enough. As the semester progressed, Olivia became more withdrawn and less motivated. She watched her grades fall steadily from "A's" to "C's." The final straw for Olivia was receiving an "F" for a missed exam because she wrote the wrong date in her appointment calendar.

Olivia also remembers feeling socially awkward in class. She felt as if she was only getting bits and pieces of the lecture. Lectures in high school were usually shorter and, if important points were missed, the material was reviewed the next class period. In college, however, the lectures were longer and material flowed at a faster pace. Olivia refrained from participating in class discussion out of fear that she would say something inappropriate, or would participate in discussion at the wrong time. Her instructors interpreted her failure to participate as evidence of lack of preparedness.

In spite of being accepted by a highly selective college, Olivia questioned whether she was truly suited for college. She wondered what had happened to the smart, self-assured, high school honors student who had walked onto the ivy-covered campus less than two months earlier.

Effects of the College Experience on AD/HD

The young adult experience is a series of transitions—changes in roles, and in definitions of self. The process of redefining oneself from a teenager into a young adult is a significant stressor during this period of transition. Many students are living away from home for the first time, dealing with a roommate or roommates in very tight living quarters, and having to juggle adult responsibilities such as paying bills, doing laundry, and shopping for necessities.

Less Structure

The structure of college also differs significantly from high school. Students have more unstructured time, more intensive and demanding classes, higher expectations both in terms of quantity and quality of work, fewer scheduled contacts with professors, and an increase in the number of opportunities for extracurricular activities. The nature of the college environment requires students to adopt more sophisticated time management skills and study habits. Students must learn early on how to balance their academic responsibilities with newly imposed adult obligations. Successful young adults with AD/HD usually develop special study methods and spend more time studying—essentially working harder and longer—to achieve the same level of success experienced by their non-disabled peers.

Increased Stress

The effects of transitioning to college can be stressful for any student. Students with learning disabilities and attention deficit disorders, however, may be at greater risk of having problems adapting to college and managing the stress associated with being in an academically demanding environment. The complexity of responsibilities that students with disabilities assume when they enter college can be overwhelming to the most savvy student. Student must learn to "navigate within a complex academic and administrative bureaucracy, identify their needs and communicate them effectively, advocate on their own behalf for accommodations, overcome obstacles, compensate for challenges presented by their disorder, and manage the stress that often accompanies these challenges" (Hatzes et al., 2001, p. 67).

Greater Demands

Women with AD/HD, whether recently diagnosed or having lived with the knowledge of their diagnosis for some time, must make a rapid transition to college life. The very characteristics of AD/HD (i.e., failure to give close attention to detail, difficulty sustaining attention, failure to follow through on instructions or complete tasks, difficulty with organization, avoidance or reluctance to engage in activities of limited personal interest, and being easily distracted and forgetful of daily activities) make the transition to college especially difficult.

Greater Need for Organization

Olivia was aware that she needed to organize her days so that she could transition with ease from classes to meals to her on-campus job to studying. She bought daily planners, wall calendars, and color-coded her notebooks. Usually, after a few days, the newness of each time management strategy wore off and she was back to "flying by the seat of her pants." Missing deadlines, losing important pieces of paper, misplacing syllabi, and leaving a notebook or textbook in the dining hall or library had a direct impact on Olivia's beliefs in her abilities as a student and as an adult. Her lack of confidence and her devalued self-concept eroded her motivation to achieve a college degree. While she had experienced similar difficulties in high school, she had always been able to push through and achieve above average grades.

Olivia's first experience in college is not unique. College students undiagnosed with AD/HD throughout elementary and high school typically have a feeling that there is something wrong. Young women with AD/HD often report a history of inconsistent performance in school, and strained relations with instructors due to the frequency of late or misplaced assignments. Young adults with AD/HD also describe feeling that they are not living up to their ability. The "history" that follows young women with AD/HD into college can have a significant impact on their personal and cognitive growth and development. Brown (1994) determined that the adult personality of an individual with AD/HD is shaped by a sense of grief and loss from a perceived inability to live up to his or her potential. These students are often able to get into college due to their intelligence, ability to compensate for areas of weakness, support at school and from family, and internal drive. It is often only when undiagnosed students enter college and encounter unexpected academic and personal difficulties that they recognize that they have struggled with a lifelong disability (Silver, 1992).

Secondary Psychological Struggles

Olivia's emotional health and academic record began to suffer. The problems she experienced in class were starting to spill over into relationships with her roommates, friends, and with her new boyfriend. Olivia withdrew socially from her friends at school and missed class on a regular basis. Olivia recalled feeling a significant loss of family support when she started college. Before, Olivia's mother served as a source of both emotional and organizational support. Now, without this support, Olivia felt as if she had lost the key that kept her life under control.

When a person experiences repeated failure or perceives their performance as inadequate, their sense of autonomy and competency decreases, while feelings of being unable to control the surrounding environment increase. Once the perceived locus of control has shifted from internal to external, psychological well-being diminishes.

Rucklidge and Kaplan (2000) studied attribution styles of women with AD/HD and their perceptions of childhood in terms of satisfaction with relationships and how much control they felt they had over their lives as children. As a result of this research, they assert that low self-esteem and learned helplessness in women with AD/HD results from a history of multiple failures, a lack of support systems, and ineffective problem-solving skills. Early learning experiences and perceptions of childhood, both in terms of relationships and autonomy, also affect a person's confidence in problem-solving abilities. In this study, women with

AD/HD perceived childhood relationships with parents and teachers more negatively than did women without AD/HD. The women also reported feeling less in control when faced with difficulties as a child and later, as an adult.

While Olivia had positive memories of family relationships, she attributed her academic success solely to her mother's ability to keep her on track. Olivia began to experience increased interpersonal difficulties in college, where she felt less in control. Interpersonal problems faced by adults with AD/HD can include frequent mood swings, having a "short fuse," appearing selfish or immature to others, lacking tact in social situations, and failing to follow through on commitments to others (Brown, 1994).

Comprehensive Treatment Plan

At the recommendation of family members and friends, Olivia took a semester off from school. Olivia felt that some time away would help her to reassess her decision to go to college, and provide her with time and space to identify the underlying causes of her current emotional and academic problems. Olivia was evaluated and received a diagnosis of attention deficit disorder. Previously, she had received a variety of labels ranging from major depression to borderline personality disorder.

AD/HD symptoms, such as not being able to concentrate, being distractible, sleep disturbances, feeling depressed or anxious, and being hyper- or hypo-responsive, can lead clinicians to an inaccurate diagnosis (Ratey, Miller, & Nadeau, 1995). Coupled with feelings of inadequacy, guilt, and a reduced sense of personal control, women with undiagnosed AD/HD may present symptoms of depression (Rucklidge & Kaplan, 2000; Shea, 1998). The winding path that some women must take to eventually arrive at a correct diagnosis of AD/HD may increase their symptoms of anxiety and depression. Whether AD/HD contributes to a greater risk for mood disorders remains open to debate (Barkley, 1998).

Olivia met once a week with a psychologist who had experience working with adults with AD/HD. Her goals for therapy were to understand her diagnosis and to learn how to live successfully as an adult with AD/HD. As part of her treatment plan, Olivia worked with a psychiatrist who prescribed a long-acting D-amphetamine and Prozac, a selective serotonin reuptake inhibitor (SSRI). For Olivia, the combination of a stimulant medication and an antidepressant was helpful in managing the core symptoms of AD/HD and the coexisting depressive symptoms (Wilens, Spencer, & Biederman, 1995).

Olivia's participation in a comprehensive treatment plan provided her with the tools necessary to learn about her disorder and to manage the full spectrum of AD/HD from both a psychological and psychopharmacological approach. Increased understanding of one's disability involves learning about what the disorder is and what it is not, and learning how the disorder affects mood and performance at work, and in social situations. Psychotherapy can make it easier for the adult with AD/HD to deal with the cognitive, emotional, and self-esteem problems that are intrinsic to the disorder (Faigel, 1995; Hallowell, 1995). A critical part of the therapeutic process involves the recognition and acceptance of individual strengths and weaknesses. Realistic goal setting, self-monitoring, confidence, and follow-through contribute to the general success of adults (Wallace, Winsler, & NeSmith, 1999).

Taking Charge of AD/HD

Olivia returned to college with a renewed sense of motivation and self-esteem. She reported feeling more confident in understanding her strengths and weaknesses and was excited about returning to college full-time. Olivia believed that she had a foundation on which to build, and that with continued work, she would be able to achieve her academic goals.

The terms *self-determination* and *autonomy,* in the eyes of many, are seen as only the latest "buzzwords" in the field of disability services (Weymehyer, 1996). Yet, self-determination and the development and sustainment of autonomy are critical to self-motivation. Research by Deci and Ryan supports that self-motivation is central to creativity, responsibility, healthy behavior, and lasting positive change. Self-determination theory postulates that an individual's innate psychological needs are the basis for self-motivation and personal development. Environmental factors can either promote or hinder development and psychological well-being (Ryan & Deci, 2000). In order to be self-determined, people must first feel competent. Competency is achieved when an individual can act and interact effectively within her environment (Deci, 1975). Ryan and Deci's (2000) research has shown that feeling competent, however, does not enhance intrinsic motivation without a sense of autonomy. "People must not only experience competence, they must also experience their behavior as self-determined for intrinsic motivation to be in evidence" (Ryan & Deci, 2000, p. 70).

Events such as receiving feedback on an assigned paper and attributing that success to one's own efforts promotes feelings of competency. The feeling of competency and the belief that it is the direct result of autonomous behavior results in motivation and lasting change. External motivators, such as deadlines, imposed goals, pressure, fear of failure, or being focused on receiving a particular grade may result in the desired result, but they ultimately undermine intrinsic motivation and diminish an individual's enthusiasm and interest. Intrinsic motivation implies that individuals feel that their behavior and the results of their behavior are truly the result of their ability, efforts, and the choices that they have made, rather than due to external control. Deci and Flaste (1995, p. 30-31) argue that while "this is a rather subtle point the significance is quite profound. The implication that a person has a need to feel autonomous is that failure to satisfy the need leads to decreased well-being—to a variety of maladaptive consequences." Intrinsic motivation is central to the success of young women with AD/HD. Women with AD/HD are more likely to thrive in college when they believe that they are capable of attaining their goals. Women with AD/HD who are self-determined stay focused on their goals and are more proactive in the management of the self.

My first contact with Olivia, as director of disability services, highlighted the importance of promoting autonomy when working with students with disabilities. Olivia recalls registering for disability accommodations with trepidation. She was concerned about what her instructors and her friends would think if they knew that she had attention deficit disorder. At first, Olivia did not want to avail herself of in-class accommodations out of fear that using accommodations, such as extended time, would be taking the easy way out.

I recalled a lecture by Priscilla Vail, Ed.D., on how emotion is the on/off switch to learning. Ms. Vail spoke about a successful young woman with a learning disability describing her experience in college. The young woman, Sarah, had spent numerous hours during her time as a college student explaining the nature of her disorder, describing how it impacted her in class and out of class, and negotiating in-class accommodations for exams and papers. Sarah had encountered professors who were welcoming of students with disabilities, and professors who conveyed their doubt in the validity of a learning disabilities and the equity of providing accommodations. Regardless of the type of professor Sarah encountered, each time she spoke about her need for accommodations, she concluded the conversation with the following statement, "I have a disability. I am not looking for an easier way out, I'm just looking for a different way in."

Olivia faced a critical task on her path to academic success—to reframe her feelings about her use of accommodations—so that she would come to view accommodations and support as a "different way in," and not the "easy way out."

Factors Associated with Student Success

For many, academic success is narrowly defined and limited to receiving a particular grade in a course. A successful college experience, however, is more than a high grade point average or earning a diploma to hang on the wall. A broader and more meaningful definition of academic success is to acquire a depth and range of knowledge, to increase understanding of oneself and others, to learn critical thinking skills, and to explore one's creativity. This latter definition of academic success values the process of learning and the individual differences of learners. This definition also embraces the importance of self-determination as an educational outcome (Wehmeyer, 1996). In order to be aware of factors that contribute to the success of women with AD/HD in college, it is helpful to understand factors that promote academic excellence for *all* students.

Although colleges and universities have information available to them—academic transcripts, SAT scores, writing samples, and letters of recommendations that can be used to predict academic potential—this information does not illuminate the path or the means students took to achieve past academic success. Nor does the information provide colleges and universities with insight into what supports students will need once they are in a more academically demanding environment.

The impact of the college experience on a student's development is important to understanding what supports colleges must provide to enhance academic excellence on their campuses. Astin (1993) conducted a comprehensive longitudinal study to measure the impact of college attendance on students' personal, social, academic, and vocational development. Not surprisingly, results from the study show a positive increase in students' sense of intellectual development and intellectual self-confidence during the time spent in college. While these factors could be attributed purely to maturational effects, positive educational outcomes for both men and women were highly correlated with overall student involvement, measured both quantitatively and qualitatively by the frequency of student contact with faculty and other students, the frequency of student engagement in student groups and organizations, and the frequency of which students were actively engaged in their learning. The ability to think critically, to look at the world from a global perspective, and to have confidence when interacting with others, are positive outcomes of the college experience. The chart that follows shows factors that contribute to academic success at the postsecondary level (Astin, 1993), and lists ways in which students with AD/HD can maximize their potential for success.

Factors that Contribute to Positive Student Outcomes (Astin, 1993)	Ways of Maximizing Positive Outcomes for Students with AD/HD
Number of hours and quality of time spent studying	▶ Identify a study schedule that fits your personal, academic, and social needs and responsibilities—build it into your daily routine and stick with it. ▶ Approach studying in ways compatible with your personal style (i.e., time of day, location, opportunity for breaks, presence or absence of food)—this will make your time more productive. ▶ If using medication, schedule your studying periods around your medication times. ▶ Make use of time immediately before and after class to review notes, skim reading assignments, and generate a list of questions for the next class period. ▶ Identify a set time each day to go over your syllabus for each class and identify what you need to do the following day.
Frequency and quality of contact with instructors	▶ Go to class! ▶ Sit front and center. ▶ Ask questions in class—most instructors factor in 10-20% of your grade on class participation. ▶ Attend office hours at least once every two weeks—instructors really do want to talk with their students. ▶ Meet with your instructor regularly before exams and papers are due.

Factors that Contribute to Positive Student Outcomes (Astin, 1993)	Ways of Maximizing Positive Outcomes for Students with AD/HD
	▶ Meet with your instructor after exams and papers have been returned. ▶ Attend supplemental study sessions.
Frequency of courses taken that emphasize writing, scientific inquiry, and historical analysis	▶ Take at least one writing-intensive course across disciplines each semester—choose classes that are of interest to you. ▶ Seek out academic support services, such as writing skills centers, peer tutoring, and quantitative literacy centers, to improve writing, critical thinking, reading, and math skills. ▶ Meet regularly with your academic advisor—select a balanced course load that is reflective of your strengths and interests. ▶ Select courses that build on prior knowledge and experience.
Number of courses that involve active engagement by students	▶ Take an active role in class—passivity leads to increased distractibility. ▶ Select courses that include a discussion section. Discussion sections are typically smaller and provide more opportunities to participate. ▶ Consider courses that include a fieldwork or experiential component.

Factors that Contribute to Positive Student Outcomes (Astin, 1993)	Ways of Maximizing Positive Outcomes for Students with AD/HD
Frequency of student-to-student interaction and opportunities for peer learning	▶ Participate in group projects. ▶ Study with a partner or study group (i.e., share notes, talk about lecture material, readings, paper assignments, exams). ▶ Make use of peer tutoring resources. ▶ Become a peer tutor!
Frequency and quality of student engagement on campus	▶ Attend campus lectures. ▶ Join a student group or organization that interests you. ▶ Do anything that is safe and legal that will help you feel connected to your campus community.

Gender differences in Astin's study accounted for nearly two-thirds of the eighty-two measures used to evaluate student development and change in life goals, self-ratings, attitudes, behaviors, and expectations. Some of the largest gender effects were reported in the area of psychological well-being and cognitive development. Women reported feeling depressed and overwhelmed more often than did their male peers. Astin contends that increased feelings of stress can be traced to the growing number of responsibilities that students must face during their four years in college. While this time is not necessarily traumatic for all college women, it is a time of heightened stress and anxiety (Graber & Brooks-Ginn, 1996). "Women enter college already differing considerably from men in self-rated emotional and psychological health, standardized test scores, GPAs, political attitudes, personality characteristics, and career plans, and most of these differences widen during the undergraduate years. Many of these, but not all, can be directly attributed to the college experience" (Astin, 1993, p. 405-406).

Factors that Promote Academic Success for the Young Woman with AD/HD

Self-determination is reflected in terms of autonomy, self-regulating behavior, self-realization, and empowerment (Wehmeyer, 1996). These four characteristics of self-determination "represent attitudes (psychological empowerment and self-realization) and abilities (autonomy and self-regulation) which must be present if a person is to be self-determined" (p. 24).

Self-regulation involves being able to cope with the environment and to make decisions on how to respond to the environment. It entails strategies such as self-monitoring, self-instruction, self-evaluation, and self-reinforcement (Wehmeyer, 1996, p. 26). Self-realization involves knowing oneself and being able and willing to acknowledge strengths and limitations. Finally, empowerment evolves from autonomy and an internal locus of control.

Succeeding in college with a disability can be profoundly challenging. Students must not only learn how to compensate for deficiencies and adapt their environment to fit their needs, but they must also learn how to articulate their disability-related needs to others and be able to respond to common questions and misperceptions about their disability (Klein, 1998). Self-regulating behavior for students with AD/HD can be promoted by making use of student services and accommodations in a proactive and responsible manner. Autonomy for the young woman with AD/HD is enhanced when she feels connected or related to others and is able to identify and build a support network, both on and off campus.

At the recommendation of the director of disability services, Olivia joined a peer support group at her college for students with learning disabilities and attention deficit disorder. The peer support group had nine members (seven women and two men) who were at various stages of their academic program.

The disproportionate number of women to men in the group may reflect gender differences in coping strategies of college students with symptoms of AD/HD. Turnock (1998) found that women with AD/HD seek out greater levels of social and peer support than their male peers during periods of difficulty or transition. Peer support groups provide a valuable network of support for students, whether they have lived with a diagnosis for years or have just recently been evaluated as an adult. Common issues addressed in such groups include emotional issues (i.e., relationships, family, self-esteem, self-advocacy) and educational issues (i.e., accommodations, legal issues, confidentiality, medication) (Guthrie & Klein, 1998). Through the group process, students recognize that the difficulties they experience, while unique, are similar to the experiences of other college students with AD/HD. The relatively simple function of recognizing a common experience can help students feel less isolated during their time at college.

I just feel like I can talk openly, like I don't feel like I have to hide a part of me that sometimes I feel like I have to hide from others. I never knew there were so many people like me—students that are smart, funny, and talented—just kidding. Really, though, everyone always thought I was stupid or lazy. I don't remember actually thinking that, but I was told to believe that. (Guthrie & Klein, 1998)

Support groups also parallel the way individuals form relationships outside of the group. "As members form connections and relationships within the group, they learn to identify feelings as they occur, and perceive their own actions" (Klein, p. 37). As one student astutely points out:

> *I think I am becoming more aware. I'm taking more risks—asking people [questions], saying 'I don't understand' in class, knowing that it's my difference, and that if other people don't accept it, that's OK—instead of feeling nervous about making mistakes, I mean I still do, but I know that it is important and necessary for me to try. (Guthrie & Klein, 1998)*

Doubts about one's ability, striving for perfection, experiencing exhaustion, fear of exposure, or being caught off-guard all contribute the hidden costs of living with a learning disability [attention deficit disorder] (Feri, 2000). The need for an appropriate and effective emotional outlet is very important to overall psychological development for women with AD/HD. A peer support group can serve as emotional support, as well as provide young women with opportunities to discuss issues related to their AD/HD that might be too difficult to discuss with family members, friends, and significant others.

> *For Olivia, the difference between thriving rather than just surviving involved using both in-class accommodations and out-of-class support services, and recognizing when it was important to ask for help.*

Researchers have identified several common characteristics of college students with AD/HD (Jones, Kalivoda, & Higbee, 1997; Richard, 1995; Quinn, 1997). Students with AD/HD typically experience:

1. Underachievement and poor or inconsistent academic performance;
2. Difficulty organizing academic and personal life;

3. Problems with prioritizing and inconsistency with follow-through;

4. Problems with identifying effective study strategies and implementing them independently;

5. Forgetfulness;

6. Procrastination, followed by frustration;

7. Difficulty with reading and writing, both in terms of comprehension and perseverance of task; and

8. A pattern of using the pressure of the "11th hour" to start the assignment.

In accordance with the provisions of the American's with Disabilities Act and Section 504 of the Rehabilitation Act, colleges and universities are obligated to provide and coordinate reasonable and effective academic accommodations, modifications, auxiliary aids, and services not of a personal nature to qualifying students with disabilities. In response to the needs of students with AD/HD, accommodations, auxiliary aids, and services commonly include, but are not necessarily limited to:

1. Priority registration and course advisement to help the student select a well-balanced course schedule that meets her individual interests and needs;

2. Program modifications such as a reduced course load;

3. Extended time on exams, with the option of taking the exam in a private room with fewer distractions;

4. Notetaking services to supplement the student's personal class notes;

5. Receiving written assignments earlier so that the student can plan and prioritize accordingly;

6. Receiving extensions on assignments with advance notice; and

7. Making use of library support services such as assistance with library search engines, copying privileges for non-circulating material or class reserve readings, and extended loan periods for books.

Other Services to Promote Academic Success

Accommodations alone are typically not sufficient to make the difference between thriving and merely surviving. The everyday symptoms of AD/HD and the history of academic struggles that often accompany a young woman to college require a comprehensive approach to services in terms of academic and personal support.

In addition to working with a therapist off-campus, Olivia worked with an academic coach.

Academic coaching is emerging as a critical support service for college students with AD/HD. Attention Deficit Disorder Coaching is a "collaborative relationship that is designed to help college students with AD/HD develop the awareness, cognitive processes, behavioral patterns, and environmental structures needed to overcome performance deficits caused by their disability" (Quinn, Ratey, & Maitland, 2000). An AD/HD coach helps students by "providing support, structure, supervision, and feedback before, during, and after performing the skills being worked on" (p. 11).

Lasting change occurs when the person sees a relation between her behavior and a desired outcome. For coaching to be effective, the coach must support the individual's autonomy by providing choice and respecting the individual's role in the coaching process. People are more likely to reach their goals when they are proactively involved in the establishment and development of goals and strategies. Supporting autonomy is achieved when the coach:

▶ explores options in self-management strategies with the student and involves the student proactively in assessing the effectiveness of the strategies on an on-going basis;

▶ establishes goals that are individualized to the student's needs and take into account the student's perspective;

▶ establishes limits with the student;

▶ helps the student understand the usefulness of limits and encourages her to think through why she is being asked to do something in a particular way;

▶ makes limits as wide as possible and allows choice within them; and

▶ encourages the student to evaluate her performance on an ongoing basis.

Promoting autonomy by engaging the student proactively in the process can lead to enhanced intrinsic motivation. Failure to promote autonomy creates inappropriate stresses and make unreasonable demands (Deci & Flaste, 1995, p. 153).

Olivia found that it was useful to meet with her coach for half an hour on Mondays and follow-up with email exchanges several times throughout the week to help her plan and prioritize. The weekly office appointments and the email exchanges

provided a structure for organizing her academic and personal life and served as a system of accountability. Participating in academic coaching also helped Olivia view past and present academic success as an indicator of her ability and efforts, not solely as the result of chance. At the end of the academic year, Olivia reported a greater sense of ownership of her learning and of her improved ability to manage her life effectively.

Conclusion

Adapting to a new environment and understanding a new diagnosis or how an old disorder reveals itself in new ways are challenging issues for the young woman with AD/HD as she enters college. For all college students, including women with AD/HD, academic success should be defined by the knowledge gained in a particular field of study, as well as by the experiences that contribute to personal, social, and academic development. By broadening one's definition of academic success, young women with AD/HD can move beyond the goal of receiving an "A" or striving toward an unrealistic standard of perfection. Instead, the young woman with AD/HD can experience the freedom of taking chances, exploring new areas, and developing her talents, strengths, and interests. Careful attention to the relationship between personal, academic, and social development and the college experience can mean the difference between *thriving* or just *surviving* in college.

References

Astin, A. (1993). *What matters in college? Four critical years revisited.* San Francisco, CA: Jossey-Bass Inc.

Barkley, R.A. (1998). *Attention deficit hyperactivity disorder: A handbook for diagnosis and treatment (2nd ed.).* New York: Guilford.

Brown, B. (1994). *Adults with ADHD: At school, at work, at play.* Paper presented at the 6th Annual Postsecondary LD Training Institute, Farmington, CT.

Deci, E., & Flaste, R. (1995). *Why we do what we do: The dynamics of personal autonomy.* New York: G.P. Putnam's Sons.

Faigel, H.C. (1995). Attention deficit disorder in college students: Facts, fallacies, and treatment. *Journal of American College Health, 40,* 147-155.

Ferri, B.A. (2000). The hidden cost of difference: Women with learning disabilities. *Journal of Learning Disabilities, 10,* 129-138.

Guthrie, B., & Klein, A. (1998, March). *Communication + awareness = empowerment: Successful support groups for students with learning disabilities and attention deficit disorder.* Session presented at the LDA International Conference, Washington D.C.

Hallowell, E.M. (1995). Psychotherapy of adult attention deficit disorder. In K.G. Nadeau (Ed.), *A comprehensive guide to attention deficit disorder in adults: Research, diagnosis, and treatment* (pp. 144-167). New York: Brunner/Mazel, Inc.

Henderson, C. (1999). *College freshman with disabilities: A biennial statistical profile.* Washington, DC: Heath Resource Center.

Jones, G.C., Kalivoda, K.S., & Higbee, L. (1997). College students with attention deficit disorder. *National Association of Student Personnel Administrators, 34,* 262-274.

Klein, A. (1998). Becoming accessible to learning. *Literacy Harvest, 7,* 34-39.

Quinn, P.O. (1997). *Attention deficit disorder: Diagnosis and treatment from infancy to adulthood.* New York: Brunner/Mazel, Inc.

Quinn, P.O., Ratey, N., & Maitland, T. (2001). *Coaching college students with ADHD: Issues and answers.* Silver Spring, MD: Advantage Books.

Ratey, J.J., Miller, A.C., & Nadeau, K.G. (1995). Special diagnostic and treatment considerations in women with attention deficit disorder. In K.G. Nadeau (Ed.), *A comprehensive guide to attention deficit disorder in adults: Research, diagnosis, and treatment* (pp. 218-235). New York: Brunner/Mazel, Inc.

Richard, M. (1995). Students with attention deficit disorders in postsecondary education: Issues in identification and accommodation. In K.G. Nadeau (Ed.), *A comprehensive guide to attention deficit disorder in adults: Research, diagnosis, and treatment* (pp. 284-307). New York: Brunner/Mazel, Inc.

Ryan, R.M., & Deci, E. L. (2000). Self-determination theory and the facilitation of intrinsic motivation, social development, and well-being. *American Psychologist, 55*, 68-78.

Rucklidge, J.J., & Kaplan, B.J. (2000). Attributions and perceptions of childhood in women with ADHD symptomology. *Journal of Clinical Psychology, 56*, 711-722.

Shea, L.C. (1998). Gender and comorbidity issues: Consideration for service providers. In P. Quinn, & A. McCormick (Eds.), *Rethinking AD/HD: A guide for fostering success in students with AD/HD at the college level* (pp. 57-66). Silver Spring, MD: Advantage Books.

Silver, L.B. (1992). *Attention deficit hyperactivity disorder: A clinical guide to diagnosis and treatment*. Washington, DC: American Psychiatric Press.

Turnock, P. (1998). Academic coping strategies in college students with symptoms of AD/HD. In P. Quinn, & A. McCormick (Eds.), *Rethinking AD/HD: A guide for fostering success in students with AD/HD at the college level* (pp. 76-84). Silver Spring, MD: Advantage Books.

Wallace, B.A., Winsler, A., & NeSmith, P. (1999). *Factors associated with success for college students with ADHD: Are standard accommodations helping?* Paper presented at the Annual Meeting of the American Educational Research Association, Montreal, Canada.

Wehmeyer, M.L. (1996). Self-determination as an educational outcome: Why it is important to children, youth, and adults with disabilities. In P. Sands, & M.L. Wehmeyer (Eds.), *Self-determination across the life span: Independence and choice for people with disabilities*. Baltimore, MD: Paul H. Brook Publishing.

Wilens, T.E., Spencer, T.J., & Biederman, J. (1995). Pharmacotherapy in adult ADHD. In K.G. Nadeau (Ed.), *A comprehensive guide to attention deficit disorder in adults: Research, diagnosis, and treatment* (pp. 168-190). New York: Brunner/Mazel, Inc.

CHAPTER
17

Single Women
with AD/HD

Kathleen G. Nadeau, Ph.D.
and Tanya Shuy, B.S.

W hile little has been written about women with AD/HD in
general, even less has been written about single women
with AD/HD. Sari Solden, in her book *Women with Attention Deficit Disorder*, makes barely a mention of issues for single women,
and *ADDvance*, a magazine for women with AD/HD, has published only one article on single women over the course of four
years. Neither Gaub and Carlson's (1997) meta-analysis of research
on gender issues in AD/HD nor Gershon's (2000) more recent review of gender issues reports any research on single women. Clearly,
this is an unexplored AD/HD population.

The concerns of single women have been largely ignored by
researchers, perhaps because it remains the cultural norm for
women to marry (Newtson & Keith, 1997). Single women with
AD/HD, of course, share many of the same concerns as those of
single women in general, ranging from financial security to
emotional issues such as loneliness, friendships, family, and

313

intimacy. Issues for single women with AD/HD may be more pronounced, at times overwhelming, because of AD/HD-related difficulties in creating and maintaining structure in their lives.

Most issues discussed in this chapter are also pertinent to formerly married women who have established lives as single women, as well as for those who have never married. However, the aftermath of divorce or widowhood, and the challenges of single motherhood are beyond the scope of this chapter. The challenges of AD/HD for a young unmarried female are different, yet again, from those of a single woman with an established single life-style. For a young woman, the most prominent issues are to separate appropriately from her parents and to learn to rely upon herself for life management and decision-making. A separate chapter in this text has been devoted to the challenging transition to independent living (see Chapter 15).

This chapter will focus on issues unique to single women, without reiterating issues of diagnosis and treatment that have been extensively addressed in other chapters of this volume. Because clinical experience has preceded much-needed research on the issues of single women, this chapter addresses the issues of single women based on the author's clinical experience, as well as the reports of single women with AD/HD.

Single Women with AD/HD

Whether a woman with AD/HD has consciously chosen a single life-style, has not married due to failed relationships, or is included in that growing group that chooses to marry far later than in previous generations, she faces issues of "singleness" that are impacted by AD/HD. While single women share much in common with those who are married, there are issues that are specific to this group that warrant consideration. One woman with AD/HD summarizes her experience of being single in the following way:

. . . no one will hold your hand while you stumble in the ADD fog, but no one will laugh at you either. You need to learn to be your own best friend and to take good care of yourself— there's no one else there to notice when you are running on empty. On the other hand, you have the freedom to live as it suits you and to develop the best in yourself.

(Brown, 1999, p. 22)

The single life can provide both advantages as well as great challenges for a woman with AD/HD. She doesn't face the pressures typical for most married women with AD/HD—the overwhelming demands of running a household, keeping track of children's schedules, organizing family meals, and keeping up with family laundry. Nor does she face the daily challenges of negotiating and communicating with a spouse that may not accept or understand her AD/HD. On the other hand, the single woman is more challenged by her internal disorganization. Living alone, she doesn't have the structure or support of living with others. AD/HD patterns of messiness, disorganization, night-owl habits, avoidance, and escape may dominate her existence. It's easier for her life to become out of control when no one else is there to counteract the chaos.

After a single woman receives a formal diagnosis of AD/HD, one of her most important tasks is to learn more about herself, how she is affected by AD/HD, and what sorts of life changes she needs to make in order to create an AD/HD-friendly life for herself. In addition to medication and other forms of therapy, she needs to understand her particular issues as a single woman with AD/HD.

The Importance of Work for Single Women

Although workplace issues are significant for all women with AD/HD who are employed outside the home, typically, work plays a more primary role in the lives of single women. For a single woman, work is often a primary source of meaning in her life, as well as the place where she is most often reinforced and valued. As a result, finding work that is well-matched to her strengths and interests (see Chapter 19) is a tremendous benefit for a single woman, enhancing the social and emotional aspects of single life as well.

Financial Security for Single Women

Unlike her married counterpart, a single woman with AD/HD must rely solely upon herself for her financial security. The best preparation for her to achieve economic security is to complete higher education, as earning power is strongly linked to educational attainment (Costello, Miles, & Stone, 1998). Research suggests that the educational level of adults with AD/HD tends to be less than that of non-AD/HD adults (Weiss & Hechtman, 1986; Manuzza et al., 1993), although this research is based on adult male outcomes and may not be accurate in describing women with AD/HD.

Because financial management skills are often an area of weakness for women with AD/HD, a single woman may need to make extra efforts to receive professional guidance regarding financial management and retirement planning.

AD/HD-friendly Life Choices for Single Women

When you live alone, there's no one to blame but yourself! When you're out of milk, when the rent wasn't paid, when the place is a mess, it's all up to you to take care of it. You can do what you like, but you have to take full responsibility for the outcome.

In general terms, an AD/HD-friendly life is one that:

> ◗ provides optimal levels of stimulation and stress;

▶ includes supportive relationships with friends and family;

▶ provides the structure needed to function effectively as a woman with AD/HD; and

▶ allows a woman with AD/HD to operate from her strengths on the job.

Life choices are often difficult for adults with AD/HD. The number of possibilities can seem overwhelming; often the easiest decision is to maintain the status quo. At other times, decisions may be reached very impulsively—a quick fix for the agony of indecision. Although a single woman can seek the advice of friends and family, she may have no daily, intimate connection with another person who can help with decision-making, and no one but herself to blame when the decisions don't work out well. Sometimes, this burdensome responsibility becomes paralyzing and decisions are made by default—allowing circumstances to dictate important life choices.

On the other hand, a single woman can make choices with much more freedom. She can go back to school, change jobs, spend her income as she likes, and live where she chooses. The more she understands how she is impacted by her AD/HD, the more accurate picture she has of her strengths and weaknesses, the better she understands the elements of an AD/HD friendly life-style, then the better able she is to make good decisions. While habit development and organization are often best approached through coaching, important life decisions are typically best made with the guidance of a psychotherapist who is expert in working with women with AD/HD. With the structure of regular therapy sessions, a woman with AD/HD can begin to explore options and take the individual steps (so often difficult for a woman with AD/HD) that are required to travel from wish to reality.

Social Connections and AD/HD

Some women with AD/HD become socially isolated out of shame, hiding their chaos behind closed doors. Often, a choice to live alone results from the chronic low self-esteem that is so common among women with AD/HD (Rucklidge & Kaplan, 1997). Other issues related to AD/HD can lead to lack of social connections as well. Maintaining social connections, especially between women, requires planning, consistency and follow-through—all of which are difficult for most women with AD/HD. Responding to letters, remembering birthdays, making long distance phone calls, and making plans are all part of maintaining relationships. Many women with AD/HD report that out-of-sight is out-of-mind. They discover, with regret, that they are no longer in touch with important people in their life once they've left the context of the friendship—the school, the job, the neighborhood.

Social Isolation and the Single Life

Many single women with AD/HD find that they become increasingly isolated and withdrawn in adulthood. While feelings of "not fitting in" with other females are common for girls and women with AD/HD, a woman is automatically surrounded by age-mates during high school and college years. Though she may not feel comfortable with the majority of her peers, she can often find a group of friends who are more accepting.

When school years are over, the more spontaneous social patterns of high school and college—cooking up plans on the spur of the moment, walking down the dorm hallway to strike up a conversation, hanging out all night with a couple of friends—fade away. Suddenly, she is more isolated. If she has temporarily returned to her parents' home, she finds that most of her old friends have moved away. If she has an apartment, her ready social life is reduced to a roommate (if she has one), coworkers (most of whom may be older and married), and an acquaintance here and there. Post-school social life requires taking *initiative*—something that may be difficult for a woman with both self-esteem issues and poor planning skills. Charlotte, a woman with undiagnosed, primarily inattentive AD/HD in her mid-thirties, had become increasingly isolated in her post-college years:

Now in her mid-thirties, "Charlotte" lived alone in an apartment. She had been shy throughout her life, with only one or two close female friends in high school and college. While Charlotte had been involved in several short-lived romantic relationships, issues of intimacy and sexuality felt very threatening, leading her to end each relationship before it became physical. Her pattern of self-soothing through late-night snacking had begun around puberty and had led to a significant weight problem.

Undiagnosed AD/HD had also contributed to academic struggles in college. Even after studying for many hours, Charlotte was only able to earn mediocre grades. Now, employed as a research assistant, under the supervision of a research librarian, the writing demands of her job nearly overwhelmed her. Yet, she took pride in her work and felt she'd found a quiet niche where she could avoid the stress and pace of other people's lives.

Late night was her favorite time of day, just as it had been during adolescence. Giving in to the temptation to stay up watching TV, she was often late for work in the morning, for which she compensated by working into the evening. This pattern also helped her cope with loneliness. By the time she returned home, picking up carry-out dinner and snacks along the way, it was often after 8 PM. No one ever entered her apartment to see her unmade bed, the floors covered with piles of newspapers, magazines, and unopened mail, or the mounds of unfolded laundry. No one witnessed her late-night eating. Once or twice a month, she made a trip to visit her mother, who nagged her about her weight and asked if she'd met "any nice young men." Charlotte had long ago given up on any hopes of finding a relationship.

Even this quiet, isolated life felt overwhelming to Charlotte—and overwhelmingly lonely. Her coping mechanisms—self-medicating with food, losing herself in the fantasies of television shows and romantic novels only served to further her isolation.

Socializing as an Escape

While Charlotte was a shy, quiet introvert with primarily inattentive type AD/HD, "Sandy" was an extrovert, with combined type AD/HD. In contrast to Charlotte, who withdrew into food and television, Sandy self-medicated with alcohol and escaped into a driven social life.

Sandy's high energy level and outgoing nature had been her hallmark in high school and college. She was the "party-hearty" girl who hid feelings of shame and low self-esteem behind a social facade. Her drinking began in high school, but became much heavier a few years later, after the supports in her life caved in. Her parents announced their separation just at the time when her grades were plummeting in college. With both parents suddenly feeling financial strain due to their divorce, they were unwilling to continue to pay for college in view of Sandy's low grades. Suddenly thrown into adult life with little preparation, Sandy's drinking increased. She never invited anyone into her chaotic apartment, but rather escaped to bars, restaurants, and social gatherings, where she was the life of the party. Only when Sandy was home was she forced to see how chaotic her life truly was.

A Balance that Works

Not all women with AD/HD who live alone do so from shame or defensiveness. Some choose to live alone out of a healthy appreciation of their need to manage stress. Chris was one of these women:

"Chris" was a dynamic woman in her early forties. She related that she had earned only mediocre grades in college, but had found her groove in the business world after graduation. She had been working in marketing and public relations for many years and was seen as a very creative person whose skills lay in reading people accurately and in building strong business relationships. At work, Chris had always had the insight to pair herself with people of complementary talents. She was appreciated for her abilities, and was not expected to manage the details of client relations.

Chris offered no apology for her lack of domestic skills. Housekeeping duties were performed by a cleaning service. Chris enjoyed the calm of her quiet apartment after a busy day at work. She reported, however, that she enjoyed having a "surrogate family." Her college roommate, Sally, had opted for the life of a stay-at-home mom. "Aunt" Chris enjoyed taking Sally's girls on special outings, and was included in their family's holiday celebrations. Chris admired Sally, describing her as the perfect mother and homemaker, but was clear that these were roles for which she was not suited.

Chris had achieved a balance in her life through a realistic assessment of the interpersonal responsibilities and life-management tasks she could comfortably maintain. She made no apologies for her use of bookkeepers, cleaning ladies, and concierge services to keep the practicalities of her life on track. Chris had a strong sense of her strengths, and had achieved career success through staying focused on her goals.

Building a Support System

A single woman with AD/HD needs to consciously build a social support system around her as an essential component of an AD/HD-friendly life-style. While certain supports are built into married life, a single woman must consciously create similar supports, asking herself: Who will look after me if I'm sick? Who should have a key to my house or apartment? Where will I spend the holidays if parents are deceased or family is too distant? With whom will I vacation? Whom can I call when I'm just feeling lonely or upset? Often, single adults band together, serving these functions in one another's life— forming a loose-knit surrogate family.

Women with AD/HD, however, may feel more reluctant to enter into such relationships, ashamed of allowing others intimate access to the chaos of their lives. "I'd never give anyone a key to my apartment," remarked one woman with AD/HD, "I'd hate to think of anyone seeing my mess." Other single women might fear that they are more needy, less "together" than their friends without AD/HD. "They wouldn't understand. They'd just think I'm a flake."

The Shelter of Support Groups

One solution to this AD/HD dilemma is to seek out the company of other women with AD/HD. Some have found online women's AD/HD support groups to be very helpful. One woman who had been socially isolated for years found that the purchase of a computer opened a whole world to her—a world that understood and accepted her AD/HD. Online relationships blossomed into in-person relationships with several women. Gradually, she came out of her isolation and was able to speak of her AD/HD foibles with humor rather than shame.

Out of the same need for connection, women's AD/HD support groups have sprung up across the U.S., providing a place for understanding, support, and coping skills. In some cases, these talking groups have become active support groups in which group members help one another to reorganize their homes or apartments. Others have organized around mutual AD/HD coaching— scheduling regular telephone sessions with one another to help stay on track toward meeting goals.

The Need to Build a Social Life

Single women with AD/HD need to actively build a social life. Defensiveness and low self-esteem may work against reaching out to others. Planning and organizing are difficult for women due to the executive functioning challenges of AD/HD. Often the most AD/HD-friendly way to build a social life is to join groups, clubs, or organizations that have automatically scheduled meetings and organized events, eliminating the pressure of initiating and planning social contacts.

Phyllis, a woman in her late thirties, was diagnosed with AD/HD after years of treatment for depression, anxiety, and overeating. She identified herself as the "black sheep" in a family of high achievers. For years, her only social outlets were self-help groups—Overeaters Anonymous, and a depression support group.

As she began to learn about AD/HD and to take charge of her life, she gradually identified less and less with other women in these support groups, but feared total isolation if she left them. In therapy she learned how her AD/HD made the organizational aspects of social life more difficult for her. Her therapist suggested that she gradually substitute other groups for the problem-focused groups that she had attended for so long. Phyllis became active in her church choir. A few months later, she decided to volunteer in a local political campaign.

She began to make healthier connections with others, not based around mutual struggles, but around mutual interests. As she came to feel more comfortable with her AD/HD, she learned to explain with humor, but without apology, how she was affected by AD/HD. "If you don't hear from me, it's not because I don't want to see you!" she'd explain. "Please call me again—sometimes there's just a black hole in my memory bank." She learned to do special things for friends— send an email greeting card, purchase a small surprise gift—to let her friends know she valued them, even when she wasn't always reliable in extending invitations or making plans.

"Now," Phyllis reported to her therapist, "I choose people because I like them, because they're fun, not because they have as many problems as I do. I've learned to be a good friend, in my own way, and have learned to explain my AD/HD patterns so that people aren't put off when I'm late or forget something. I make sure my friends know how much I value them, and they are happy to overlook my occasional glitches."

Romantic Relationships for Single Women with AD/HD

What's the "right" match for a woman with AD/HD? Seeking an answer is often a tumultuous quest for a single woman with AD/HD. In the stories of the women described earlier, each had reacted differently. Charlotte, shy and with low self-esteem, had chosen loneliness over potential hurt and rejection. Sandy found a different route to self-protection. Although always romantically attached, she actively avoided men who "had their act together," as she described it. Instead, she chose men who were more attracted to her than she to them, men whose lives were as chaotic as her own. Sandy ended each relationship at the first sign of discord, usually dating a man for only a few weeks or months. By contrast, Chris had been involved in several long-term relationships over the years. While she cared about the men she dated, she placed limits on these relationships, enjoying weekend dates, but keeping her weekdays free to focus on her career. Each of these relationships had ended when her partner began to want more involvement and commitment. Each of these women had opted for self-protection, and none of them had found a deep, long-term romantic connection. How can a single woman with AD/HD move beyond such costly emotional compromises to find a relationship that works?

"Lisa," a dynamic, outgoing woman in her early thirties with hyperactive/impulsive tendencies, entered psychotherapy when her most recent romantic relationship ended in disaster. She had actively dated since high school. After fifteen years of relationships that never worked out, she wanted to better understand her AD/HD patterns and how they impacted her romantic involvements. Lisa strongly desired a committed relationship. She was tired of the emotional roller coaster she'd been on for years.

Her psychotherapist, only a few years older than she, was a great match for Lisa. Because her therapist was both an expert in AD/HD, as well as a member of her generation, Lisa felt, for the first time, that she had found someone who could help her understand her relationship patterns and make better choices. In therapy, Lisa described her long history of relationships, none of which had worked out. Some men had been exciting; however, the volatility of these relationships had been their undoing. Pairing herself with an equally volatile and reactive partner had created fun times punctuated by volcanic arguments, some even physically violent. Recognizing this pattern, Lisa had, on a couple of occasions, chosen to be with men who were quiet, and introverted—a recipe for a different type of frustration since these men were incapable of meeting Lisa's need for interaction and stimulation. Jokingly, she described her dilemma as being a little like the "Three Bears." This one was too hot, this one was too cold, but she hadn't found one that was "just right."

Over the next year in psychotherapy, Lisa came to better understand that her intense self-doubts, covered over by a convincing veneer of confidence, was intimately related to her choices of partners. Although highly intelligent, she had never finished college—a fact about which she felt very defensive whenever she interacted with men who had law or graduate degrees. And, although successful in her work life, her home environment was chaotic. Thus, she tended to only choose men who had achieved less than she had, men whose own life-management difficulties would never lead them to criticize hers.

She came to realize that until she focused on herself—her self-esteem issues, her life-management skills—and could come to a place where she felt less defensive and more in control of her life, she would continue to go from one dysfunctional relationship to the next. After a year in AD/HD-focused psychotherapy, Lisa felt calmer and more self-accepting. Rather than seeing her lack of a college degree as a badge of failure, she began to seek career-related training that would strengthen her resume. Coaching from her therapist had helped her to gain better control over life-management tasks, so she was no longer embarrassed to invite someone to her home.

Through one of her business contacts, Lisa met a man for whom she felt a growing attraction as she came to know him. Like her, he had experienced many struggles in his life, and like the "new Lisa," he was clearly committed to taking his life goals seriously. For the first time, Lisa was involved with a man who could understand and accept her AD/HD tendencies, who was stimulating without being hot-tempered, and who encouraged *her to move toward her own goals. Only after she had come to terms with herself had she been able to choose a relationship that supported her personal growth.*

Life-management Resources

AD/HD Coaching to Develop Habits

Often an AD/HD coach or psychotherapist who provides "coaching" as an integral part of the psychotherapy can be very useful for a single woman with AD/HD as she learns to better manage her habits of daily living. Developing better self-care routines is essential to learning to manage AD/HD. A coach can help a single woman to develop regular sleep habits, exercise habits, good nutrition patterns, and stress-management techniques.

Professional Organizing to Gain Control

Sometimes, to gain better control over her life, a single woman with AD/HD needs more active assistance than can be provided by coaching or psychotherapy. This can often be accomplished by working with a professional organizer. An organizer can rapidly help a woman with AD/HD to "clear the decks." Trained to look at a home environment, suggest and assist in the selection of storage units, shelving, etc., an organizer can help a single woman with AD/HD to clear out her living space—sorting, discarding, and ordering her paperwork and belongings.

Of course, organization is a daily process, not an event. Crash organizing, like crash dieting, never works for long. But an organizer can help a single woman rapidly create a more ordered, livable environment. Then it becomes her task to develop the habits, with the help of a coach, organizer, or therapist, that will allow her to maintain order in her life. However, she doesn't have to do it alone. Often the expense of a cleaning service is money well-spent and will lead to a better quality of life than spending the same money on other discretionary expenditures. Some women build the expense of a professional organizer into their annual budget, planning to have repeat visits at regular intervals throughout the year. For women whose income does not allow for professional organizers, similar support can be found among friends and other women with AD/HD. Many women with AD/HD have bartered services with other women to get help with organizing. For example, one woman offered her services as a computer expert to a highly organized friend with limited computer experience. This became an enjoyable and mutually supportive relationship.

Financial Advice for "Checks and Balances"

Sometimes, the services of a professional are necessary to gain control of one's life in the financial arena. Managing finances and staying within a budget are often difficult for adults with AD/HD. As a single woman with AD/HD, there are no built-in checks and balances—no one to help maintain financial records, or to remember when bills need to be paid, and no one to help put on the brakes when impulse spending patterns spin out of control.

"Sonya" entered the workforce after college, intending to pay off her student loans before applying to graduate school. Almost ten years later, her plans for graduate school had faded into the distance. She was more in debt than ever having succumbed to the siren call of the shopping mall. Very attractive, with a figure made for the latest fashions, Sonya had fallen into the habit of impulsive and compulsive shopping. As other aspects of her life crumbled, she managed to exit from her apartment each morning carefully groomed, wearing stylish clothes. Her flawless image belied the financial chaos in her life. Bills went unpaid. She had not filed income tax returns for several years, and student loan payments were delinquent. As her anxiety over finances grew, so did her spending habits. A new outfit was a reliable "quick fix," helping her feel better while she avoided the looming problems that weren't so readily fixed. Acutely ashamed of the situation that she had created through

overspending and chaotic record-keeping, Sonya told no one, least of all her parents.

Sonya is not alone. A single woman with AD/HD may need the advice and support of a professional with financial expertise to gain control of her money issues. It is important, however, that she seek help from someone who understands the particular challenges of AD/HD. A complex filing and/or bill-paying system won't work for her. Likewise, if she is given the advice to carefully track each and every expenditure (common advice given by many financial advisors), she is almost sure to fail.

Financial advice needs to be AD/HD-friendly. For example, one simple way to gain better control of daily expenditures is to have a weekly "allowance"—a regular day to withdraw a preset amount from an ATM. Then, daily decisions become more concrete. She can simply check the cash in her wallet as she decides whether to bring lunch or buy it, whether to order a "designer" coffee or a regular. Her goal is simply not to run out of money until the next allowance day.

If she is an impulse buyer, perhaps she needs to stop her habit of window shopping, finding other ways to relax or entertain herself. If she purchases makeup, clothing, or jewelry to boost her spirits, she needs to find other, less expensive ways to feel better—calling a friend, taking a hot bath, renting a video. If her financial chaos is due to late bill-paying, she can work with her coach or therapist to develop better ways to store her bills and develop a reliable system for payment. She may find that online bill paying is more AD/HD-friendly because there is no need for envelopes, stamps, and trips to the post office or mailbox.

Her debt may be the result not of impulse purchases, but of other costly AD/HD-related patterns—unpaid parking tickets that double or triple, speeding tickets that lead to higher insurance rates, neglected car maintenance that results in very costly repairs, or late tax returns that result in interest and penalty payments. A careful analysis of the patterns that have led to financial chaos need to be undertaken to understand the AD/HD-related patterns that are the source of her financial problems before advice can be given.

Conclusion

Whether a woman with AD/HD is single by choice or circumstance, the realities of life as a single person impacts upon AD/HD issues, in both positive and negative ways. She has fewer responsibilities for others, but less support for herself. She isn't required to accommodate the needs and schedules of others, but must learn to provide her own structure to keep her daily living patterns from spiraling into dysfunction. Through working to gain a better understanding of the special challenges of being a single woman with AD/HD, she can gain the tools, and seek the resources and supports that will allow her to function at her best.

References

Brown, D. (1999). The challenge of freedom—living as a single woman with ADD: An interview with Dale Brown. *ADDvance, 2(3),* 19-22.

Costello, C., Miles, S., & Stone, A. (1998). *The American woman, 1900-2000: A century of change. What's next?* New York: W.W. Norton, & Co.

Gaub, M., & Carlson, C. L. (1997). Gender differences in ADHD: A meta-analysis and critical review. *Journal of the American Academy of Child and Adolescent Psychiatry, 36,* 1036-1045.

Gershon, J. (2000). *A meta-analytic review of gender differences in AD/HD. Journal of Attention Disorders, 5, (3),* 143-154.

Mannuzza, S., Klein, R., Bessler, A., Malloy, P., LaPadula, M., & Addalli, K. (1993). Adult outcome of hyperactive boys: Educational achievement, occupational rank, and psychiatric status. *Archives of General Psychiatry, 50,* 565-576.

Newtson, R.L., & Keith, P.M. (1997). Single women in later life. In J.M. Coyle (Ed.), *Handbook on women and aging.* Westport, CT: Greenwood Press.

Rucklidge, J. J., & Kaplan, B. J. (1997). Psychological functioning in women identified in adulthood with attention-deficit/hyperactivity disorder. *Journal of Attention Disorders, 2,* 167-176.

Solden, S. (1995). *Women with attention deficit disorder: Embracing disorganization at home and in the workplace.* Grass Valley, CA: Underwood Books.

Weiss, G., & Hechtman, L. (1986). *Hyperactive children grown up.* New York: The Guilford Press.

The Challenges of Motherhood for Women with AD/HD

Kathleen G. Nadeau, Ph.D.
and Chris Adamec

T oday, women with AD/HD are faced with some of the greatest mothering challenges ever. But before these challenges and the impact of AD/HD are addressed, a quick review of what life is like for most contemporary mothers is warranted.

Challenges for Mothers Today

Working full-time outside the home, while being a hands-on mother and homemaker inside the home is no longer called being a superwoman, now, it's just called "life." After a long day at the office, so much is expected of contemporary mothers. No matter how tough her day has been at work, she still must be "up" and ready to fulfill her child's needs, whatever they may be. Carpooling, tutoring, attending athletic events, and helping with homework are all part of the daily mix.

In previous generations, homework was the child's work. There might have been punishments or admonishments if grades faltered, but few parents felt it was their nightly duty to help their children struggle through lengthy assignments. Today, many mothers feel they should monitor, supervise, and even participate in their child's homework, special projects, and test preparations night after night.

Adding to the pressure on women, the divorce rate has grown so that nearly half of all mothers today can expect to not only work full-time while raising children, but must also cope with single parenting under these demanding circumstances. Although paternal custody of children is on the rise, it still remains customary that the mother receives physical custody of children following a divorce, even in "joint custody" cases.

If this review of contemporary mothering challenges is not already completely daunting, the picture can be complicated further by adding in the possibility of raising a child with AD/HD. Demanding homework monitoring and assistance increases, intensified by their child's frequent resistance to doing homework. A mother's already crushing schedule becomes more crowded as she tries to meet her child's special needs through school conferences, tutoring, and AD/HD treatment. With their traits of hyperactivity, disorganization, messiness, argumentativeness, forgetfulness, emotional reactivity, and difficulty falling asleep at night, these children can prove difficult for even the best of parents.

Challenges for Mothers with AD/HD

And what if a mother has AD/HD herself? This may be the case far more often than is commonly recognized. One recent study of parents of children with AD/HD found as many mothers as fathers exhibited AD/HD symptoms (Walker, 1999). A recent study (Weinstein, Apfel, & Weinstein, 1998) found that mothers with AD/HD are more likely to have neuropsychiatric disorders, and to experience problems with daily living compared to mothers without AD/HD. The great majority of women with AD/HD did not grow up understanding that they had a treatable disorder, but instead blamed themselves for the difficulties they experienced throughout their lives (Rucklidge & Kaplan, 2000). Most grew up with a pervasive sense of shame from the cumulative effect of negative messages (Solden, 1995).

When women become mothers, they are often compared, and compare themselves to an impossible ideal, the "perfect mother." Who is this paragon of perfection? The perfect mother knows where everyone's jacket is; has the laundry washed, neatly folded, and put away; has the time and date of each soccer practice and dental appointment noted on her kitchen calendar; and arrives home from work every night prepared to whip together a delicious, nutritionally balanced meal. She never yells or forgets to make sandwiches for school lunches, and never fails at anything.

Presented with this impossible set of expectations, any woman would wilt. Women with AD/HD may feel even more overwhelmed—sinking into an abyss of self-reproach and despair, losing their sense of self as they constantly strives to meet standards that seem out of reach (Ratey et al., 1995).

Sari Solden (1995), author of *Women with Attention Deficit Disorder*, refers to the role of homemaker as "the job description from hell" for a woman with AD/HD:

> *Woman wanted to coordinate multiple schedules in very unstructured, distracting atmosphere. Must be able to process great numbers of details quickly and maintain very neat and well-organized environment. Must keep track of all important occasions, including social obligations, birthday cards, and thank-you notes to many people as well as be responsible for all subtleties and niceties of life. Must be able to choose quickly and easily from a great number of options. Applicant will be responsible for all record keeping and for maintenance of all systems in the organization, as well as the upkeep on all equipment. For those interested, please call (911) n-o-t A-D-D-D. (p. 81)*

What's a Mother (with AD/HD) to Do?

This description of the multiple challenges facing mothers with AD/HD is presented not to overwhelm and discourage, but to convince both clinicians and women with AD/HD to give priority to the mother's treatment. AD/HD must be addressed as a *family* issue rather than a child issue when a mother has AD/HD. Recent parent training research has begun to emphasize the importance of supporting the mother's needs as an integral part of helping children with AD/HD (Fallone, 1998).

Although little research has been done to date on women with AD/HD, recent studies have shown that the simple fact of diagnosis can be a very positive and empowering experience, providing a woman with validation and a reason for her differences and struggles (Rucklidge & Kaplan, 2000). Many newly diagnosed mothers emerge from the experience determined to spare their children the struggles that they faced as undiagnosed, misunderstood girls.

Make Mother's Treatment a Priority

Many mothers with AD/HD will go to almost any lengths to find help for their children with AD/HD, expending limited family funds on psychotherapy, tutoring, medication, private school tuition and the like. And yet, they leave their own AD/HD untreated, acknowledging, with a smile and a shrug, that they "have it too," not feeling the same urgency to make their own treatment a priority. Professionals, more familiar with treating children, may largely ignore the mother's symptoms.

This pattern of neglecting the treatment needs of mothers with AD/HD has negative consequences for both mother and child. When a mother has untreated AD/HD, her child's AD/HD patterns can exacerbate her symptoms, leading to a downward spiral of chaos and emotional overreactions (Dixon, 1995). Because of the potential damage caused by this powerful, negative synergy, there is no more important step that a mother with AD/HD can take to help her child with AD/HD than to seek the support and treatment that will assist her in taking charge of her own AD/HD.

By getting the help she needs to simplify her life, to better order her environment, and to learn good time-management tools, she can serve as a role model for her child on how to develop habits and patterns that will minimize the negative impact of AD/HD. Research shows that mothers with AD/HD involved in parent-training significantly improve their child management skills when prescribed stimulant medication (Evans, Valano, & Pelham, 1994). Children with AD/HD need structure, consistency, patience and support. Yet most AD/HD specialists don't place emphasis on treating the mother, and on making AD/HD-friendly parenting recommendations, so that a woman with AD/HD can be calmer and more consistent in creating the home environment that can help her child thrive.

Much of the well-being and functioning in any household depends heavily upon the mother, whether she is married or single. The effects of AD/HD don't disappear once a girl with AD/HD is grown and out of school. In fact, running a household and raising children are, arguably, more challenging than academics were for these women. Children, especially children with AD/HD, need their mother to feel and function at her best. Her mood and stress level set the tone for the family.

Several studies have shown that mothers of children with AD/HD report higher levels of depression, lower confidence in themselves as parents, and greater self-blame (Barkley, 1990; Mash & Johnston, 1983). These patterns reflect the stress related to raising a child with AD/HD. Another study finds that among mothers of children with AD/HD, those who have AD/HD themselves are at much greater risk for depression than are mothers without AD/HD (Rucklidge & Kaplan, 1997). A depressed, highly stressed mother is more likely to distort or overreact to her child's problems (Chilcoat & Breslau, 1997), and less able to be an effective parent. Treatment for mothers with AD/HD must be given equal priority to treatment for her child so that she can meet her child's needs.

Get Support and Validation

Mothers with AD/HD have a strong need for their own support groups, where they can find the understanding and validation that is so crucial to their emotional well-being and growth toward leading a more effective and satisfying life. Langner (2002) writes very persuasively about the pervasive negative impact of social pressures upon women with AD/HD and their need for validation and acceptance. Solden (1995) writes that when women with AD/HD feel that they are unacceptable because they have failed to meet the cultural standards about how to behave appropriately, they often feel ashamed and withdraw from others, isolating themselves to prevent others from seeing the disorder and chaos in their physical environments. A support group for women with AD/HD can provide such women with perhaps their first supportive and accepting social environment, a place where they can learn how to take the positive steps necessary to help themselves and their children.

Set Realistic Expectations

A mother with AD/HD needs to set realistic expectations—realistic in terms of her own situation, not in comparison to non-AD/HD mothers. Setting realistic expectations is not making excuses, but is making a responsible, informed adjustment. It is the first crucial step toward creating a home environment in which she and her child can function better.

Most mothers without AD/HD live highly stressed lives—holding down full-time jobs while straining to provide their children with all of the "advantages"—often as a single parent. Women *with* AD/HD should not use these already stressed non-AD/HD mothers as models. Through therapy, support groups, and reading about other women with AD/HD, the concept of a more realistic, manageable life-style needs to emerge.

"Fran" found that she had functioned better as a single parent of two sons than she functioned following her remarriage. As a single parent, she worked only during school hours. She also received some parenting support from her ex-husband, who cared for the children two evenings a week, giving her time to relax or spend with friends. She lived in a two-bedroom apartment that required little upkeep. Laundry and housekeeping were relaxed. Suppers, several times a week, consisted of fast food takeout.

Then Fran married a successful physician. Just like Cinderella, she was transported from her modest life-style to a huge house. Within a year of being "rescued" by Prince Charming, Fran was anxious and frazzled. The expectations had gone up—way up. Her new husband, Charles, had no understanding of his wife's AD/HD, and didn't seem to "believe" in the condition. Charles had much higher expectations of his wife than she was capable of fulfilling. For example, he assumed that since Fran "didn't have to work," she should be able to manage the very complex household. He expected carefully planned meals, a beautifully kept home, and well-mannered children.

After the marriage, Charles' expectations of Fran's children increased as well. He paid private school tuition for them, and constantly pressured them to try harder to earn good grades. A year after their marriage, Fran was miserable in her new, AD/HD-unfriendly life.

This family didn't "live happily ever after" because very unrealistic expectations were suddenly imposed upon both Fran and her sons. Her new husband had no understanding of AD/HD and was unable to accept her AD/HD challenges. His approach was to repeatedly criticize Fran and her children, urging them to live up to his expectations.

Not all mothers with AD/HD live with the pressure that Fran's husband imposed on her. But, sadly, many women with AD/HD, impose unrealistic expectations upon themselves, feeling ashamed and blaming themselves for being unable to live up to these standards of perfect achievement, order, and life management. The first and most important step toward learning to manage, as a mother with AD/HD, is to step back and assess what tasks can be reasonably accomplished and to reduce expectations that will lead to certain overload.

Bring the Whole Family into the Process

If members of the family aren't part of the solution, then they are part of the problem. A family needs to work together to create an "AD/HD-friendly family" (Nadeau, 1998).

An "AD/HD-friendly family" . . .

- ▶ celebrates the best and can see humor in AD/HD foibles;
- ▶ can creatively problem-solve rather than criticize;
- ▶ looks for ways to simplify routines and solve problems;
- ▶ is patient when people are short-tempered, and accepts sincere apologies;
- ▶ focuses on the big picture and doesn't over-focus the details;
- ▶ is one in which it's OK to be yourself;
- ▶ chooses AD/HD-friendly furnishings—casual, sturdy, easy-to-maintain;
- ▶ develops reminder techniques that work for them—a family message center, sticky notes, and voice mails;

> spends time enjoying each other's company; and

> understands the need for down time and quiet
  time to counteract the stresses related to AD/HD.

Only when a mother, father, and their children all come to understand AD/HD, can they become an "AD/HD-friendly" family.

Learn to Deal with Stress

Stress is a fact of life for a woman with AD/HD. It is essential for women with AD/HD to identify stressors in their lives that can be eliminated, and to learn to anticipate high stress times and develop techniques to reduce stress.

A mother with AD/HD should familiarize herself with stress-management and stress-reduction techniques, and appreciate the importance of stress reduction as an essential method for managing AD/HD patterns in her life. She needs to give herself permission to take breaks, and to find ways to arrange those breaks. This is, of course, most difficult for single mothers. Building a support group of friends, relatives, and other mothers with AD/HD should become a priority, so that she can build breaks into her schedule.

Learn to Deal with PMS

Many women with AD/HD report that their highest stress times are related to premenstrual syndrome (PMS). PMS symptoms can sometimes become so severe that they interfere with functioning. In a woman with AD/HD, who already struggles with a compromised self-regulatory system, the "endocrine storm" caused by fluctuations in estrogen and progesterone during the PMS phase of the menstrual cycle tends to make AD/HD symptoms worse (Ratey, 1995). In addition, some women may also experience severe mood swings, irritability, and depression during this time as well. In these extreme cases, the possibility of the diagnosis of Premenstrual Dysphoric Disorder (PMDD) should be discussed with a therapist. Medication regimens may need to be altered to offer relief from increased depression, anxiety, or AD/HD symptoms during the premenstrual phase of the cycle.

Potential for Child Abuse during High Stress Periods

A mother with AD/HD may become so overwhelmed by prolonged struggles with a child, especially a child with AD/HD, that verbal or physical abuse may occur (Dixon, 1995). Many of these incidents may not be primarily triggered by the child's behavior, but rather are the result of overload in the life of the mother. Self-neglect often increases chronic stress which can, in turn, lead to emotional explosions, and even physical overreactions.

"Suzanne" had AD/HD as well as severe PMS symptoms. She was a full-time parent, raising three children, two of whom also had AD/HD. After entering treatment for her AD/HD symptoms, Suzanne tearfully and guiltily reported that she engaged in frequent verbal abuse and even occasional physical abuse of her two AD/HD children. This pattern was most likely to occur during her premenstrual week.

After long hours alone with her three children, two of whom were quite intense and insistent, Suzanne found herself yelling at the slightest provocation and locking herself in her bedroom in order to avoid spanking or slapping her children when they were provocative. Her child without AD/HD had learned to stay out of Suzanne's way when she was in a reactive mood, but her two children with AD/HD frequently became locked in a ricochet of reaction and counter-reaction with their mother. This pattern had the potential to escalate into an abusive situation.

When the gravity of the situation was explored in therapy, several approaches were suggested that Suzanne found helpful. The dosage of her antidepressant medication was increased during the latter half of her menstrual cycle to better control her PMS symptoms, as recommended by her psychiatrist.

Afternoons were Suzanne's most trying times. All three children were home together at that time, and Suzanne tended to be more tired and especially in need of a break in the afternoon. One recommendation that greatly helped Suzanne was to switch her five-year-old to afternoon kindergarten. With this arrangement, Suzanne could enjoy some relaxed time with her kindergartner in the mornings, while her nine-year-old was at school and her three-year-old was at preschool. At noon, her five-year-old went off to kindergarten as her three-year-old returned, ate lunch, and lay down for a nap. Naptime became an opportunity for Suzanne to rest for an hour. At 3:30 PM, the two older children returned from school. Suzanne was more rested and able to more calmly be "on duty" with all three children until her husband came home from work at 6 PM.

During her PMS week, Suzanne took care to arrange for an after-school mother's helper, pro-actively avoiding the increased potential for frustration and emotional explosions during this more emotionally reactive phase of her menstrual cycle.

Suzanne's husband was brought into the therapy to help him better understand the situation and his wife's urgent need for his support. During her PMS week, he agreed to come home from work early to give his wife a break. Suzanne's mother became part of the solution as well. As a result of educating her entire family about AD/HD and its impact upon her, Suzanne's mother agreed to stay over, whenever possible, during those times that Suzanne's husband had out-of-town travel. Thus, Suzanne was spared the frantic, overtired feeling of single parenting for several days at a time.

Mothering Challenges from Birth through Adolescence

A well-informed mother with AD/HD is a mother who can anticipate the particular challenges of each developmental stage, and who is aware of the community supports and resources that can help her and her child to function best in each stage.

Challenges of Being a New Mother

Before I knew I had AD/HD, I blamed myself horribly. I'd wanted children desperately and when they arrived, I felt like I was the worst mother because I couldn't handle the crying, the whining, the tugging, and the constant neediness that's involved in raising children (Adamec, 2000, p. 100).

As one mother with AD/HD recalls, "The hardest part of having a new baby is that you're always 'on'." Women toward the hypo-active end of the AD/HD continuum may find that they are especially in need of time to de-stress and to "recharge their batteries." A naturally lower energy level combined with the fatigue of caring for a newborn calls for extra support.

My AD/HD is of the non-hyperactive variety. For me, that means that I need a lot of down time. I also crave quiet and calm. If you have been blessed with a sweet-tempered, easy baby, you are indeed lucky. My babies were not "easy" babies. One had colic for three months. The other didn't sleep through the night till she was seven months old.

If such women are denied "down time," day after day, nerves can become dangerously frayed. New mothers with AD/HD who struggle with chronic stress may feel depressed, tearful, and overwhelmed, wondering if they are "terrible mothers" or if they should have had a baby at all. Regular, built-in breaks from being the "on call" parent 24 hours a day are necessary for new mothers with AD/HD in order to manage their stress level.

Postpartum Depression

Postpartum depression may be a significant risk for women during the early weeks of motherhood. During the postpartum period, estrogen levels plummet from the previous high-estrogen state of pregnancy. Women with AD/HD may be particularly vulnerable to depression, bipolar, or even psychotic episodes during this period. A woman needs to recognize the early warning signs of depression and to work with her physician to treat it before it progresses to a dangerous state.

Chronic Sleep Deprivation

Another danger for new mothers is chronic sleep deprivation,

. . . what I consider one of the toughest parts for an AD/HD mom when it comes to babies: lack of sleep!

Lack of sleep is hard on all new mothers, but sleep deprivation is especially hard on women with AD/HD. Recent research has documented that sleep deprivation, even short-term sleep loss, significantly reduces frontal lobe functioning. During such times, AD/HD symptoms may increase, along with feelings of stress that may build into full-blown depression and anxiety.

A new mother with AD/HD needs regular, frequent downtime, and a spouse who pitches in on the night shift, the early morning shift, or whatever shift will help his wife to get adequate sleep. Baby-sitters or mother's helpers are not just "nice" to have—they are *essential* for new mothers with AD/HD. A new mother can seek support through family members, cooperative childcare arrangements, and, if married, support from her spouse. It is crucial that the new mother not wait to seek support until she feels depressed, anxious, and overwhelmed—entering into motherhood with full awareness of her need for downtime is critical if motherhood is to be the positive experience that it should be.

Preschool

The preschool period can be very challenging for women with AD/HD, especially if their toddler has AD/HD as well. The "terrible twos" are a time when most new mothers experience self-doubts.

The key to raising toddlers is to learn effective parenting tools and then to use them consistently—tools such as praising good behavior, recognizing when the toddler is misbehaving due to hunger or fatigue, structuring the toddler's activities so that he does not become overstimulated or overtired, judicious use of time-outs, and anticipating potential battles so that many of them can be averted.

A woman with AD/HD may need help and guidance to develop routines, and learn effective parenting techniques. Regular meals and bedtimes are important to establish, but may pose an extra challenge for a mother with AD/HD who may have had little regularity in her daily life prior to motherhood.

While it can be very difficult for a woman with AD/HD to be consistent and focused in applying behavior management strategies, it is equally true that some of the traits associated with AD/HD can be very effective in raising toddlers. Who is better than a mother with AD/HD at coming up with surprising, unexpected behavior that can interrupt misbehavior? For example, one mother with AD/HD suddenly and impulsively stood on her head during her child's prolonged tantrum. The headstand instantly captivated the child's attention, distracting her from her tantrum. Distractions and diversions are an intrinsic part of being a mother with AD/HD—and mothers can learn to use them to their benefit.

One of the most important issues for mothers with AD/HD is to give herself guilt-free breaks from being the "on duty" parent. Many women who do not work outside the home feel that they "shouldn't" use regular day care, preschool, or baby-sitters. But, each woman differs in her ability to cope with the stress of parenting preschoolers. And some children are much more challenging than others. Each mother should work to build supports into her daily life, and give herself permission to use them!

Elementary School

As a child enters school, structured patterns become increasingly important. If a child has been in preschool, the mother with AD/HD may have already had to struggle with getting her child ready and out the door on time each morning. As a child enters elementary school, more demands are placed on both mother and child. The school arrival time is more strict, and there are lessons, sports activities, many papers to be signed and returned, and homework to be supervised.

If morning, homework, and bedtime routines can be developed and ingrained early, the middle and high school years will go more smoothly. However, such routines are difficult for women with AD/HD to establish. The mother with AD/HD needs to develop an established rising time for herself, and an organized way to prepare for *her* day before she can successfully structure her child's morning and evenings in a more predictable way.

Homework assignments become part of the pattern of daily life during elementary school years. And, if both mother and child have AD/HD, homework struggles often become "homework wars." If mother with AD/HD has difficulty structuring and supervising homework, it may be better for the child's father or a tutor to take on this responsibility. The assistance of a tutor may be particularly helpful if the child has AD/HD and experiences greater than usual difficulties in completing homework within a reasonable period of time.

Middle School

Entering middle school is often a time of greater stress and challenge for children. As the demands for academic performance increase, the demands placed on their mothers with AD/HD increase accordingly.

Middle school is challenging for other reasons as well. As a child goes through puberty, with changing hormone levels, interest in the opposite sex begins to develop as a major distraction from academics, along with the numerous lures of the teen subculture. Mother-daughter battles, influenced by fluctuating hormonal levels in each of them, tend to intensify. A mother with AD/HD should not hesitate to get all the support that she can from women's AD/HD support groups, coaches, and family therapists, as she works with her child to make the difficult transition to adolescence.

High School

The mother with AD/HD may find, as do many parents, that her child's teen years are the most frustrating and challenging. She may need help to create the structure and set the limits that her adolescent needs. Often, her greatest struggle is to maintain emotional control during conflicts with her rebellious adolescent. She may find herself reacting impulsively, making unreasonable threats, only to forget the threatened consequences once the argument has passed. If such patterns are frequent, she risks losing credibility with her teenager, with the result that setting limits becomes increasingly difficult.

A mother with AD/HD may benefit from working with a therapist around reasonable expectations and limit-setting. A therapist can help her pick her battles wisely rather than being emotionally reactive to the issue of the moment. Therapy can also be a place where she can discuss implementing reasonable consequences in a consistent fashion when her teenager is defiant or refuses to comply with limits that she has set.

High school years are fraught with many "at risk" behaviors—sexual experimentation, alcohol and drug use, cigarette smoking, and dangerous driving habits, among others. The more sources of self-esteem that a high school student has, the less likely he or she is to turn to substance abuse and sexual experimentation to achieve the social acceptance that may seem lacking elsewhere. Supervised, structured activities such as church-sponsored social groups, school clubs, competitive sports, and lessons of all kinds can be helpful in structuring their time, allowing them to socialize with their peers while still receiving adult supervision.

Raising a Child with AD/HD

Many parents of children with AD/HD blame themselves for their child's difficulties, feeling that if they were "good" or at least "good enough" parents, then their child wouldn't act the way he or she does. This pattern of self-blame is often reinforced in the community, by grandparents, other relatives, school personnel, neighbors, and other parents of children without AD/HD. It's all too easy for the parents of a non-AD/HD child to congratulate themselves for their child's compliant behavior, taking undeserved credit for their child's inborn temperament.

While mothers with AD/HD cannot avoid all misguided criticism from those around her, it is essential that she avoid destructive self-blame. Research (Barkley, 1997a) confirms that the severity of AD/HD symptoms in children has little to do with the home environment or child rearing methods, and is primarily the result of genetic endowment. As parents who have children both with AD/HD and without AD/HD know, and as researchers have well-documented (Rutter et al., 1964; Thomas, Chess, & Birch, 1968; Thomas & Chess, 1977), children arrive in this world with temperaments that differ markedly, even at birth. Studies have shown that children who are temperamentally difficult as infants are likely to develop behavior problems in toddlerhood (Earls, 1981).

Getting Professional Help

When a mother has a challenging child, such as one with AD/HD, she needs professional help to meet the challenge. Studies have also shown that treatment of children with AD/HD can have a positive impact on the mother-child relationship, and that stimulant medication can help children be more compliant. This allows mothers to be less controlling and demanding, improving the relationship for both mother and child (Barkley, Karlsson, Pollard, & Murphy, 1985).

When her child is struggling, a mother with AD/HD needs to work closely with a therapist to better understand her child and the ways in which she can be helpful. Some specific parenting skills (Edwards, 1998) have been useful in helping children with behavioral difficulties. Working with a professional can help her to maintain perspective, to not blame herself, and to learn new attitudes and parenting techniques that will help both herself and her child. It is essential for the mother of a child with AD/HD to understand that, even with her best efforts, raising a child with AD/HD is a task that would try the patience of virtually any parent. She needs to guard against expecting the impossible of herself *or* her child.

Understanding without Over-identifying

There are both advantages and special challenges when a mother with AD/HD raises a child with AD/HD. When she has AD/HD herself, a mother has a special understanding of what her child experiences and can be more empathic. Having grown up with AD/HD, she may be fiercely determined that her child with AD/HD does not experience the same struggles, criticisms, and rejections that she suffered as a child. Such strong, determined parental advocacy can be very advantageous for a child.

Some mothers with AD/HD educate themselves, in depth, about their child's educational rights and needs. They offer their child a tremendous advantage by making sure that their child's educational needs and needs for treatment are met. However, if the mother's empathy for her child crosses the line to over-identification, she may be prone to poor limit setting, to making excuses, and to giving her child the message that he or she is not responsible for misbehaviors (Nadeau, 1995).

Single Parenting

Single parenting is never easy, and a mother with AD/HD faces a double challenge as a single parent. She should look for all the supports that she can find—parent and family counseling, as well as a mother's AD/HD support group, if one exists in her community.

She should also look for creative solutions to build support systems. One mother with AD/HD shared a house with another single mother and child. That way she had adult support, someone to share cooking and childcare, and a playmate for her child. Another single mother with AD/HD arranged for a young woman to live in her home—helping with childcare, meal preparation, and carpooling.

The rule of thumb is to *try not to do it all alone.* The more support the single mother with AD/HD can find, the better off both she and her child will be.

Special Gifts that Women with AD/HD Can Bring to Motherhood

Although much of this chapter has focused on the multiple challenges of being a mother with AD/HD, it is also very true that women with AD/HD can bring much that is positive to parenting.

Because they have experienced AD/HD themselves, these mothers are often very supportive and understanding of their child with AD/HD—serving as fierce and effective advocates for their child in the school setting. They often meet the challenges of parenting, determined to raise their child with a level of understanding and acceptance that they probably didn't receive when they were growing up. While there is a danger in over-identification with the child with AD/HD, the mother who can keep her empathic responses in perspective can have a powerful, supportive, and growth-promoting influence on her child with AD/HD.

Mothers with AD/HD are often playful and creative—able to enjoy the moment with their child and to create a safe place where their child can feel nurtured and understood. One child of a mother with AD/HD said, "My mother's really cool. One day, she let us eat breakfast in a tree in the backyard. We pulled up our breakfast in a basket! My friends always like to play at my house because my mom lets us do cool stuff." Another mother with AD/HD described with glee the enjoyment that she and her children shared when she decided to wrap their Christmas gifts in highly creative ways. Her goal was to keep her sons, normally pre-Christmas snoops, utterly baffled about the contents of each package. Her sons enjoyed the game so much that they almost didn't want to end the fun by opening their gifts. Yet another mother with AD/HD describes, with pleasure, her role of confidant to many of her daughter's friends who appreciate her non-judgmental wisdom.

It can be easy for a mother with AD/HD to over-focus on her difficulties, and forget to appreciate her strengths—the warmth, acceptance, spontaneity, and creativity that she can bring to the parenting experience.

Conclusion

Mothers with AD/HD face special challenges. If she is to succeed in her multiple roles, each mother with AD/HD must develop a more AD/HD-friendly family life-style, one that takes her AD/HD-related challenges into account. Because she is likely to encounter a world of healthcare professionals inexperienced in treating women with AD/HD, she must learn to advocate for herself, seeking a professional who is open to new information, and helping to educate her therapist about the issues of women with AD/HD. Whether in individual counseling, or child and family therapy, her AD/HD must be taken into account if treatment is to be helpful. By giving priority to treatment for her AD/HD, and by learning child-management approaches that suit her, a mother with AD/HD can be a responsive, effective parent—bringing warmth and sensitivity to the challenging task of raising children.

References

Adamec, C. (2000). *Moms with ADD: A self-help manual.* Dallas: Taylor Publishing.

Barkley, R. A., Karlsson, J., Pollard, S., & Murphy, J. V. (1985). Developmental changes in the mother-child interactions of hyperactive boys: Effects of two dose levels of Ritalin. *Journal of Child Psychology and Psychiatry, 26,* 705-715.

Barkley, R. A. (Ed.) (1990). *Attention deficit hyperactivity disorder: A handbook for diagnosis and treatment.* New York: Guilford Press.

Barkley, R.A. (1995). *Taking charge of AD/HD: The complete authoritative guide for parents.* New York: Guilford Press.

Barkley, R.A. (1997). *ADHD and the nature of self-control.* New York: Guilford Press.

Barkley, R.A. (1997a). Parents as shepherds, not engineers. *The ADHD Report, 5 (6),* 1-4.

Chamberlain, R.W. (1974). Authoritarian and accommodative child-rearing styles: Their relationships with the behavior patterns of 2-year-old children and with other variables. *Journal of Pediatrics, 84,* 287-293.

Cohen, C. (2000). *Raise your child's social IQ.* Silver Spring, MD: Advantage Books.

Dixon, E. (1995). Impact of adult ADD on the family. In K. Nadeau (Ed.), *A comprehensive guide to attention deficit disorder in adults: Research, diagnosis and treatment* (pp. 236-259). New York: Brunner/Mazel

Earls, F. (1981). Temperament characteristics and behavior problems in three-year-old children. *Journal of Nervous and Mental Disease, 169,* 367-373.

Evans, S.W., Valano, G., & Pelham, W. (1994). Treatment of parenting behavior with a psychostimulant: A case study of an adult with attention-deficit hyperactivity disorder. *Journal of Child and Adolescent Psychopharmacology, 4,* 63-69.

Fallone, G.P. (1998). Parent training and AD/HD. *The AD/HD Report, 6(2),* 9-12.

Horner, B.R., & Scheibe, K.E. (1997). Prevalence and implications of attention-deficit hyperactivity disorder among adolescents in treatment for substance abuse. *Journal of the American Academy of Child & Adolescent Psychiatry, 36*, 30-36.

Huessy, H.R. (1990). *The pharmacotherapy of personality disorders in women*. Paper presented at the 143rd Annual Meeting of the American Psychiatric Association (symposia), New York.

Ingersoll, B. (1998). *Daredevils and daydreamers: New perspectives on attention-deficit/hyperactivity disorder.* New York: Doubleday.

Jones, C.B. (1989). Teachers' corner. In *Kids getting you down?* (Newsletter). San Diego: Learning Development Services.

Langner, H. (2002) The importance of social acceptance and validation for women with AD/HD. In P. Quinn, & K. Nadeau (Eds.), *Gender issues and AD/HD: Research, diagnosis, and treatment*. Silver Spring, MD: Advantage Books.

Mash, E.J., & Johnston, C. (1983). Parental perceptions of child behavior problems, parenting self-esteem, and mothers' reported stress in younger and older hyperactive and normal children. *Journal of Consulting and Clinical Psychology, 51*, 68-99.

Milberger, S., Biederman, J., Faraone, S.V., Chen, L., & Jones, J. (1997). AD/HD is associated with early initiation of cigarette smoking in children and adolescents. *Journal of the American Academy of Child & Adolescent Psychiatry, 36,* 37-44.

Murphy, K.R., & Barkley, R.A. (1996). Attention deficit hyperactivity disorder in adults: Comorbidities and adaptive impairments. *Comprehensive Psychiatry, 37,* 393-401.

Ratey, J., Miller, A., & Nadeau, K. (1995). Special diagnostic and treatment considerations in women with attention deficit disorder. In K. Nadeau (Ed.), *A comprehensive guide to attention deficit disorder in adults: Research, diagnosis and treatment* (pp. 260-283). New York: Brunner/Mazel.

Nadeau, K. (1998). *Help4ADD@HighSchool*. Silver Spring, MD: Advantage Books.

Quinn, P. (1997). *Attention deficit disorder: Diagnosis and treatment from infancy to adulthood*. New York: Brunner/Mazel.

Roizen, N.J., Blondis, T.A., Irwin, M., & Stein, M. (1994). Adaptive functioning in children with attention-deficit hyperactivity disorder. *Archives of Pediatric and Adolescent Medicine, 148,* 1137-1142.

Rucklidge, J. J., & Kaplan, B. J. (2000). Attributions and perceptions of childhood in women with AD/HD symptomatology. *Journal of Clinical Psychology, 56,* 711-722.

Rutter, M., Birch, H., Thomas, A., & Chess, S. (1964). Temperamental characteristics in infants and the later development of behavioral disorders. *British Journal of Psychiatry, 110,* 651-661.

Shaywitz, S.E., & Shaywitz, B. (1988). Attention deficit disorder: Current perspectives. In J.F. Kavanagh, & T.J. Truss (Eds.), *Learning disabilities: Proceedings of the national conference* (pp. 369-523). Parkton, MD: York Press.

Solden, S. (1995). *Women with attention deficit disorder: Embracing disorganization at home and in the workplace*. Grass Valley, CA: Underwood Books.

Thomas, A., Chess, S., & Birch, H.G. (1968). *Temperament and behavior disorders in children*. New York: New York University Press.

Thomas, A., & Chess, S. (1997). *Temperament and development*. New York: Brunner/Mazel.

Walker, C. (1999). *Gender and genetics in ADHD: Genetics matter; gender does not*. Presentation at the National Attention Deficit Disorder Association conference, Chicago.

Weiss, G., Minde, K., Werry, J. A., Douglas, V. I., & Nemeth, E. (1971). Studies on the hyperactive child, VIII: Five-year follow-up. *Archives of General Psychiatry, 24,* 409-414.

Weinstein, C.S., Apfel, R.J., & Weinstein, S.R. (1998). Description of mothers with AD/HD with children with AD/HD. *Psychiatry, 61,* 12-19.

Willerman, L., & Plomin, R. (1973). Activity level in children and their parents. *Child Development, 44,* 854-858.

ISSUES AND CHALLENGES FOR WOMEN WITH AD/HD

CHAPTER 19

Women with AD/HD
in the Workplace:
The Glass-Block Ceiling

Wilma R. Fellman, M.Ed., LPC

A D/HD is a life-span condition, with major implications for all areas of life functioning, including the workplace. Research to help us understand the impact of AD/HD on workplace functioning and the strategies, accommodations, and career choices that can optimize functioning at work is clearly needed. Statistics demonstrate that, among the college population, AD/HD is one of the most commonly reported conditions (Henderson, 1999). Four short years after entering college, this wave of college students with AD/HD enters the workforce. Many more never enter college, or complete only a few courses before dropping out. As these young adults with AD/HD enter the workplace, they have little information or assistance to guide them in making a good career choice, and their employers have even less information available to help them appropriately place and supervise them. Older adults with AD/HD also abound in the workplace, often undiagnosed, never understanding the reasons for their chronic under-functioning, or frequent job-hopping.

This chapter will explore the issues and challenges faced by women with AD/HD in the workplace, as well as ways in which they can empower themselves to identify and overcome workplace challenges, while building on their strengths and positive attributes. As is true in most aspects of working with adults with AD/HD, the information in this chapter is based on the clinical experience of the author, and of those few other authorities in the field who have written about adult AD/HD workplace issues.

Women with AD/HD who experience workplace difficulties often begin a career consultation by asking, "What is a good job for someone with AD/HD?" The answer to this simple question, however, is complex. There is no single solution that will fit all women with AD/HD. Women with AD/HD are wonderfully unique individuals with varying combinations of strengths and challenges. Solutions will be as diverse as the women who seek them, tailored to each woman's specific areas of strength. With some attention to understanding herself better, a woman with AD/HD can move forward from a position of both greater strength and comfort. "Marisa" expresses many workplace concerns common to women with AD/HD:

"I worry about my career. I've always tried to do a good job at work, but I think I'm a duck out of water! I hide how much time everything takes me to do. It makes me feel totally inadequate. I have poor memory-retrieval skills. I'm ashamed when my boss asks me a simple question about recent work, and I can't even remember having done it! I do try hard, but I think I'm not suited for being an executive assistant. They expect me to organize them! What a joke! I need a different job that allows me to be me, without always feeling stupid and totally inadequate."

"Marisa" is a bright, 31 year-old female with AD/HD. Try

as hard as she may, she cannot seem to rise above the barriers that prevent her from doing her best at work. She is frustrated, which has led her to the erroneous thought that she wouldn't be good at anything. She concludes that she might as well just stay in her current job and continue to "play the losing game." Marisa thinks she has no other options. She sees the glass ceiling above her, and believes that she'll only be able to go up "just so far."

The Glass-block Ceiling

The "glass-block ceiling" is a concept that refers to subtle, invisible barriers that often prevent females in the workplace from moving up as far as their male counterparts. Because of the traditional roles of wife and mother, and the expectations that come with these roles, women have been fighting the home vs. career balancing act probably since Eve attempted to leave the cave to help bring home the bacon! For women with AD/HD, the potential workplace barriers are far from subtle, and oftentimes appear overwhelming. Many women with AD/HD experience constant frustration, with little hope of penetrating through the "glass-block ceiling" that prevents them from reaching their true potential.

The Changing Workplace Environment

Jeremy Rifkin (1995) explores what it takes to be successful in our rapidly changing workforce. He indicates that work as we knew it, 40 hours a week for one company for a lifetime, is being phased out. Instead, we find that many more people have what he calls, "a portfolio career." Increasing numbers of people are choosing to work 20 hours at one place and perhaps 10-20 hours somewhere else. Rifkin refers to this shift in the workplace as "the beginning of a great social transformation and a rebirth of the human spirit." The very thought of workplace structures opening up to accommodate individual differences is a comforting idea for women with AD/HD.

What Do Employers Look for in the People They Hire?

While being comforted by Rifkin's view that the corporate world is becoming more flexible, it is still important for individuals to understand what it will take to be successful in this rapidly changing workforce. Below is a list of the 20 most valued qualities that employers seek in an employee (adapted from the New York State Employee Survey of Workplace Skills, 1996).

1. Excellent communication skills
2. A positive attitude
3. A good work ethic
4. Honesty
5. Motivation for continued learning and development
6. Good problem-solving skills
7. Creativity
8. Intelligence and education
9. High energy and stamina
10. A team player who works well with others
11. A flexible/adaptable worker
12. Reliability
13. Punctuality
14. High productivity
15. Accuracy
16. Good common sense
17. Good balance of responsibilities

18. Above-average performance

19. Attention to detail

20. Good attendance

In the process of thinking about a good job match, a woman with AD/HD can benefit by using this list to assess herself in terms of these qualities. It is helpful to keep a record of this self-assessment, along with examples, for future reference and self-esteem building. The qualities that she believes she lacks are the very ones that she should begin to develop. Such a self-assessment can often be best accomplished by working with a therapist, coach, or career counselor. Such support can help a woman work on one quality at a time and work at it until success becomes automatic. Few individuals possess all of these qualities, and the woman with AD/HD should not despair if she finds herself lacking in several of them. She should simply work on developing those "good employee" qualities that may be weak, while emphasizing her strengths more than her failings.

One Woman's Story: Finding a Job that Matches Her Strengths

"Clara" is a 38-year-old mother of two daughters. When her youngest child was diagnosed with AD/HD at age six, Clara's AD/HD was also diagnosed. At that time, Clara began to understand why the struggle to balance her life caused her so much burnout. She expected that she could be the perfect wife, mother, daughter, friend, neighbor, school helper, and paralegal. Clara's balancing act resulted in total frustration on all fronts. She had little energy left to be an engaging wife; she could barely keep things organized enough to get her two daughters out to school everyday; and her work as a paralegal suffered badly from her lack of skills in organization, attention to detail, and memory. Clara always felt like a fake. She had trouble focusing on any of the areas of her life, and couldn't see a way out of this downward spiral.

While she sought counseling for her AD/HD issues, it was suggested that Clara work with a career counselor in an effort to evaluate the degree of match between her job and her strengths/challenges. She did so, and discovered that her job wasn't exactly a bad match. However, it appeared that the environment in which she was working as a paralegal required her to excel in the very areas that she felt most deficient. At the end of each workday, she was totally spent, with no energy to face the responsibilities of home and family.

Clara learned that she worked best if she were under fewer time restraints in order to allow herself more leeway to remember, plan, organize, and carry out her duties. Moving from a highly competitive law firm to a nonprofit organization allowed her the breathing room she needed. Without such emphasis on rapid turnaround, Clara felt more relaxed, more self-assured, and much more capable of doing her job as she had been trained. Her self-esteem benefited from the switch. She learned that sometimes a small change can be all that is needed in order to feed her energy at the end of the day instead of drain it. While it didn't solve all of her problems at home, it did leave her with more fuel to deal with them, and she felt that progress had definitely been made.

Traditional Jobs for Women Are Often Poor Matches for Those with AD/HD

According to the U.S. Department of Labor and Statistics (1999-2000), women comprise between 46 to 48 percent of the current workforce. While women continue to be employed in traditional work settings, including administrative support, nursing, or teaching, a myriad of options are open today for women to consider. Many women still enjoy more traditional careers, especially when they are in keeping with their strengths. But when traditional careers aren't a good match, an expanded menu of choices is available to women, including "non-traditional" job titles typically held by men, such as truck driver, electrician, plumber, physician, and CEO. In fact, the term "non-traditional" has less meaning today, as women move into every possible area of the workplace. For women with AD/HD, making the right choice has less to do with tradition than it does with finding a good match for her strengths that allows for individual challenges.

AD/HD, according to the *Diagnostic and Statistical Manual of Mental Disorders: Fourth Edition (DSM-IV)* (1994), often results in problems with distractibility, inattention to detail, disorganization, difficulty following through on tasks to completion, and difficulty paying attention when listening, to name but a few. In considering these symptoms as they relate to jobs traditionally held by women, such as administrative support staff, nurse, or teacher, it is easy to understand why these jobs may not be a good match for a woman with AD/HD. To excel in these careers requires outstanding skills in organization, attention to detail, and a good memory.

It was once thought that, by virtue of being a female, one would automatically possess these qualities and excel in these fields. What happens when the female has AD/HD and finds it a nightmare to organize herself, not to mention someone else? What happens when the price for being detail-oriented means that a woman with AD/HD is devoid of energy by the end of each day, and her strenuous efforts only enable her to do a less than average job? What happens when memory issues can be a matter of life and death, as they are in some aspects of health care? The stress and strain that results from forcing a square peg into a round hole is what happens when it is assumed that a female with AD/HD should still be a "great little gal Friday," and needs to struggle to cover up her failures. Sari Solden (1995) has written extensively about the high price paid by women with AD/HD as they struggle to conform to roles for which they are ill-suited.

Unrecognized Pluses of AD/HD for Women

It is often thought that AD/HD is not only accompanied by challenges, but brings strengths as well. Lynn Weiss (1996), an author and AD/HD expert, has written extensively on this topic. For example, one woman, self-described as "the poster-woman for AD/HD," was able to hyperfocus so well (a capacity reported by many individuals with AD/IID) that she became a very successful corporate accountant. She was able to tune out the world while she mentally dove into her work, achieving a flawless accounting reputation. Another woman, who grew up feeling "flaky" because she wasn't able to focus on projects for long periods of time, found that she worked very well at the creative end of a major advertising company. Her campaigns were described by upper management as some of the most "out-of-the-box" ideas the company ever presented to a satisfied client. (No one needed to know that she had enlisted the help of a coach to keep her on a timeline track. All they saw was a most successful result, and everyone was happy!) It is important that women with AD/HD explore how they are affected by AD/HD, and how those qualities may even become assets in the right work setting.

Finding Solutions: Three Levels of Change

Nadeau (1995) writes that when an individual with AD/HD encounters difficulty on the job, she has several options:

1) better adapt to the job that she has, 2) look for a different job within the same career path, or 3) search for a different career that better matches her strengths and challenges.

Making a Current Job More AD/HD-friendly

A career counselor can work with a client to make her current job more AD/HD-friendly. Often, by learning coping strategies and engineering certain changes at work, a woman with AD/HD can learn to function much more effectively.

Nadeau (1995) also lists a number of strategies that can be helpful in creating AD/HD-friendly changes on the job:

1. Becoming informed about AD/HD;

2. Making an accurate AD/HD self-assessment;

3. Seeking appropriate help for AD/HD;

4. Learning techniques to minimize AD/HD symptoms;

5. Recognizing and using positive traits; and

6. Learning how to appropriately self-advocate.

The last strategy, self-advocacy, may be particularly difficult for women with AD/HD. Solden (1995) writes about the difficulty that many women with AD/HD experience in advocating for themselves due to feelings of shame or guilt. When this is the case, counseling may be important in helping her overcome these self-doubts and move forward to make the changes that she needs.

Wrong Job, Right Career Path

In the case of Clara, her role as a paralegal was often described to her as the "gal Friday of the legal world." She was expected to research and focus on several cases, keep all details straight, synthesize the data into reports, and provide timely results to those who competed in a high-profile law market. Clara had undergone extensive paralegal training and was disheartened to think that she had made a terrible mistake in her career choice. In working with her career counselor, she discovered that the major difficulties she encountered had less to do with her career path than with the current work environment. After she changed jobs, to work in a charity-oriented legal service, she found that the people she supported were more understanding of individual differences and gave her more time in which to complete her tasks. For Clara, this made all the difference. As her stress level was decreased, she had more success in compensating for her AD/HD-related challenges.

A career counselor can help a woman with AD/HD to evaluate the barriers to success that she experiences in her current job. Together, they can consider whether a similar job in a more AD/HD-friendly setting may be the solution to her workplace dilemma.

Changing Career Paths

What happens, however, when a woman with AD/HD finds that it's not just her particular job, but her career field in general that is a bad fit? The degree of match between a woman and her career can be evaluated systematically. The best approach is to begin by considering what is "right." A career counselor can assist a woman with AD/HD to list her strengths. Then, using the systematic approach outlined below, they can work together, evaluating the degree of match between her profile of strengths and challenges and several alternate career choices.

Some women begin with the assumption that they should stay away from any kind of job that requires sitting still, doing detailed work, or utilizing memory. Eliminating options using such a broad brush approach might rule out some wonderful career opportunities. The most consistent thing about AD/HD is its inconsistency. AD/HD can manifest quite differently in individual women. Therefore, it would be a mistake to eliminate career choices that may, on the surface, seem a bad match for someone with AD/HD.

Breaking through the Glass-block Ceiling

To break through the glass-block ceiling and make choices that can help you reach your true potential, four critical steps are involved:

1. Identify areas of strength.

2. Identify areas of challenge.

3. Identify potential accommodations, modifications, or adaptations.

4. Assess the degree of match with each career being considered.

Identify Areas of Strength

Each individual is multi-faceted. When considering areas of strength, a woman with AD/HD should consider all facets of herself, including her:

- interests and passions—(What "lights me up?");

- aptitudes and abilities—both innate and learned;

- personality factors—(What personality type am I and what jobs are matched with the needs of that personality type?);

- energy patterns—(Do I work in spurts or plod along?);

- accomplishments—(What have been high points for me so far?);

- skills acquired from life and from other jobs; and

- values—(What are my driving forces, personally and professionally?).

Identify Areas of Challenge

Each woman should take a look at any special challenges, including those symptoms related to AD/HD that are the most limiting. Nadeau (1995) provides a detailed list of potential AD/HD workplace difficulties that can assist in this assessment process. A woman with AD/HD should add to this list any of the qualities that she feels she are lacking when comparing herself to the list of traits most sought by employers, discussed earlier.

Identify Potential Accommodations, Modifications, or Adaptations

Once a woman with AD/HD has made a list of her challenges, she should allow her support professional to help her examine these potential problem areas, evaluating whether there are accommodations/modifications that can offset each challenge. She should not discount a career option until she's taken the time to see if her areas of challenge can be minimized or even erased by suitable strategies.

"Lindsay" had always imagined herself as a physician. She worked hard in school and earned good grades. An adult with AD/HD, Lindsay found life increasingly difficult once she finished school and began to practice medicine. She was suddenly required to juggle the multiple roles of business owner, practitioner, employer, and member of the medical society. Her self-esteem dropped to an all-time low. She began to believe she had chosen the wrong field and dreaded the idea of admitting this to her parents, who had sacrificed to help her get through medical school. After working with a career counselor, Lindsay found that by adopting simple strategies in her everyday work routine, she could manage all aspects of her chosen profession . . . and be good at it!

With the proper modifications to her workday, Lindsay began to relax and enjoy the practice of medicine. Building in the structure and support she needed, her career could work for her. Strategies she used included:

- choosing her office management staff carefully, selecting someone with those qualities that Lindsay herself lacked;

- using a beeping watch—to compensate for poor time-management skills;

▶ taking 15 minutes at the start and end of each day for reflection and planning;

▶ delegating tasks that were most efficiently handled by staff; and

▶ using an executive coach, who kept Lindsay on-track with short and long-term strategic planning.

Lindsay considered the fees paid to her executive coach part of "the cost of doing good business." She saw this person as a type of business partner, and did not consider herself weak for benefiting from this level of support.

Self-esteem can be enhanced with the proper framing of a situation, or it can suffer from an erroneous assumption that to accept help is to be less than strong. The truly strong recognize that supports can help to break through the glass-block barriers that women with AD/HD face every day.

Test Out the Degree of Match

When a woman with AD/HD and her career counselor determine that her job is a good match, then support services should be put in place. Such was the case with Lindsay. She found that with the proper support, she could soar to her greatest potential. What would have happened if she had discovered that even with accommodations, modifications, and strategies, the glass-block ceiling would never shatter? Then she would have had to consider other options.

The most helpful approach, when a woman realizes that she has made a poor job match, is to begin at the assessment process and consider other options. When a woman with AD/HD is poorly matched with a job in terms of her strengths, her self-esteem suffers doubly—from her initial decision-making error and also from her inability to make things work. It's helpful for a woman with AD/HD to remind herself of all of the positives—things that are going well—and begin to build upon them. Successful feelings build upon themselves and soon, new career options that present themselves can be considered.

A great way to "try out" a potential career match is for a woman with AD/HD to immerse herself in that career environment to see how it feels. Perhaps she can work as a volunteer to learn more about the environment. An internship can also provide invaluable information about whether or not the career being considered will allow her to lead with her strengths. If there is insufficient time to do either of the above, she should observe as much as possible and talk to people in similar positions, who can give her realistic information.

Identify and Secure Needed Support Systems

Once a career decision has been made, it's important to insure that it will work in the long run by analyzing support systems that may be needed to maintain the optimal quality of work. Not everyone needs the same supports, however, the following list represents supports that can make or break long-term success on the job:

1. **Ongoing accommodations/modifications and strategies—** These will help take the barrier out of the task. (These include memory aids, "white noise" devices, taking frequent breaks, watches that beep as reminders, etc.)

2. **Coaching**—Coaching can often make the difference between success and failure. If professional athletes, who are talented and gifted in their job, require a coach, why shouldn't women with AD/HD? Coaches frequently operate over long distances by phone or email to keep their client on-track. This is often very affordable and should be considered a long-term support system. There are many web sites that

give information on coaching and how to locate a coach that may work well with the individual woman with AD/HD.

3. **Counseling**—If a woman with AD/HD finds that she struggles with feelings of inadequacy and low self-esteem due to previous failures, she can give herself a wonderful gift by entering into counseling or therapy. This can clear out "old business" and allow her to move ahead as a much stronger person.

4. **Mentoring**—Nearly every successful career woman states that there was at least one influential person in her life. Such positive forces are powerful guides that direct us toward our strengths, and help us deal with our challenges. For women with AD/HD, the idea of a mentor is especially helpful. Such an individual can teach a woman to avoid the pitfalls that she may not be able to see from where she sits.

Working from a Position of Strength and Comfort

Dr. Lynn Weiss (1996) writes that to be successful in the workplace, a woman with AD/HD should keep in mind that:

- As many assets as liabilities come from AD/HD.

- Not everyone with AD/HD is the same. You'll have your own special combination of AD/HD traits.

- Knowing how your AD/HD affects you is empowering.

- Appreciate your AD/HD, and it will work on your behalf.

- You can be responsible for your AD/HD.

- It's helpful to find someone to help you plan and structure your life.

▶ You shouldn't be afraid to follow your dreams, even when they are big ones.

▶ You can have AD/HD and be successful.

▶ Everyone has innate talents and gifts that the world and the people in it need.

With knowledge comes power. With self-knowledge comes understanding, acceptance, and forgiveness. Once a woman with AD/HD identifies her strengths, she can build upon them, and move forward with a sense of calm—making career decisions that are appropriate for her. As she feels better about herself, she can begin to tackle the glass-block ceiling. With better self-knowledge, she'll be able to move ahead with enough self-assurance to reach her true potential. The task for a woman with AD/HD is to collect as much information as she can, make a good decision, and then, put in place those support systems that will enable her to carry out her career goals with fewer barriers.

References

American Psychiatric Association. (1994). *Diagnostic and statistical manual of mental disorders* (4ᵗʰ ed.). Washington, DC: Author.

Fellman, W. R. (2000). *Finding a career that works for you.* Plantation, Florida: Specialty Press, Inc.

Henderson, C. (1999). *College freshman with disabilities: A biennial statistical profile.* Washington D.C.: Heath Resource Center.

Morrison, A. M., White, R., & Velsor, E. (1988). *Breaking the glass ceiling.* Cambridge, MA: Perseus Publishing.

Nadeau, K. (1997). *ADD in the workplace.* New York: Brunner/Mazel.

New York Association of Training and Employment. (1996). *New York state employee survey of workplace skills.* Albany, NY: Author.

Rifkin, J. (1995). *The end of work.* New York: Putnam.

Solden, S. (1995). *Women with attention deficit disorder: Embracing disorganization at home and in the workplace.* Grass Valley, CA: Underwood.

U.S. Department of Labor, Bureau of Statistics. (1999-2000). *Occupational outlook handbook.* Washington, DC: Author.

Weiss, L. (1996). *ADD on the job: Making your ADD work for you.* Dallas: Taylor Publishing.

CHAPTER 20

Back to School for Women with AD/HD

Joan Shapiro, Ed.D.

For many women with AD/HD and/or learning disabilities (LD), school years were often completed without benefit of diagnosis and treatment. Because they did not understand the nature of their problems, many of these women were academic underachievers, either never attending college or never graduating from college. However, several very positive changes have occurred in recent years, leading to increased opportunities for women to earn a college or postgraduate degree.

First, there is a significant increase in the number of adults returning to college or university to further their education, including increasing numbers of women with AD/HD and/or LD. In response, most colleges and universities now have programs for students with disabilities that offer a range of supports and accommodations that are considered to be critical for success. Second, courses are available in the evening hours to accommodate women who work or who care for children during the day. To-day, in many parts of the country, it is possible to earn all of the credits for a college degree by taking evening courses, and now the computer age has generated online courses as well. Finally, as AD/HD and LD in adults and in women are recognized and understood, it is easier for women to address these issues and explore treatment options, including counseling, tutoring, coaching, medication, and psychotherapy. These supports help women better understand their struggles and equip them with effective coping strategies that allow them to return to school and experience a new level of success.

This chapter focuses on the issues and opportunities for women with AD/HD and/or LD who desire to return to school in order to increase their career opportunities and earning capacity as well as their self-esteem and personal fulfillment.

Changing Educational Goals for Women

In more advanced industrialized societies such as the United States, education and achievement are held in high regard. A college degree is considered critical to professional advancement and improved job status, especially in an information-based, highly technological society.

The value placed on education influences both men and women as they look to pursue educational goals and the right careers. But do these values affect women differently than men? It seems they do. Marriage and raising a family have been traditional goals. As such, women have been expected to fulfill the cultural stereotype of the competent wife and mother. However, particularly during the last quarter-century, many women are rejecting this stereotyped role as too limiting. Instead, many women are taking the initiative to attain new levels of independence and competency at home, in school, and in the work force. For example, increased numbers of women are returning to college or graduate school (Digest of Education Statistics, 2000). Of this group, many are helping to support families or themselves as single women. More and more women are striving to achieve academic and occupational success as well as personal satisfaction.

The Challenges of Returning to School for Women with AD/HD or LD

Returning to school as an adult is a difficult step, requiring risk-taking and the ability to meet new challenges. These challenges mean that one has to juggle multiple responsibilities while taking on the role of a student. Returning to school involves learning new, challenging material and coping with a demanding schedule. In many cases, adults must relearn mathematical rules or formulae, or brush up on rusty writing skills. Just keeping up with course material, examinations, and written papers can be overwhelming. While women succeed in these endeavors, they often have to reach out for a support system, even though asking for help may seem difficult.

Returning to school for women with attention deficit/hyperactivity disorder (AD/HD) is often further complicated by a history of underachievement, attentional problems, and academic difficulties, and in many cases learning disabilities (LD). Those who attend college may become overwhelmed by the work demands and withdraw from school. Many do not understand why they feel afraid, why tasks are so difficult, or why work takes them so much longer than it does for their friends. Many of these women have not yet been appropriately diagnosed, and therefore have little understanding of the nature of their problems.

In addition to school-related issues, heightened anxiety and low self-esteem are often seen in women with AD/HD and/or LD. Discouragement and frustration from persistent failure often erodes a woman's confidence and negatively affects her motivation, making it difficult to initiate and sustain the effort needed to reach her goals. Some women with AD/HD report that they have particular problems with self-confidence and family relationships. There are data pointing to a higher incidence of depressive episodes and associated low self-esteem in females than in males (Rucklidge & Kaplan, 1997). The added burden of a learning disability certainly contributes as well to a woman's negative estimate of her competence

Lack of self-confidence is also related to what researchers have identified as passivity or "learned helplessness" (Deshler, Ellis, & Lenz, 1996). Learned helplessness is strongly associated with persistent and negative early experiences, particularly difficulties with schoolwork. These experiences are in many cases attributed to "not being smart" rather than to specific learning problems. Many women find it difficult to break through what Solden (1995) calls "internal barriers." They are reluctant to ask for help because of feelings of shame, guilt, and embarrassment, as well as passivity. As a result, many women do not reach out for help, and never receive diagnosis or treatment for their learning challenges.

The expectations and demands of family, friends, and employers can feel overwhelming. Repeated admonitions to "try harder" or "get organized" only make women feel worse, particularly when they know how much effort, caring, and time has been put into their work. This type of feedback undermines confidence, and only serves to verify negative self-perceptions. The psychological support and reinforcement that are so critical are often unavailable.

Clearly, the environment that a student lives and works in influences and helps to shape her learning patterns, behavior, and sense of self. The type and quality of support provided both at school and within the home are considered to be strong determinants of success, not only in school, but also in work and personal life. A supportive family and appropriate professional intervention may make all the difference in helping a woman compensate for learning challenges.

AD/HD and Learning Disabilities

Women with AD/HD may have problems with inattention, impulsive behavior, and feelings of restlessness. In many cases, they have experienced school-related problems such as poor reading comprehension. Often, they have not learned to approach problems strategically. A subgroup of women with AD/HD also suffer from a learning disability. Barkley (1990) reports that over 30 percent of AD/HD children have a learning disability, and more than 50 percent of children with AD/HD are considered to be underachievers in school. AD/HD is also reported to be a secondary pattern among dyslexics (Pennington, 1991). AD/HD and LD are different disorders with distinct symptom clusters. Both disorders persist into adulthood, though the pattern and severity of the symptoms change. While one does not cause the other, they are often seen together in the same individual. In fact, LD is the most common condition coexisting with AD/HD.

A learning disability is an umbrella term that includes different subsets of problems. These may include difficulty with reading decoding, reading comprehension, written expression, mathematical reasoning or calculations, and oral language. A learning disability is caused by specific dysfunction in the central nervous system.

A core problem common to both AD/HD and LD is weak "executive functioning" that contributes to poor self-regulation. It is suggested that each of us has our own "executive" centered in the frontal cortex of the brain that directs and controls cognitive actions and regulates behavior, much like a CEO of a large corporation. If the "executive" is efficient and aware of the skills and strategies needed to accomplish a task, the appropriate plan of action can be put into effect. If a plan is unsuccessful, then the "executive" re-evaluates and initiates a new or modified course of action.

Individuals who have AD/HD and/or LD have a less efficient "executive," and are therefore less able to generate and use effective strategies in their personal and professional lives. For example, many women with AD/HD are disorganized and have difficulty planning ahead. Planning involves the ability to determine the outline of a task and the skills it will require to reach a known goal. Planning helps us generate strategies and know when to ask for outside help. When tasks are new or complex or when there are competing demands, active planning is needed.

Poor self-regulation also shows up as an inability to manage one's time effectively to accomplish something on schedule. For example, many college students do not leave sufficient time to research and write a term paper, and find themselves frantically completing it the night before it is due. At work, one may delay writing a budget or marketing report, finding it hard to begin. At home, one might find it hard to plan and coordinate children's schedules or to anticipate or delegate tasks.

A weak executive function leads to problems with initiation and control of learning and behavior. Such problems tend to be persistent. While many individuals get by in high school, college represents a significant shift in overall demands, including greater academic competition and significant increases in the level of difficulty and amount of work. There are also limited support systems, along with the loss of a protective environment. These changes place more demands on the student, requiring her to be more independent and shoulder more responsibility. The need for and use of "executive" planning is critical. But given the complex set of psychological and learning problems, women with AD/HD or LD cannot always manage and cope with these demands effectively. To succeed, she must be able to talk to professionals and look for appropriate help.

Assessment

The first step in getting appropriate help is an assessment for learning and attentional problems. An assessment includes a range of tests needed to determine the nature of the problem(s). This data helps professionals target problems and recommend the right type of support. The assessment explains why one's performance may be inconsistent, why reading comprehension and writing may be weak, and why planning and organization are such a struggle.

Such an assessment is necessary if a woman plans to return to school and requires documentation for accommodations. An assessment is particularly important for women with AD/HD since there are lower rates of identification in girls. Typically, girls with AD/HD are not always brought to the attention of school personnel; only those with more severe attentional and academic problems are targeted for help (Biederman et al., 1999). While there is heightened awareness of this disparity, many girls still fall between the cracks. Thus, for many women, their AD/HD is not diagnosed until adulthood when they seek assessment for learning problems in preparation for college level work.

While the diagnosis and recommendations for intervention are essential features of the assessment, the process also helps an individual become educated about her disability as well as the more subtle problems that may interfere with learning. Evidence strongly points to the fact that such knowledge is critical if one is to be proactive, take control, and develop a sound and realistic set of personal goals. These goals are different for each individual and range from working toward an academic degree, seeking advancement at work, participating in a support program, or just developing specific skills and strategies.

Goals of the Assessment Process

1. To develop a current profile of strengths and weaknesses to determine whether an individual has a disability.

2. To recommend appropriate supportive intervention.

This includes instruction geared to the development of skills and strategies or referral to other professionals. Most professionals agree that one of the major roles of assessment is the recommendation of needed interventions.

3. To evaluate and monitor progress following the assessment.

Types of Assessment

Psychoeducational and neuropsychological assessments have traditionally been used for both children and adults. Although the neuropsychological approach is gaining in popularity, the psychoeducational approach is used more often. Both approaches look at a range of behaviors, abilities, and skills and use the pattern of strengths and weaknesses to diagnose a learning disability or associated problems. A psychologist or learning disabilities specialist, or the two working as a team, performs a psychoeducational assessment.

The assessment includes both standardized and non-standardized tests. Psychological testing typically includes a test to measure intelligence or cognitive abilities, such as verbal reasoning, vocabulary knowledge, memory, and perceptual-motor skills. The Wechsler Adult Intelligence Scale—III (Wechsler, 3rd Edition, 1997) is the most widely used intelligence scale for adults.

The psychological evaluation may also include tests to evaluate problems in psychological functioning that may negatively impact academic success. Often, a general screening test is used, and if test responses suggest areas of concern, more in-depth psychological evaluation may be recommended.

The educational part of the assessment includes a broad array of tests to measure skill development in the academic areas as well as the ability to process and use language. Academic skills include: reading (word recognition, phonological processing, vocabulary knowledge, and comprehension of text) and written expression (organization of content, use of vocabulary, grammar, and spelling). Language tests tap auditory comprehension needed to process classroom lectures, verbal directions, as well as knowledge of vocabulary and the ability to understand and use grammatical structures and rules.

Professionals involved in the assessment process analyze and synthesize the information in order to develop a profile of strengths and weaknesses that is used to determine whether an individual has a learning disability. The discrepancy formula is the most commonly used criterion for diagnosing a learning disability. This criterion requires a significant difference between one's ability, measured by an intelligence test, and one's level of achievement.

Information from the test profile is used to develop recommendations for instruction or other types of intervention. To be effective, recommendations must be a "good fit" with an individual's needs and goals. Two types of recommendations are generally provided. The first type focuses on specific guidelines for instruction or accommodations: suggestions for material, or techniques for teaching skills and strategies. Accommodations might include the use of a tape recorder for meetings or lectures, or extended time for tests or work projects. The second type of recommendation provides referral information that might include a support program within a college setting or referral to other professionals.

The assessment helps a woman understand the nature of her learning problems. For example, she might learn that reading problems, such as phonological errors, which result in sound substitutions or difficulty blending, or problems with reading comprehension are at issue. Certainly, her difficulty in comprehending and retaining facts becomes more critical in a college setting where the language and meaning of the text is more complex, when tasks are lengthy, and when she does not use strategies to help construct meaning and improve her comprehension. Problems with reading comprehension can interfere significantly with college or graduate level work or job responsibilities.

An assessment might show, for example, that a woman with AD/HD has difficulty processing information in lectures or meetings. She may have trouble initiating a writing task, because she does not organize her ideas before beginning. Often, her ideas are not well-developed, vocabulary is repetitious, and spelling and/ or grammatical errors may be evident. Problems with mathematics may show up as well in an assessment.

Reading problems are often found in women with AD/HD as well as those with LD. Reading is a complex, dynamic process. The successful reader must be a motivated problem-solver, actively engaged in constructing meaning. To comprehend what she is reading, a skilled reader uses her background knowledge and experience as a framework for integrating new information. In order to perform this complex activity, she must use appropriate strategies to identify the words and comprehend the text. All this requires adequate levels of attention and concentration. Skilled readers can flexibly vary their strategies, depending on the type and complexity of the material. For a woman with AD/HD, the variability in attention and inadequate use of reading strategies can significantly interfere with success. For those with learning problems, the pattern is similar, although there are often specific deficits that also contribute to poor performance.

Finding out that one has a learning disability or subtle learning problems does not mean that one is not intelligent or capable. Women with learning disabilities have average to above-average intelligence, as well as abilities and strengths that can be used in pursuit of a college or graduate degree or personal goals. The diagnostic process helps a woman begin to understand her disability and find compensatory strategies and appropriate goals. For example, a disability in mathematics might preclude her from succeeding in a college major or career that depends on mathematical skills. But she might also learn that her reading comprehension and written expression are strong, but limited by inadequate use of strategies. With the right kind of support, she might consider a graduate program in law or medicine.

Support

There are a range of supports and accommodations that can be very helpful to a woman with AD/HD and/or LD. Federal laws described below mandate some of those supports. Others are not legally mandated, but may be available on campus, through private professionals in the community, through private clinics or public agencies.

Disability Law

Individuals with AD/HD and/or LD are protected by the regulations of two important Federal statutes: Section 504 of the Rehabilitation Act of 1973 and the Americans with Disabilities Act (ADA) (1990). Section 504 prohibits discrimination of individuals with disabilities by educational facilities, including colleges (all public colleges and most private colleges) that receive federal financial assistance. ADA extends Section 504 to include facilities, whether or not they receive federal assistance.

Section 504 defines a handicapped person as one who has a physical or mental impairment that substantially limits one or more major life activities, such as learning. Both AD/HD and LD are considered "handicaps" under this law. Facilities receiving federal monies must ensure that all their programs and activities are accessible to otherwise qualified handicapped individuals. "Otherwise qualified" has been interpreted to mean that, when provided reasonable accommodations, an individual is able to meet academic requirements for admission or participation in a program or activity. Colleges and universities require documentation for both AD/HD and LD. Documentation is needed to determine eligibility for services, and relies on the results of a full neuropsychological or psychoeducational test battery and diagnosis by qualified professionals. A diagnosis of LD is typically made by a psychologist or educational specialist and AD/HD by a psychiatrist, psychologist, or neurologist.

Accommodations

What are reasonable accommodations? Accommodations are considered to be reasonable if they do not fundamentally alter the nature of the program. Generally, the college must provide services necessary for coursework and examinations and make the activities accessible. While colleges provide note-takers and test accommodations free of charge, supplementary fees are charged for services considered being over and above legal requirements, such as a remedial tutor.

Examples of reasonable accommodations for students with AD/HD and/or LD in college settings might include: reduced course-load, taped textbooks, tape recorders, course adjustments, tailored assignments, note-takers and readers, extra time when taking exams, readers, exams in a separate room or in a different format, and use of computers or other technical aids.

A woman with AD/HD or LD should be aware that these accommodations are not provided automatically. She must inform the institution of her condition and make a request for aid. The college is not required to provide accommodations if a disability is not disclosed and documented. A woman with AD/HD or LD may elect to disclose her disability either before or after admission if she wishes to request accommodations.

College Support Programs

Colleges will require documentation for the disability and may specify that an assessment be recent, that it have been performed by a professional, that it include specific tests. Such assessments are typically not provided by the educational institution and must be paid for by the student or some other agency such as the Department of Rehabilitative Services.

While more and more programs for college students are emerging, the degree and nature of support varies. For example, support programs are designated as "structured" or "coordinated services" or "services," each label identifying the extent to which support is available. A structured program is the most comprehensive. A woman with AD/HD or LD needs to determine whether there is a good match between the programs a school offers and her particular needs. In evaluating a school, she should determine the extent and nature of the tutoring, related services, such as therapy or career counseling, and, of course, the experience and training of staff members. Additional questions she might ask include:

▶ Are special courses available, such as a study strategies course, a writing course, or a remedial mathematics course?

▶ Is a special orientation provided for students with learning disabilities?

▶ How many learning disabilities specialists are on staff?

▶ What is the maximum number of hours of service given to each student each week? Are these services required?

Remediation

Remediation or tutoring involves working individually with a special educator trained and experienced in working with individuals who have AD/HD and/or LD. These interventions focus on basic reading, writing, and mathematical skills as well as instruction in the use of strategies for problem solving, time management, note taking, organization of written material, and textbook reading. The information from the assessment is used to develop an individualized instructional plan. The test profile helps both the tutor and the student to develop instructional goals that are appropriate to her needs and academic demands. Some of these goals might involve teaching her strategies such as note-taking to improve her reading comprehension. Her textbooks or work-related materials would be used as content while developing these skills. For writing, a process approach is used which consists of prewriting, drafting, revising, and editing.

Individuals who have AD/HD without coexisting LD can also benefit from this type of support. Working on strategies to improve planning and organization, and learning to schedule time for study and writing papers can be a significant help to a woman with AD/HD whose papers, file cards, and notes tend to be haphazardly and randomly organized. This type of support is often available on a flexible schedule, such as evenings, lunch hours, or weekends.

Other Types of Support

There are a number of "therapies" available to help women with AD/HD or LD change their self-perceptions about success and failure, and help them to master social skills. In addition, psychotherapy or counseling is used to help women who have AD/HD and/or LD understand and deal more effectively with their issues and problems. The approach a woman chooses—whether with a psychiatrist, psychologist, or social worker—should be dictated by the nature of her problems as well as her goals. In some cases, family therapy is indicated, particularly since AD/HD and/or LD affect all family members.

The impact of having AD/HD and/or LD differs at each stage of development. Adulthood has many stages, each with its unique challenges. Satisfaction or dissatisfaction, success or failure at one stage does not determine the degree of adjustment or success that will occur at another life stage. At one point, a women might focus on self-identity, at another on returning to school, employment, or economic independence, and at other stages, with personal responsibilities and relationships. Often, as a woman with learning disabilities matures, she develops coping skills that increase her chances for success.

Success Factors and Risk Factors for Returning Students

What can help a woman with AD/HD or LD to juggle her many demands and still be able to achieve personal and professional goals? Studies have shown that while the problems associated with a learning disability persist, there are adaptive and positive changes that increase with age. In a longitudinal study, Emmy Werner (1993), a psychologist, followed subjects (learning disabled and controls) from birth through early adulthood and found that by age 32, individuals with disabilities were as successful in their marriages, family life, and work as the control group. Werner suggests that several factors contributed to this success. These include positive temperamental characteristics, the ability to use compensatory strategies, realistic goal setting, and the help of supportive adults. She also notes that at critical turning points, these individuals had the advantage of opportunities such as education and employment. Other studies (Spekman, Goldberg, & Herman, 1993; Vogel, Hruby, & Adelman, 1993) have also been helpful in identifying both risk and protective factors that enable some adults who have learning disabilities to be resilient while others are more susceptible to stress and failure.

Vogel and colleagues (1993) list among *risk* factors: the type or nature of the learning disability, the degree to which the symptoms are chronic or severe, comorbidity with attention deficit/hyperactivity disorder, and other psychiatric problems. Poor social skills, unemployment, and divorce are also thought to make it harder to compensate for and cope with one's learning disability.

Using broad definitions of success, researchers (Spekman, Goldberg & Herman, 1993; Gerber, 1991) have consistently identified self-determination, control, and the ability to set and pursue realistic goals as critical *protective* factors. Other protective factors include well-developed metacognitive insight, or the realistic assessment of our knowledge and skills as well as acceptance and understanding of one's disability, good communication skills, and the ability to call on family, professional, and community support systems. Studies that define success as related to academic achievement and degree attainment suggest that factors such as socioeconomic status, higher ability level, motivation, and the ability to use support systems are important. Also, strong grade point averages in college preparatory courses, well-developed reading and mathematical skills, above average intelligence, and extracurricular involvement in high school correlate highly with success in college (Vogel et al., 1993).

As Werner (1993) reported, some problems soften with age. Others may surface as risk factors change over time. At one stage, an individual may have to deal with the stress of schoolwork, while at another must face the responsibility of maintaining a home and raising a family. While it is difficult for any woman to maintain control and resilience in times of stress, having AD/HD and/or LD adds to this burden.

Self-determination is a characteristic often linked to college success (Field, 1996). It refers to an individual's ability and willingness to assume responsibility for defining her own goals, for taking the initiative to implement these goals, and accepting the responsibility for accomplishments and setbacks. Self-determination is not easy to develop. Lack of self-awareness, a passive and ineffective approach to learning, and low self-esteem—too often by-products of years of struggling with AD/HD and learning problems—can create barriers to self-determination. Self-advocacy—taking action on one's own behalf—helps to promote self-determination. In addition, success on all levels is strongly dependent on the ability and willingness to work hard, persevere, and reframe the experience of having AD/HD and/or LD in a more positive manner. This means being proactive, asking for help, and using the available support systems and interventions that help one learn new and better ways to compensate and succeed.

Conclusion

Along with the internal factors that have been identified as critical for success, there are now many more opportunities for women with AD/HD and/or LD in both academic settings and the workplace. Today, support programs are in place in most colleges. These programs provide a range of services and accommodations to meet the varied needs of women returning to school. For example, there is help with time management and organizational skills, as well as tutoring to strengthen academic skills. Counseling and psychotherapy, easily available options, help one deal with the psychological pressures that go along with the demands of college, work, and family.

Returning to college is certainly a difficult step to take. However, as a group, adults are less conflicted and more goal-directed, and therefore better able to sustain the effort and meet this challenge. Other data indicates that in many cases, the symptoms of AD/HD and/or LD decrease with age, making it somewhat easier to begin college or start over a second time. Increasing numbers of women with AD/HD are enrolled in and are graduating from college programs, leading to success in a range of career settings as well as personal satisfaction and self-fulfillment.

References

Americans with Disabilities Act of 1990 (ADA). 42 U.S.C. 12101 et seq.

Barkley, R.A. (1990). *Attention-deficit hyperactivity disorder: A handbook for diagnosis and treatment.* New York: The Guilford Press.

Biederman, J., Faraone, S.V., Mick, E., Williamson, S., Wilens, T.E., Spencer, T. J., Weber, W., Jetton, J., Kraus, I., Pert, J., & Zallen, B. (1999). Clinical correlates of ADHD in females: Findings from a large group of girls ascertained from pediatric and psychiatric referral sources. *Journal American Academic Child Adolescent Psychiatry. 38,* 966-975.

Deshler, D.D., Ellis, E.S., & Lenz, B.K. (1996). *Teaching adolescents with learning disabilities: Strategies and methods.* Denver, CO: Love Publishing.

Digest of Education Statistics (2000). http://nces.ed.gov/pubs2001/digest.

Field, S. (1996). Self-determination instructional strategies for youth with learning disabilities. *Journal of Learning Disabilities. 29,* 40-52.

Gerber, P. (1991). *Successful adults with learning disabilities: Factors of risk, elements of resilience.* Paper presented at the Frostig Center and Borchard Foundation Meeting on Risk and Resilience in Individuals with Learning Disabilities: An International Focus on Intervention Approaches and Research, Missillac, France.

Pennington, B.F. (1991). *Diagnosing learning disorders: A neuropsychological framework.* New York: The Guilford Press.

Rucklidge, J.J., & Kaplan, B.J. (1997). Psychological functioning of women identified in adulthood with attention-deficit/hyperactivity disorder. *Journal of Attention Disorders, 2,* 167-176.

Section 504 of the Rehabilitation Act, of 1973 , 29 U.S.C. 794.

Solden, S. (1995). *Women with attention deficit disorder: Embracing disorganization at home and in the workplace.* Grass Valley, CA: Underwood Books.

Spekman, N.J., Goldberg, R.J., & Herman, K.L. (1993). An exploration of risk and resilience in the lives of individuals with learning disabilities. *Learning Disabilities Research and Practice, 8,* 11-18.

Vogel, S.F., Hruby, P.J., & Adelman, P.B. (1993). Educational and psychological factors in successful and unsuccessful college students with learning disabilities. *Learning Disabilities Research and Practice, 8,* 35-43.

Wechsler, D. (1997). *Wechsler Adult Intelligence Scale-III, 3rd Edition.* New York: Psychological Corporation.

Werner, E.E. (1993). Risk and resilience in individuals with learning disabilities: Lessons learned from the Kauai longitudinal study. *Learning Disabilities Research and Practice. 8,* 28-34.

CHAPTER 21

Sexuality for Women with AD/HD

Barbara A. Cohen, Ph.D., MFT

Sexuality is often confused and conflicted for contemporary women. Rather than feeling comfortable with their own natural sexuality, they are influenced by strong and often contradictory messages from the media and from society about female sexuality. If a woman today is also challenged by AD/HD, her sexual experience might be further complicated by patterns of inattentiveness, hyperfocusing, impulsivity, and/or hyperactivity. This chapter will present the effects of broader societal issues on female sexuality, as well as the impact AD/HD has on female sexuality.

Portrayal of Sexuality in the Media

"Normal" or "appropriate" sexuality, as described in various magazine articles, movies, or television is sexuality in which the woman is always ready and responsive. Women are depicted as lusty, ripping off their clothes, and ready to go at a moment's notice. In these media presentations, sexual or sensual encounters always result in great satisfaction for both parties with complete attention focused on one's partner. If a woman measures her sexual relationships against these media depictions, she may feel that she or her partner is inadequate because her level of sexual desire and degree of sexual satisfaction is very different from these extreme fantasy models presented by the media.

Idealized Body Image

Sexuality is further complicated by the variety of "idealized body images" against which women have been measured throughout history. Such idealized images have varied widely at different times in history and seem to be strongly influenced by political and economic forces (Cohen, 1984). For example, in eighteenth century America, the "ideal" colonial woman was tough, big, muscular, strong, and fertile (Valentine, 1984). Her fertility was important because the more children she could produce, the more free labor the family would have to work the land. By the nineteenth century, the ideal woman was sickly, frail, pale, wan, and prone to frequent fainting (Valentine, 1984). Valentine hypothesizes that the ideal woman was viewed as being frail and in need of help as part of the white male's justification of slavery. Ironically, this ideal effectively made slaves of women, too—slaves to the restrictive clothing they were expected to wear and to the limited life-style they were allowed to live. The corset came into fashion during this period and remained in fashion until the 1920s. Some women went to the extreme of having ribs surgically removed in order to corset themselves into the desired image of a hand-span waist.

Later, at the turn of the twentieth century, the Greek ideal of physical beauty—broad waists and Venus de Milo figures—came into fashion, and during the twentieth century the idealized female form changed many times. Most significant was the idea that women, by their very nature, were now considered sexual and should show their sexuality by looking sexy (Hynowitz & Weissman, 1978).

What has remained constant, however, throughout these extreme changes in the image of the ideal feminine form is the pressure that women feel to conform to the image of the moment. In our contemporary society, women are given very mixed and confused messages about their sexuality. While the media depicts women as sex objects, parents, schools, and religious teachings demand female chastity and a childlike asexual innocence. It is easy to understand why so many women today respond to this conflict by becoming too fat or too thin; these women either starve or overeat, damaging their minds and bodies to the point that sexual activity may no longer be a part of their lives.

Styles of Sexual Expression

Another important issue to consider is the sexual style of each partner. When partners have different sexual styles, and do not understand one another's style, the likelihood of sexual dissatisfaction is greatly increased. According to one theory of sexuality, there is both "emotional" and "physical" sexuality (Kappas, 1992). We each have elements of both, with one tending to be more dominant in its expression than the other. Neither style of sexual expression, either "emotional" or "physical," is better. Each is just a different style of becoming aroused and of experiencing sex. Clinical experience has shown that assisting women, especially "emotional" females, to better understand their sexual style can provide them with a strong identification with their sexual pattern and a tremendous sense of relief that they are not sexually dysfunctional, but simply different from "physicals."

A woman's sexuality is an important part of her sense of identity, the experience and expression of herself as a woman. Sex, on the other hand, is the engaging in certain behaviors that may be physically, emotionally, and spiritually satisfying. First, this chapter will address the complexities of sexuality and sex with and without AD/HD, and then AD/HD will be considered in greater depth. In the following discussion of sexual styles, extreme examples are used to contrast women who are "emotionals" and those who are "physicals." Most women fall into a more intermediate ground, with some aspects of both.

"Physicals"

A "physical" female's sexuality is one in which sexual desire begins in the body rather than in the mind or emotions. "Physicals" use their body to feel comfortable in the world. They like to have frequent physical contact, and need physical reassurance in order not to feel abandoned or rejected. In case of an argument, a "physical" woman might seek to make up by having sex or intimate time together first, before she is ready to talk about the argument. Touch needs to come before talk because verbal expression of emotions is an area of great vulnerability. Sometimes, it is even difficult for "physicals" to find the words to express what they are feeling emotionally. Their awareness and vocabulary focuses more on what they are feeling physically. The primary love relationship is the number one priority for them, and when they cannot connect physically in that relationship, their life as a whole is out of balance. They may even experience physical pain when their primary relationship causes them emotional pain. This pain extends to all aspects of their life and creates a distraction in their daily life.

"Emotionals"

For more women, sexual desire begins in the mind and emotions first, rather than in the body. This is true for approximately sixty percent of the female population (Kappas, 1992). "Emotionals" use their emotions first in order to be comfortable in the world. They need to feel safety and comfort in the relationship emotionally before they can be sexual or physically intimate with a partner. For an "emotional" woman, her most vulnerable aspect is her physical body. She needs to protect her body from any potential hurt, and feel a sense of trust with a someone before she will consider moving forward toward physical contact. The partner of an "emotional" who is in distress will not be allowed to approach her physically until the emotional issues have been resolved. An "emotional" needs to discuss the issues of a disagreement before she can move forward to physical intimacy. And, if her emotional hurt was severe, she might shut down for an extended period of time, withdrawing physically. Such behavior is often interpreted as "frigid" by a rejected "physical" partner.

Sexual Abuse and Sexual Style

If a woman has experienced any sexual abuse, whether physical, emotional, or spiritual, she may develop a sexual overlay, hiding her true sexual style, as a defense. For example, a woman may be a "physical" by nature, but because of physical abuse, she no longer feels safe as a true "physical." As a defense against overwhelming anxiety, her behavior changes to resemble that of an "emotional" female. Internally, she still reacts as a "physical," however, because she lives in fear for the safety of her body, she behaves externally as an "emotional." Such an overlay may further complicate her ability to be sexually satisfied and must be dealt with in therapy.

Sexual Style . . . "The Approach"

"Physicals"

Typically, this woman wants to be with a man who really understands her body. She longs for her body to be touched in ways that are deeply arousing, for extended periods of time. Through such physical affirmation, her self-esteem is strengthened and she feels alive. This type of woman enjoys physical foreplay and is likely to encourage her partner to stimulate her erogenous zones much sooner than the "emotional." Touching of erogenous zones or any specific sexually sensitive area is completely acceptable to them and is welcomed immediately. Touching that moves in the direction "toward" sexually sensitive areas is pleasurable for her. These women enjoy the sexual tension that builds as their partner strokes their thighs in the direction of their genitals in happy anticipation of intercourse. Snuggling after intercourse is deeply satisfying. These women typically enjoy talking during sex about what they are experiencing and often encourage their partner to do the same.

"Emotionals"

Typically, this woman wants to be with a man who is not sexually assertive early in the relationship, but rather takes time to allow her to get to know him. Since sexuality begins in her mind, not her body, it is very important that the mood be set and that trust is generated before her partner embarks on the sexual journey. A romantic environment (e.g., music, candles, and comfortable conversation) help to set her mood. A back massage or foot massage is relaxing for her. Women with this sexual style will pull back from any immediate touching of their erogenous zones or any specific sexually sensitive areas. Such an approach is too abrupt in transitioning from the nonsexual moment and is not welcomed. Stroking directed away from sexually sensitive areas is appreciated by an "emotional" until her body is relaxed and receptive to sexual stimulation in a more direct fashion. "Emotional" females typically do not enjoy the building sexual tension caused by stroking toward their genitals, unless they feel completely emotionally safe with their partner. Snuggling, for an "emotional," tends to be brief, and then she wants to move away from physical contact and on to other activities, which might include verbal connection. An "emotional" does not enjoy talking during sex (talk is distracting, especially if she has AD/HD) because she needs to focus on her physical sensations.

For an "emotional," it is the anticipation of the sexual interaction that creates greater interest than the act itself. For the "physical," the sexual act itself is most satisfying. Actual intercourse for
a "physical" is truly a joining together, a union of two individuals, first physically and then emotionally. For the "emotional,"
the union needs to occur first on an emotional level before moving to a physical union through intercourse.

Sexual Style—Overview

Women need to be encouraged to understand their sexual style
and that of their partner in order to promote the greatest degree of
sexual satisfaction for both. Because opposites tend to attract, it
is highly likely that an "emotional" will be with a "physical" partner. However, it is also possible that two "physicals" will come
together, especially when AD/HD is an added feature. Women
with hyperactive/impulsive AD/HD who are "physicals" may be
attracted to other "physicals" because of the high levels of excitement and stimulation that tend to occur between two "physicals." It is less likely, however, that an "emotional" woman with
AD/HD will join with another "emotional," unless she has primarily inattentive type AD/HD and is easily overwhelmed by
stimulation. An "emotional" who is hyperactive/impulsive would
almost never choose another "emotional" because the slow pace
and tentative nature of their relationship would lead to boredom
and frustration.

In the newness of a relationship, all people tend to act more
"physical" than their true nature. "Physicals" become even more
physical and "emotionals" behave like "physicals" during the
early, intense phase of a romantic relationship. However,
"emotionals" can only sustain this level of physicality for a limited time. When the honeymoon phase of the relationship is over,
everyone reverts to their true nature—which can result in a feeling of rejection or abandonment for a "physical" who is in a relationship with an "emotional." This transition often begins the

downfall of a relationship if it is not understood. For couples in therapy, it is important to review this material on sexual style within the context of their relationship. Typically, the couple quickly identifies who is the "emotional" and who is the "physical" and can begin to understand what has gone wrong. This understanding alone helps to begin to strengthen and heal the relationship.

One of the biggest problems that can occur to complicate the sexual experience is the woman seeing herself as a victim. Rather than understanding that her partner is different and that they each need to understand the other, she interprets any negative experience as intentional. "They are doing it to me." "It's personal." "They're rejecting me." "They're hurting me." "They set me up." A woman needs to understand that she may be misinterpreting the motivation of her partner's behaviors. A therapist may need to help each partner explore whether there are issues in the relationship that are leading to troubled sexual encounters, or whether it is primarily an issue of different sexual styles.

The E & P Dance ("Chase")

Many couples come into therapy seeking help for sexual problems. Typically, the "physical" partner reports feeling rejected and/or abandoned and the "emotional" partner describes feeling smothered. Since about sixty percent of the female population is "emotional" (Kappas, 1992), more often it is the woman that feels smothered. Her partner, typically the "physical," has been giving her so much attention that she is feeling trapped, smothered, and overwhelmed. These women report that they need their partner to understand their need for personal space and downtime. This feeling is especially intense for women with AD/HD who often feel overwhelmed by life in general. In these relationship patterns, when the woman pulls away in order to get a little space and regain a sense of balance, the chase begins.

In chasing her, the "physical" male is saying, "Don't go away! I'm feeling rejected. I'm feeling abandoned. I need you. I need to touch you. I need to be physical. I need to have physical contact." The "emotional" female responds by saying, "I'm feeling smothered. I'm not emotionally comfortable. I need more space." The "physical" advances again toward the "emotional," seeking physical contact, and the "emotional" pulls away, retreating. This pattern of approaching and pulling away continues, until, eventually, the "emotional" female is driven out of the relationship. Strategies that women use to gain space include going for a walk, going out for a drive, taking refuge in a separate room and locking the door, or actually leaving the relationship.

In order to facilitate the rebalancing of a relationship in sexual crisis, in which the "emotional" woman no longer feels safe in trusting her partner, the "physical" needs to be encouraged to back away. Often, the "physical" is too impulsive to give the "emotional" the space she needs to reestablish balance in the relationship. If an agreement of cooperation is reached, trust begins to rebuild, and the relationship can flourish again. However, the relationship will continue to suffer if the "physical" becomes impulsive as the "emotional" comes closer, reacting too intensely. If the "physical's" approach is too rapid, the "emotional," feeling smothered again may retreat.

Not all women are "emotionals," however. Forty percent of females are "physicals" (Kappas, 1992). The "physical" female will chase just as aggressively as the male. She needs physical attention and interaction, and will do what she must in order for her needs to be met. A woman with AD/HD who is a "physical" will need to work especially hard to control her needs and impulses if she is partnered with an "emotional."

Sexuality and AD/HD

In addition to the complications that can occur in sexual relationships due to differences in sexual style, certain symptoms of AD/HD can introduce another set of complicating factors.

Inattention and Daydreaming

Particularly for the "emotional" female, if inattention and day-dreaming are primary issues, resulting in a tendency to fade in and out, she will not consistently track what's going on in the interaction with her partner. Some women report making a grocery list in their head while they are engaged in a sensual or sexual encounter. This disengagement is much easier for women to hide than for men. A woman with inattentive type AD/HD may find that her mind wanders, especially if the sexual interaction has become stale or routine.

Tendency to Become Bored

An AD/HD mind seeks stimulation. Since sexual arousal begins in the mind for an "emotional," it's easy for her to become distracted when what she's doing isn't holding her attention. It's important for these women to feel interested in the interaction between themselves and their partners. Sexual intimacy is not automatically interesting, especially for a woman with AD/HD. She may also need variety and a degree of emotional intensity in order to remain engaged and focused. Stimulant medication can help to reduce distractibility and disengagement, if the woman chooses to include medication as a part of her treatment plan.

Short Attention Span

Some women with AD/HD have very short attention spans, and even when they want to focus, they find it very difficult to maintain focus for more than a few minutes. If medication is not being used, or has not proved helpful in decreasing distractibility, a variety of problems related to short attention span can develop. Distractibility has an impact on the relationship, both in verbal communication and in sexual relations. Some women with short attention spans, who either do not use medication or are not helped by medication, may not be able to enjoy prolonged sexual encounters. Potential distractions, such as a ringing telephone or distracting noise, should be eliminated before beginning a sexual encounter. It is important that her partner be able to understand how she is impacted by AD/HD and not misinterpret this pattern as a reflection of lack of interest or attraction.

While it is important for women to seek to understand their partner's sexual style, such conversations should be brief, frequent, and held at nonsexual times, if the AD/HD partner is highly inattentive. When discussions are too lengthy, the woman with AD/HD loses focus and she will retain little memory of the discussion. Then, a frustrating cycle can ensue, with long discussions leading to forgetting, frustration, and repeated long discussions.

Hyperactivity

If a woman with hyperactive type AD/HD is a "physical," her hyperactivity and impulsivity may lead her to treat her "emotional" partner like a "physical," wanting to have the sexual experience move more quickly than it can in a relationship with an "emotional." Too hyper can become too aggressive and lead to discomfort in the relationship. It is important for her to learn to slow down in order to attend to her partner's responses. Her "emotional" partner needs time to become comfortable in order to fully participate. Although typically such "physical" patterns are associated with male behavior, it's important to remember that roughly forty percent of the female population is "physical" as well.

Hyperfocus

In contrast to the problems caused by short attention span, it is also possible to become so hyperfocused on the sexual interaction that a woman with AD/HD overlooks important cues from her partner. She may become so focused on what she is feeling or doing that she develops a tunnel vision that excludes her partner's responses. Engrossed in her own sensations and reactions, she may unintentionally hurt her partner or touch her partner in ways that are irritating rather than pleasurable, resulting in her partner pulling away rather than coming closer for more intimacy.

Missing Social/Sexual Cues

Many different sorts of "cues" are sent by one's partner during an intimate encounter—emotional, physical, vocal, visual, kinesthetic, as well as others. Both hyperfocusing or a state of distractedness can lead a woman with AD/HD to miss social cues. Medication may help a woman with AD/HD to focus and pay attention to details.

If a "physical" female with AD/HD is out of touch with her "emotional" partner's feelings and reactions due to hyperfocusing, the "emotional" male may pull back because he is being overstimulated or touched in a way that is not pleasurable. The "physical" female then feels rejected by his withdrawal and tries even harder to engage him sexually. The harder she tries, the more he pulls away. Finally, feeling rejected and abandoned, she quits approaching her male partner and the relationship dissolves into a nonsexual state with minimal physical closeness.

In contrast to hyperfocusing, there are women with AD/HD whose attention is so scattered that they find it difficult to track words and meaning in a conversation. In the excitement of the sexual moment, these women may be completely unaware of the needs of their partner. This can be frustrating and demoralizing. The woman with AD/HD realizes the importance of attending to her partner's feelings and reactions, yet, in the moment, she overlooks the partner's cues that communicate a desire to pull back or that something in the sexual interaction is uncomfortable.

Rapid Shifts in Mood and Interest

Another AD/HD pattern that can negatively impact sexual relations is rapidly shifting moods and interests. Moods can swing from intense and unrelenting desire to disinterest in very short periods of time, as something else catches the interest or attention of the woman with AD/HD. Sex was interesting for her a few minutes ago, but suddenly something else became more interesting. Such patterns are important to understand and discuss at a nonsexual time because such rapid shifts in interest can lead to great feelings of rejection and resentment in the partner.

Insatiability and AD/HD

A strongly "physical" woman with AD/HD may desire sex multiple times per day. This demand can potentially put a strain on the relationship if the partner is an "emotional" who has a lower sex drive. If the partner with a lower sex drive has poor boundaries and gives in to sexual demands, the eventual result is resentment. The partner with lower sexual desire feels disrespected in the face of repeated requests/demands for sex. A hyperactive/impulsive woman with AD/HD may feel that her requests are reasonable or infrequent, while her partner feels bombarded by her needs.

Sexual Addiction and AD/HD

The possibility of sexual addiction needs to be explored when sexual demands seem extreme and unrelenting. Clinical experience has shown that individuals with AD/HD should explore the possibility of sexual addiction. Impulsivity and the need for immediate gratification common to some with AD/HD can increase a tendency toward sexual addiction. Some women may limit their sexually addictive behavior to the relative safety of internet "encounters," but others move from virtual sex to much riskier physical encounters. When sexual behavior seems driven and continues despite risks to significant relationships, as well as health risks, sexual addiction is likely. A combination of psychotherapy and stimulant medication may be helpful to reduce impulsivity and to more clearly assess these behaviors before serious damage is done.

Additional Suggestions for Consideration

In addition to the issues of sexual style and AD/HD discussed above, it may be very useful for women with AD/HD to also consider the following suggestions.

Styles of Processing and Communication

Laying the foundation for a successful sexual relationship includes understanding the "style" of expression and communication of each partner (Kappas, 1987). People tend to express and receive information either literally or inferentially, with one style being more dominant. It is important for a woman's therapist to recognize her style of communication in order to build the greatest amount of rapport with her. Literal processors interpret information at face value — what people say is what they mean. Inferential processors read into the information—looking for the hidden message—not just what was said. Styles of expression can also be "literal" or "inferential" — either saying what you mean or inferring what you mean while leaving out information.

Applying this information in the sexual arena can assist a woman to understand what her partner is expressing as needs or desires. In addition, checking with the partner to make sure that the communication is understood can support the development of a richer connection in the relationship.

Links to Other Experiences Can Better Explain Sexual Needs

Sometimes, when a partner doesn't understand a sexual communication, it can be helpful to use as an example something that is already in the woman's memory and experience. In this way, she can form associations, and link new information to that previous experience. For example, "Bob" is sexually uncomfortable with "Joanne" because her touch is too aggressive. He decides to have a brief conversation with her about his feelings while they are taking their evening walk. He begins by affirming his love for her and then states that he has a few thoughts he would like to share with her that he feels would even deepen their love and enrich their sexual life together. Bob has done well, and Joanne is very receptive at this point.

Since Joanne is an avid seamstress and loves the feel of fine fabrics, Bob relates a brief story of one of their visits to the fabric store in which Joanne observed a woman being very aggressive with the bolts of fabric in the way she touched and handled them. This offended Joanne. Bob reminded her of how he observed her with the fabrics and felt that she was very respectful, tender, gentle, and even a bit sensual as she ran her hands over the various fabrics, as if she was making a very deep connection with the fabric. He shared with her that he even felt aroused as he watched her touching the fabrics. He expressed a wish that she would touch him that way when they were making love, so that he could again experience the depth of connection, tenderness, gentleness, and arousal he experienced at the fabric store observing Joanne. She had been unaware that Bob would like to be touched in this manner and was excited about touching and connecting with him as she would a fine fabric.

Be Open-minded in Discussing Sexual Differences

To develop a mutually satisfying sexual life, women with AD/HD should be open-minded enough to adjust their style to be in rapport with their partner, and vice versa. Taking the needs of the other person to heart and meeting them halfway is a win-win situation. Open-mindedness and rapport do not mean that the woman becomes codependent, or that she needs to give up who she is. Rapport has to do with feeling, knowing, and communicating that you understand and have been understood. Women need to understand that there is nothing wrong with their own sexual style or that of their partner. There are simply differences in the ways in which they become aroused and sustain arousal.

Improve Sensory Acuity to Enhance Sexual Response

Making efforts to develop sensory acuity and awareness can increase a woman's sexual responsiveness. One technique to increase awareness is to focus for short periods of time, on little playful exercises in which each partner tries something new, something different, and pays attention to the feedback they receive. In this awareness exercise, there are no mistakes, only feedback that can increase sexual awareness. "Wow, I never saw that about my partner before. I never saw their face look like that. I never saw them move their body like that. I never heard them say that to me. I never heard them tell me that this is not good for them, this doesn't work for them."

Trance States and Sensory Overload

Women with AD/HD should be aware that sensory overload can lead to the possibility of slipping into a state of trance, a common occurrence for many people. A trance state is natural, however, a woman who remains in a prolonged state of trance may start to feel cloudy, foggy, and/or spacey. Common activities that can create a state of trance are watching television or movies, driving for long distances on the freeway, conversations that are too lengthy or detailed, or excessive sexual stimulation. A woman in a trance state may have a glazed or faraway look in her eyes, and feel as if she is in a dream. The state of trance can be intentionally induced, and can, under the right circumstances, be a very productive state for learning and creativity. By regulating the amount of sensory input at any one time, a woman can lessen her susceptibility to slipping unintentionally into the trance state.

Conclusion

A woman with AD/HD can improve her sexual experience by learning to be compassionate and understanding toward her partner and herself. Without judgment, both partners come to accept that, "We are who we are, not good, bad, right, or wrong." As a woman learns how her sexuality is impacted by AD/HD, and comes to understand her own and her partner's sexual styles, her relationship can be enriched, leading to the increased sexual enjoyment and intimacy that she is seeking.

References

Cohen, Barbara A. (1984). *The psychology of ideal body image as an oppressive force in the lives of women.* Unpublished bachelor's thesis, International College, Los Angeles, CA.

Hynowitz, C., & Weissman, M. (1978). *A history of women in America.* New York: Bantam Books.

Kappas, J.G. (1987). *Professional hypnotism manual.* Van Nuys, CA: Panorama Publishing Company.

Kappas, J.G. (1992). *Relationship strategies, The E & P attraction.* Tarzana, CA: Panorama Publishing Company.

Valentine, M. (1984). Personal communication.

Romantic Relationships for Women with AD/HD

Jonathan Scott Halverstadt, M.S., LMFT

In considering how AD/HD impacts love relationships, there is no "typical" woman with AD/HD. Each woman is unique, not only because attention deficit/hyperactivity disorder is manifested in many ways, but also because AD/HD commonly coexists with other disorders such as depression, anxiety, obsessive-compulsive disorder, bipolar disorder, and learning disabilities. In addition, countless other factors contribute to the complexity of human nature. Keeping these caveats in mind, there are some commonalities that may prove helpful when discussing the impact of AD/HD in romantic relationships, and in the choice of a life partner.

Developmental Stages of a Romantic Relationship

First, before addressing AD/HD as it impacts relationships, it is helpful to consider the developmental stages of romantic relationships in general.

The Honeymoon Phase

The early phase of a romantic relationship—the "Honeymoon Phase"—is typically characterized by a rush of neurochemicals that result in feelings often interpreted as "true love." This feeling of "falling in love" is the result of the activation of the neurochemical reward system that consists of certain neurotransmitters, especially dopamine, and hormones, notably oxytocin in females. Oxytocin produces a warm, floaty, loving feeling that encourages pair bonding (Carter & Frith, 1998). It might be said that oxytocin truly is Cupid's hormone arrow. It is no wonder that a woman feels wonderful when this neurochemical event takes place; oxytocin is closely linked to endorphins (opiate-like brain chemicals).

The Knowing Phase

As wonderful as this honeymoon phase may feel, such feelings will soon begin to fade as the relationship moves into the second stage of a romantic relationship—the "Knowing Phase." In this phase, a woman begins to see and know the real person with whom she has chosen to form a relationship. Now that the very intense feelings that characterize the honeymoon phase have passed, she can make more rational decisions about her wants and needs, deciding whether she wants to remain with her new partner. Gradually, her partner's laugh may become more and more annoying to her, making her question her initial feelings of infatuation. Perhaps there are differences in personal values that she begins to notice about her partner. During this phase, she evaluates whether her attraction continues as she gets to know the other better. If she decides she doesn't want to spend a lifetime with this person, she can end the relationship before becoming more emotionally involved. If she likes what she sees as she gets to know this other person (and the feeling is mutual), the couple moves into the "Growing Phase" of their relationship.

The Growing Phase

To enter this phase, a couple assumes that there is some form of commitment—going steady, becoming engaged, deciding to live together, or getting married. It is during this phase that the real work of a relationship begins. Here is seen the process where two discover how to live as one. Growing pains may develop, but this challenging process is necessary for a couple to deepen their understanding of each other and strengthen their commitment. Through the growing phase, the relationship enriches the life of each, with deepening connection and commitment. The couple moves from "you and I" to "we," beginning the lifelong process of learning to live as a team while still maintaining healthy individual identities. To be in a positive long-term romantic relationship is to live a mystery that is both difficult and enchanting, a mystery in which both partners must lose themselves in the relationship in order to find themselves—both as individuals and as a couple.

While no research has yet been done on romance and marriage in women with AD/HD, many authors have discussed difficulties in intimate relationships as a major issue for adults with AD/HD (Robin & Payson, 2001; Halverstadt, 1998; Hallowell & Ratey, 1994; Ratey, Hallowell, & Miller, 1995; Whiteman & Novotni, 1995). Murphy and Barkley (1996), among others, report that adults with AD/HD, as a group, tend to marry and divorce significantly more times than adults without AD/HD.

AD/HD Traits and Romantic Relationships

With this view of the developmental stages of a romantic relationship in mind, one must consider a range of AD/HD traits that may interfere at various stages along the way.

Social Skills Deficits

In part, marital and relationship difficulties for many women with AD/HD may result from social skill deficits. While social skill deficits in children with AD/HD have been documented by several authors (Frederick & Olmi, 1994; Landau & Moore, 1991), research on adult social skills deficits remains sparse. Novotni (1999) is one of the first to focus, in detail, on the range of social skills deficits in adults with AD/HD and how those deficits impact relationships in their lives. These deficits, along with other AD/HD traits, can strongly influence the course of a romantic relationship. One long-term follow up study suggests that adults with AD/HD of the hyperactive/impulsive subtype (referred to as "hyperactives" in the study) reported both problems with both socials skills and self-esteem (Weiss & Hechtman, 1986).

Low Self-esteem

Research suggests that a woman with AD/HD is likely to struggle with feelings of low self-esteem (Arcia & Conners, 1998). Shameful feelings and messages of inadequacy are programmed very early in little girls with AD/HD (Nadeau, Littman, & Quinn, 1999). These painful, demeaning messages, internalized at a young age, can cause considerable disruption much later in life, when a woman begins to enter into romantic relationships.

Solden (1995), in her book, *Women with Attention Deficit Disorder,* describes women of the primarily inattentive subtype as struggling with low self-esteem, tending to withdraw from social relationships, to feel misunderstood, and to have difficulty maintaining long-term relationships. Solden (1995) writes, "Living with AD/HD has a great effect not just on a woman's cognitive or attentional processes, but impacts every area of her life, especially her intimate partners, friendships and relationships with family members" (p. 129).

Old Nagging Voices Cause Poor Romantic Choices

After years of internalized negative messages, upon reaching the knowing phase of the relationship, a woman with AD/HD may accept characteristics in her partner that would make a woman with healthier self-esteem choose to end the relationship.

If her self-esteem is low, she is more likely to settle for less than what she wants in a partner. Out of loneliness or from a fear that she would not be acceptable to a better partner, she may stay with a poor choice—knowing that it is not an ideal pairing, but believing that some love is better than no love at all. Although her fear is understandable, such a choice usually leads to more hurt and pain as her needs and wants are not fulfilled.

Instead of giving up on romance, or settling for a relationship that leads to further pain, she needs to invest her energy in accepting and appreciating herself. Only then will she make a more positive choice in a partner. Psychotherapy can often be helpful for women with AD/HD working on developing healthy self-esteem.

Lois was one such woman. Although she was smart, congenial, and attractive, her low self-esteem, resulting from years of undiagnosed and untreated AD/HD, had prevented her from finding satisfying romantic relationships. She reported a pattern of "settling" for men who were "second or third best." After receiving medical treatment for her AD/HD, combined with ongoing psychotherapy, Lois began feeling much better about herself. Her decisions began to change in many ways, all reflecting a much healthier and more accurate self-concept. This pattern was also reflected in the better choices of men whom she dated. As Lois developed higher self-esteem she noticed that, not only was she not willing to settle for second best, she was automatically attracting more attractive, better-adjusted men.

Romantic Addiction and Stimulation Hunger

The physiological experience that comes with falling in love—the neurochemical rush of the honeymoon phase—can be quite intoxicating, even addictive. Some women with AD/HD spend their lives moving from one relationship to another—from one honeymoon phase to another—as a means of finding high levels of stimulation. Once the neurochemical rush of the honeymoon phase wanes, such a woman quickly ends the relationship—

in search of her next neurochemical "fix." The task of the therapist in these situations is to help the woman with AD/HD understand the neurobiology of her disorder, the reasons that she is so attracted to the neurochemical high of the honeymoon phase, and the ultimate futility of chasing the dream of finding "true love," in which the neurochemical "high" never stops.

Women with AD/HD who crave stimulation need to learn to find stimulation from other sources instead of expecting their love relationship to keep them entertained forever. Further, they need to learn ways to keep their long-term relationships alive and stimulating rather than relying on neurochemicals to do the job.

Romance is only one of a number of self-destructive stimulation-seeking patterns observed in some women with AD/HD. In psychotherapy, a woman with AD/HD can come to understand her need for stimulation, and learn healthy, constructive ways to find it—both within, and outside of her romantic relationship. Only when she understands her brain chemistry and learns more reliable and healthy ways of stimulating her brain—through exercise, stimulant medication, and constructive stimulating activities—will she be able to give up the intoxicating, yet destructive pursuit of a permanent state of romantic bliss.

A Misspent Loyalty

Sometimes, a woman with AD/HD may stay in a relationship out of an intense sense of loyalty, long after she discovers that her partner is not a good choice. If she experienced rejection and abandonment herself during her childhood years, she may over-identify with the person to whom she has made an emotional commitment. While loyalty to the right person is a positive trait that can maintain a relationship through difficult times, this same trait can work against a woman if the partner she has chosen is not a good match. To justify her loyalty to an undeserving partner, such women often fantasize that they will "help" or "change" their partner, a fantasy that is unrealistic and ultimately self-defeating.

The woman with AD/HD needs to reserve her loyalty for a partner who deserves it. When directed toward a suitable partner, her loyalty will become a positive force during the growing phase of a healthy long-term relationship.

Impulsivity and Romantic Relationships

When the impulsive side of AD/HD comes into play in the early stage of a relationship, a woman with AD/HD may be unable to heed advice from her friends and family. Her impulsivity may cause her to plunge into a committed relationship, even marriage, before she has had a chance to get to know her partner realistically or learn how to communicate, to problem-solve, and establish mutual goals. Acting on impulse, she ends up with a poor match.

Therapy can help a woman with AD/HD recognize her pattern of impulsivity. Though these patterns may persist, and she may be just as sure she's found "the right one" next time, therapy can help her learn not to act on those impulses too quickly, giving herself time to test her feelings and improve her judgment.

Conflict-seeking Behavior

Conflict is frequently another way that stimulation-craving women with AD/HD use to maintain interest in their relationship. Arguing, for some, is very stimulating—more interesting than the low daily hum of life. And then, there is the excitement of making up after the argument. Unconsciously, some women may look for conflicts in order to keep their relationship satisfying. They may quickly learn, however, that their partner finds such constant conflict exhausting and hurtful. And, if they can't find a less destructive way to keep the flame alive, they may soon find themselves out of the relationship.

When Jim and Becky entered couples therapy, Jim stated that he loved Becky, adding, "But, she is driving me nuts." He related that he and Becky had been dating for about nine months and that they generally got along well and had fun together. "However," he said, "if there is ever a dull moment—even if we have had a wonderful weekend together—Becky will get this playful, little grin on her face and start picking a fight about something . . . and the next thing you know, we really are in a fight about something. I hate it when she does that—and the fight is always about something really stupid!" Becky agreed with Jim's report, adding that it wasn't Jim's fault. She related that she never meant for the fights to get out of hand. She enjoyed the verbal sparring, but didn't know how to stop herself—or the sparring—until it was too late, when both ended up with hurt feelings. Through therapy, Becky and Jim were able to identify this as conflict-seeking for the sake of self-stimulation. A medical referral was made for Becky to start a psychostimulant medication and in couple's therapy, both learned more constructive ways to connect with each other.

Disorganization and Forgetfulness

Piles of laundry and paperwork, misplaced keys, forgotten promises and late arrivals—all hallmarks of AD/HD—can take their toll on a romantic relationship. The partner of a woman with AD/HD may begin to feel that she just doesn't care enough to make the effort to be organized or on time. "Why did you stay on the phone when you knew I was waiting for you?" "You promised you'd make the reservation. I can never count on you."

If a relationship survives to the growing phase, both will need to work hard to keep the chaos of AD/HD from destroying their bond and commitment. A woman with AD/HD will need to actively work on ways to reliably respond to her partner's needs, while her partner works to understand AD/HD and learns not to misinterpret her forgetfulness or lateness.

Poor Communication Skills

In order to have a good relationship, a couple must be able to communicate effectively. Clinical experience suggests that there are several poor communication patterns common among women with AD/HD that may interfere with a relationship:

- not communicating ("I *thought* I told you.");
- always needing to have the last word;
- inability to quit arguing once it's begun;
- interrupting;
- compulsive talking that shuts out her partner's participation;
- divided attention while listening; and
- emotional overreacting rather than conversational interacting.

Robin (2001), in his paper, "Can this AD/HD Marriage be Saved?" reports that communication problems are at the heart of many difficulties in marriage for an adult with AD/HD. Attempts to communicate about or resolve the issues fail because the AD/HD partner keeps making the same mistakes and cannot communicate effectively.

The solution to this communication dilemma? Commitment to learning new communication skills and practice, practice, practice. A woman with AD/HD needs to discover what her most problematic conversational patterns are and learn to catch herself as she starts to repeat those patterns. A good marriage and family therapist can probably help both partners learn more effective communication.

Simply put, good communication is making certain that the message sent was received and interpreted correctly, thus insuring that understanding takes place. Good communication must also include understanding the meanings behind the communication and supporting the partner's sense of significance. Through learning effective communication patterns, the woman with AD/HD can help her partner gain insight into her experience—her thoughts and feelings, her wants and desires—without trying to control her partner or demand that her partner agree with her.

Diane and Leonard sought marital therapy after 15 years of marriage. Leonard was ready to leave the relationship out of pure frustration with Diane's AD/HD patterns. Leonard clearly stated that this time (their third attempt at couples therapy) was his last-ditch effort before he made a final decision to divorce. He stated that he really did not want to divorce Diane, but he could no longer tolerate Diane's untreated and unaddressed AD/HD behaviors. Diane clearly wanted to preserve her marriage, and was willing to do whatever she could to improve their relationship, though she had little notion of what changes were needed. Leonard set a deadline of three months. He stated that, after that time, if the relationship had not considerably changed for the better, he would leave the relationship.

A first step in the treatment plan was a thorough diagnostic work-up for both partners by a neuropsychiatrist who specialized in AD/HD. Although Diane had been taking a psychostimulant medication, it was determined that she also needed other medications to treat other conditions that contributed to her AD/HD symptoms. Leonard was taken aback when the psychiatrist suggested that he, too, needed medication, though he did not have AD/HD. Out of their commitment to do whatever it would take to save their marriage, both chose to follow the physician's treatment recommendations. At that point in time, with appropriate medications prescribed for each partner, each committed to an all-out effort for the next three months, over the course of which a wonderful transformation took place.

While many different psychotherapeutic interventions were used, one intervention the couple worked on continuously was something called the "couple's dialogue." This exercise, described by Harville Hendrix (1990) in his book, *Getting the Love You Want*, involves a specific template for learning how to communicate more effectively—an exercise that leads to increased emotional intimacy between partners.

Diane's AD/HD behaviors and Leonard's reactions to those behaviors had long gotten in the way of creating intimacy. Near the end of the three-month commitment to therapy—when their relationship was clearly showing signs of life and love—both partners identified that it was their partner listening to them with empathy and validation that made the greatest difference in bringing them back together as a loving couple. In that same session, Leonard, with tears in his eyes, confessed that he was falling in love with Diane, all over again.

Poor communication patterns related to AD/HD often interfere with intimate relationships. A major contributor to the restoration of Diane and Leonard's love and marriage was their improvement in communication patterns.

The Positive Side of AD/HD in Relationships

While most of this chapter has focused on the difficulties AD/HD creates in an intimate relationship—people with AD/HD have many positive traits—also related to their AD/HD—that can make them wonderful partners.

Creativity

Being creative in the little things, the daily things, can keep a relationship alive and vibrant. Creativity can also come in handy when solving relationship problems.

Spontaneity

One must look at both sides of the AD/HD coin. Women with AD/HD may not be naturals when it comes to consistency and routines, but the flip side of this trait is that they're often spontaneous—catching the mood of the moment and coming up with a reaction or idea that makes life interesting.

Loyalty

As discussed earlier, misplaced loyalty can get a woman with AD/HD in trouble, and keep her there. But when that loyalty is directed toward a loving partner, it can be the glue that keeps a relationship strong through any difficulties.

Empathy and Caring

Women with AD/HD often act from the heart, from their feelings, rather than carefully considering each and every action in advance. This trait can get them into trouble in the practical world, but it can be a very loving, open, and generous trait when a partner is in need. A woman with AD/HD has experienced hurt in her own life, and can respond in a very empathic and caring fashion when those she loves are suffering.

Intuitive Understanding

Women with AD/HD may miss details, and may not always engage in careful analysis, but many find that they become masters at intuitively sizing up a situation quickly. They can often "sense" something long before anyone else. That kind of insight can be very beneficial in a relationship. Often, such women may be able to sense, through intuition, the core issues in a conflict and use that information to negotiate resolution more quickly.

Choosing a Life Partner

People with AD/HD vary enormously. While there is no "right" partner for a woman with AD/HD, one common pairing pattern warrants discussion. People with AD/HD often seek a partner who has better organizational skills—someone who can stay organized, stay on task, keep track of time, and put things away where they belong. Consciously or unconsciously, the woman with AD/HD may feel that such a person can compensate for her areas of weakness. Likewise, people who are very organized often seek balance in their lives through pairing with AD/HD types who are spontaneous, creative, and free. This can be a great combination for couples who can maintain respect for each other's different approaches to life.

After the honeymoon phase of the relationship ends, these very different partners may begin to focus on the negative aspects of their differences, and conflicts often begin. The organized partner may become frustrated with his wife's disorganization, and may try to "organize" her. She eventually becomes resentful, feeling controlled. Conversely, sometimes a woman with AD/HD, having chosen an organized partner, later feels bored and restricted in the relationship. Ironically, the very things they found attractive in each other initially have become the reasons for their current discord.

It is not a bad combination—AD/HD and good organizational skills. In fact, it can be an incredible combination if the two partners can learn to appreciate, value, and respect each other's traits and gifts and then work together as a team. A good therapist who thoroughly understands AD/HD patterns can help the couple rediscover why they chose each other, helping them to appreciate the gifts that each brings to the relationship. The therapist also needs to help each partner come to an understanding of how AD/HD impacts their relationship and how to work with it in a constructive, cooperative way.

AD/HD Treatment and Romantic Relationships

Life works better when one's brain is functioning well and this truth also applies to love and romance. Treating AD/HD with appropriate medication and working with a good psychotherapist can help a woman who has AD/HD make much better choices in a mate. With the appropriate help, she can learn be more patient with the process of a relationship as it moves through each phase of development. Along the way, medication may help her to more thoughtfully consider whether she has made a good choice, rather than impulsively leaving the relationship at the first sign of discord.

Medication is not the only answer, however. Too often, couples in therapy think that medication will make everything better. However, medication alone will not solve problems in a relationship. Once medication helps the brain to function better, it is usually essential to engage in couples therapy with a psychotherapist who understands AD/HD. Such a therapist can help the woman with AD/HD and her partner to develop mutual understanding, to learn better problem-solving skills, and to develop more cooperative, constructive communication patterns with each other.

Once the more negative aspects of AD/HD have been addressed through medication and cooperative problem solving, the positive aspects of AD/HD—the warmth, creativity, and playfulness—can emerge. Suddenly, both partners can clearly see what attracted them to each other. Irritating problems can seem minor as the couple learns to focus once again on the positive feelings that brought them together in the first place. When the challenges of AD/HD are constructively met by both partners, the relationship can have a rich and rewarding future.

References

Arcia, E., & Conners, C.K. (1998). Gender differences in ADHD? *Journal of Developmental and Behavioral Pediatrics, 19,* 77-83.

Carter, R., & Frith, C. (1998). *Mapping the mind.* London: University of California Press, Ltd.

Frederick, B.P., & Olmi, D.J. (1994). Children with attention-deficit/hyperactivity disorder: A review of the literature on social skills deficits. *Psychology in the Schools, 31,* 288-296.

Hallowell, E.M., & Ratey, J.J. (1994). *Driven to distraction.* New York: Pantheon.

Halverstadt, J.S. (1998). *A.D.D. and romance.* Dallas: Taylor Publishing Company.

Hendrix, H. (1990). *Getting the love you want.* New York: Harper Perennial.

Landau, S., & Moore, L.A. (1991). Social skills deficits in children with attention-deficit hyperactivity disorder. *School Psychology Review, 20,* 501-513.

Murphy, K.R., & Barkley, R.A. (1996). Attention deficit hyperactivity disorder adults: Comorbidities and adaptive impairments. *Comprehensive Psychiatry, 37,* 393-401.

Nadeau, K., Littman, E., & Quinn, P. (1999). *Understanding girls with ADHD.* Silver Spring, MD: Advantage Books.

Novotni, M. (1999). *What does everybody else know that I don't? Social skills help for adults with attention-deficit/hyperactivity disorder (AD/HD).* Plantation, FL: Specialty Press.

Ratey, J.J., Hallowell, E.M., & Miller, A.C. (1995). Relationship dilemmas for adults with ADD: The biology of intimacy. In K. Nadeau, (Ed.), *A comprehensive guide to attention deficit disorder in adults: Research, diagnosis and treatment* (pp. 218-235). New York: Brunner/Mazel.

Robin, A. L., & Payson, E. (2000). *Can your marriage survive ADHD?* Presented at the CH.A.D.D. National Conference, Chicago, IL.

Solden, S. (1995.) *Women with attention deficit disorder: Embracing disorganization at home and in the workplace.* Grass Valley, CA: Underwood Books.

Weiss, G., & Hecktman L.T. (1986). *Hyperactive children grown up.* New York: Guilford Press.

Whiteman, T.A., & Novotni, M. (1995). *Adult ADD.* Colorado Springs, CO: Pinon Press.

Organizing for Women
with AD/HD

June Johnson, Professional Organizer

Disorganization is frequently one of the primary present-ing symptoms when adults seek treatment for AD/HD, but, surprisingly, the symptoms of AD/HD listed in the Diag-nostic and Statistical Manual, Fourth Edition (APA, 1994) do not include "disorganization." Being disorganized can feed feelings of inadequacy and failure, not to mention the added stress of living in a cluttered and chaotic home or office.

The most common image that comes to mind of a woman with AD/HD is that of a scattered, messy person arriving late and unprepared. While that image is not universally true, women with AD/HD report feeling out of control, overwhelmed, and not centered. If such feelings persist, and if others consistently point out her problems, it is easy for the woman with AD/HD to give up, thinking that it is not possible for her to improve. Eventu-ally, she may settle into a role as "the messy one," always misplacing things and seeing no way to get it right. She may become comfortable with the familiarity of her discomfort. As she resigns herself to her fate, her rut grows deeper. Any opportunity for control over her situation is quickly abandoned, and then she wonders why everything remains the same.

While being organized is neither natural nor gender linked, women most often bear the responsibility for "doing organization." This is true both at the office and at home. Many men who have left the corporate structure bemoan the lack of a secretary to "keep up with things." The complaint typically ends with "my assistant (female) always did that for me." Few women, with or without AD/HD, have enjoyed the benefits of having a secretary or personal assistant to provide organization and structure. However, it is possible to learn to become one's own best assistant.

Learning about being organized should begin with two affirmations:

> **Being organized is a *skill*, not a character trait.**
>
> **Being organized is a *process*, not a destination.**

These are both difficult concepts if a woman with AD/HD has spent years hearing "why can't you just . . . ," but necessary to accept in order to move beyond the belief that change is not possible. Organizational skills are part of what we *do*, not synonymous with who we *are*. Even with AD/HD, organizational skills can be learned, practiced and incorporate into daily living, despite the reality that the brain's wiring (neurochemistry) may make it a challenge.

The Pressure of Cultural Norms

As a professional organizer conducting workshops, the author often asks attendees in a mixed-gender "get organized" workshop a simple question: "How many rolls of toilet paper are in your house right now?" Most men look blank or puzzled. Women laugh and tell you the number. In some cases, men don't understand the purpose of the question—even men who live alone. The prevailing cultural norm continues to be that "Mom" keeps up with the household needs, even if that is not always reality. Mothers, who have difficulty because of their AD/HD, frequently waste precious energy in self-punishment and self-blame, unable to forgive themselves for failing to live up to a cultural ideal. Despite the lack of realism or fairness in these norms, many women are unable to let these expectations go and continue to feel inadequate and frustrated.

Understanding What Organization Is and Isn't

Before one can become organized, it is important to understand the meaning of the word. The author, in conducting numerous workshops across the country, defines organization in a simple, but limited way:

> **You are organized when you can find what you want, when you want it.**

In practical terms, being organized means that there is no morning search for car keys or the needed umbrella. Bill paying does not always start with searching the entire house for the bills, checkbook, envelopes and stamps. The school holiday schedule is accessible when needed without making a call to the school for yet another copy. That is being organized. Anything more, such as having all the paid bills filed by payee, is an extra bonus.

When women with AD/HD first begin talking about "getting organized," the military, spit-polished image typically comes into the conversation—all the corners square and everything in a straight line. These women often protest that they are too creative to be organized and that they don't want to become rigid and boring. Once they begin to redefine organization, they come to understand that organization functions in our life the way our skeleton does in our body—as the supporting structure necessary for us to stand up and move. Both skeletons and organization are essential, but something is wrong when they show! Good organization provides flexibility and efficiency, which encourages creativity and productivity. Disorganization can erode creativity and interfere with pleasure as a woman spends her time searching for needed items rather than enjoying the planned activity.

> **"Organized" is not synonymous with "neat and orderly."**

Levels of organization should meet the needs and preferences of the individual. For example, a sock drawer might appear messy because all the socks, all colors and styles, are thrown in together. However, the highest level of organization that a woman may need for her socks is that they be in one place with pairs rolled together. Because this is all that counts for her, she gives it no more effort. However, for this same woman, the organization of her costume jewelry earrings may be more important to her and would warrant far more effort—gold must be with gold, silver with silver, pearl with pearl, each in its drawer in the jewelry box. The woman who jumbles her socks is very careful with earrings because it *matters* to her. It satisfies her need to be organized and makes it easier to get dressed. Both the sock drawer and the jewelry boxes are "organized" because they meet the needs of the woman.

One function of the professional organizer, whether the client has AD/HD or not, is to assist her in determining how she defines being organized. It is very difficult to attain a goal that cannot be described clearly. A desire that can be written in twenty words or less, that has specific parameters, and that can be achieved in a step-by-step manner is a clearly defined goal. "Getting my house organized" is a wish. "Acquiring the habit of hanging up clothes and putting away clean laundry" is a clearly defined goal. The work of the professional organizer, or any professional assisting in the treatment of AD/HD, is to facilitate the process of reaching that level of clarity.

> **Tackle one thing at a time.**
> **Small successes lead to larger successes.**

Setting clearly defined goals is extremely important as an antidote to disorganization that causes confused vision and muddled thinking. Clearly defined, simple goals can penetrate confusion just as strong, tall buildings penetrate smog, rising above it and serving as guideposts. Most women want to clear away all the smog at once, but that is unrealistic. Instead, tackle one habit or one area at a time and work through to success. Small successes build the base for larger successes. With this step-by-step approach, soon the woman with AD/HD can see through the smog all the way to the horizon.

Five Steps to Being Organized

Below is a five-step plan for achieving organization that is helpful for women both with and without AD/HD. Notes and comments have been added to help the individual in adapting each step to her particular situation.

1. Set Clear Goals

   Instead of continuing to talk about "getting organized," the woman who seeks to become organized should identify one problem that leads her to feel disorganized and then devise a way to resolve the problem. For example, she may have a permanent pile of newspapers around the sofa. One possible solution is for her to put an attractive basket by the sofa to hold the papers until they can be recycled. When the container is full, she can put the contents in a recycling container or in the trash. Using this system, current and recent newspapers are easily accessible *and* her floor is clear. If the smog rolls in and newspapers accumulate again, it will take her less than ten seconds to pitch them into the basket— even a five-year-old can help.

Such a solution is long-term, earth-friendly, and creates a physical habit that the body remembers even when the brain is overloaded. As a rule of thumb, every woman with AD/HD should keep in mind that a simple solution is more likely to work than an elaborate one. When a woman achieves a small success, such as the newspaper basket, she is ready to move on to the next problem area, taking that expectation of success with her.

2. Get Physical

Practicing a physical motion, just like rehearsing the steps of a dance, can actually help teach a woman with AD/HD to be more organized. However, she should not try to learn fifty steps at a time. First, she should establish one habit, and then work on another.

Habits that help to maintain organization are similar to tooth brushing. Half asleep, rushed, alert, relaxed—no matter how she feels, a woman with AD/HD is highly unlikely to forget to brush her teeth. Physical habits such as tooth brushing become deeply ingrained and require no thought. Likewise, other physical habits can become ingrained. For example, one woman never forgets to record auto mileage when she drives because her physical routine is the same every morning—get in, put down coffee cup, start ignition, and reach for mileage book. The ignition requires the right hand and the mileage book the left, as it is in the driver's door pocket. If she doesn't reach for it, she has the *physical* sensation that something is wrong. The physical habit is a reminder of an important accounting process.

Because "being organized" is usually presented as a way of thinking instead of as a set of physical habits, most women continue doing the same physical things they have always done—reinforcing old physical habits, while waiting for their thinking to change.

It is more effective to change a physical activity to reinforce a desired habit than to attempt to remember a desired behavior without a physical reminder. For example, if a woman walks into the house and unloads everything in her hands onto the kitchen table, the following technique can help her to break this habit. She should begin, in the evening, by setting the table for the next meal. When unloading the dishwasher, instead of re-shelving the dishes, they go back on the table ready for tomorrow's dinner. Then when she returns home the next day, plates, silverware, and napkins are the first things seen instead of an inviting bare surface that tempts her to offload her belongings. It is not likely that briefcases and mail will be dumped on top of dishes that are already in place for dinner. Other members of the household will see a different surface, too, and will also change how they act. In this manner, the activity of a physical change begets a change in habits and organizational skills.

3. One Thing at a Time

It is helpful to work on one habit at a time for development—such as a consistent place to put the car keys. A woman with AD/HD should hang a key rack by the door (or a basket or a bowl—whatever feels right to her) and practice putting the car keys there until it becomes a habit. As she walks in the door, she should repeat aloud, "I will put the keys on the rack." If she forgets and finds her keys somewhere else during the evening, she should place them on the rack immediately, and continue doing this nightly until it becomes a habit.

Some women with AD/HD may need an extra reminder to help establish a new habit. For example, she might write herself a note, and post it in the kitchen, that asks, "Did you put your keys on the rack?" If she has not put her keys where they belong, this serves as an immediate reminder to do so. As she establishes this habit, she is then ready to move on to the next one.

When reorganizing her house, she should focus on one room at a time. Guiding women to select one room in their home per month for concentrated "get organized" efforts allows the work to be "on purpose" and to not become overwhelming. The circuit of all the rooms can usually be accomplished within a year, with visible results beginning from the very first month.

Scheduling the pattern of rooms in her day planner in a way that makes sense and supports her family's plans will increase the likelihood that her plan will be realized. For example, she could plan to concentrate on the family room in May before the children come home for the summer. Or, she might work on the guest room the month before the grand-parents come for their annual visit. She could focus on the master bedroom in February for a saner, more loving Valentine's Day. By taking on one room at a time, not the whole house in a weekend, the job gets done.

4. **Get Real**

The professional organizer helps a woman do what is important to her, looking at what makes her feel disorganized, out of sorts, unfocused, or unattractive. However, if a goal is not realistic for her, she will not make the consistent effort that is necessary for per-manent change to occur. For example, if she has three children under the age of eight, two dogs and two cats, and a full-time job, a professional organizer would be the first to advise her that creating a picture perfect home is not an achievable goal. A colorful basket in the family room in which toys are tossed at the end of the day is a more realistic organizational goal for a family with preschoolers. The finer points of decorative detail can be saved for more grown-up years.

Another common, but unreasonable goal, for many women is an expectation that everyone in the family will instantly become better organized. Try-ing to get others to be organized instead of focusing on one's own habits is a way of continuing a cycle of self-defeat. Instead, she should begin with her own challenges—her calendar, her closet, her kitchen counter, car or desk. This approach eliminates blam-ing others or accepting the current chaos as the only possible status. When a woman begins to change and succeed, family members and co-workers will, by example, begin to change.

5. **Celebrate Every Victory**

   Because being organized is a process, there will never be a time when all the work is done. Celebrations of each small organizing step can offer great rewards and help the woman with AD/HD to stop and take notice of her accomplishments, instead of focusing only on what remains undone. A woman might choose to wear red, buy a pair of earrings, have an ice cream float, see a movie, watch a sunset at the beach—whatever means celebration to her, every time she achieves even the smallest success. Life is sweeter when small rewards become part of her relationship with herself. And that sweetness gets passed on to those around her because she allows herself to feel joy.

Changing the AD/HD Legacy

Because current evidence shows that AD/HD occurs in families, understanding that organization is a skill is important. It is natural to become "fired up" when one is suddenly faced with multiple problems having to do with organization—an employee evaluation pointing out deficiencies, forgetting to pick up a child from school on time, or feeling that the family is drowning in kids' toys strewn in every room of the house. The way to make real changes, however, is not to start flailing in every direction at once, but to use the "fired up" energy to begin the process of organization—one issue at a time.

Develop *simple* organizing solutions.

As adults, we are responsible not only for increasing our

own skills but also for passing these skills on to our children. Part of what we pass on is the skill of developing simple solutions. Key ring + key rack = no more lost keys. Newspapers + basket = clean floor. That process can be taught by professionals working with women with AD/HD and applied even to the child areas of her house. For example, if the refrigerator is covered with artwork and more arrives every week, a mother with AD/HD can buy a large, cheap scrapbook. Then, each time a new drawing goes on the refrigerator, the old drawing gets put in the scrapbook—no more artistic chaos in the kitchen. When grandparents come to visit, they can enjoy the scrapbook while Mom enjoys less clutter in the kitchen.

If a child with AD/HD loses schoolbooks and papers almost every day, a simple plastic crate in a bright color just inside the child's bedroom door may be the answer. This same crate can hold what is needed for the next day to save time in the morning. If two children share a room, the crates can be stacked on their sides and personalized by using a different color for each child.

To Organize, Start Big

Contrary to the usual cliché, in organizing one should always start big. Organizing should begin on the "macro level" instead of the "micro level." Many women attempting to organize start too small—micro managing, to use the current buzzword. In the excitement of beginning, she may decide to create a file folder for each and every subject, a system that's too detailed to maintain. The best way is to start big and do breakouts as needed. For example, if a woman with AD/HD is always losing financial papers such as bank statements, bills, etc., she should get a box and begin putting all these papers in that box. Whenever financial papers are found anywhere else in the house, she should move them into the box. Once it becomes a habit to put all financial papers in the box, she can add a folder for each month. She then puts everything for the current month in the folder for that month. At the end of the year, the woman with AD/HD starts a new box. She should add folders for special events such as a house purchase, a birth or death, college tuition, or other major changes, only as needed. Such a system is easy to maintain and what is needed can be found in just a few minutes.

Organizing Concepts

So much of what is written about getting organized—even what is written here—emphasizes the tips and techniques. Because being organized is a skill that can be learned, beginning with techniques is usually more productive than starting with trying to change woman's way of thinking.

Change Your Behaviors to Change Your Thinking

Organizing experience has shown that a woman can act her way into a better way of thinking faster than she can think her way into a better way of acting.

Clutter Is Postponed Decisions

Barbara Hemphill, superstar professional organizer and creator of "Paper Tiger Paper Management" software, teaches this concept of clutter as postponed decisions. Things are kept because the woman with AD/HD is not sure what to do with them, and because she does not want to deal with it now. Information on what to do is obtainable if she *decides* to decide. A woman with AD/HD can buy thirty minutes of an accountant's time in order to get a clear outline of what financial papers to keep and what to discard. With that information in hand, it is possible for her to begin to clean out old stacks of paper and set up simple files of what is needed. Nothing will happen, however, as long as she sighs over the clutter because she just doesn't know what to do.

The test that Hemphill teaches us to apply to everything in the home is to ask oneself:

1. Do I think it's beautiful?

2. Do I know it's useful? (Clearly defined useful, by the way, not "well, someday it might come in handy" vaguely useful.)

3. Do I love it?

Whenever a woman can answer "yes" to one of these questions, the item should be kept. If the answer to these questions is "no," what is the purpose of keeping the item?

When Nothing Is Important, Everything Is the Same

When a woman with AD/HD has to be at work at eight o'clock in the morning, her morning activities should be clearly focused on that goal. The night before, she can set up the coffee pot and decide what she is going to wear. In the morning, she should focus strictly on those activities necessary to prepare for work. She should not try to start a load of laundry, unload the dishwasher, or damp mop the kitchen floor before she showers and dresses. When she is very clear about she wants to accomplish—being on time for work—she can voluntarily restrict her options and make it easier to accomplish the goal that she has acknowledged is important.

> **Stay focused on your top priority.**

If she doesn't have to go to work until noon, she has time for additional tasks—coffee and the newspaper, doing a load of laundry, and dropping off the dry cleaning.

Separate the Concrete from the Gravel

Concrete is heavy and immovable, gravel is smaller and can fit in almost anywhere. Appointments and events which cannot be changed—the concrete—should be written in a woman's day planner each day instead of relying on memory. Once the "concrete" is set, she now pours in the "gravel"—other flexible things that have to be done—in the planner around the concrete. For example, if her child's daycare center closes at six o'clock (concrete), she might decide to patronize the dry cleaner (gravel) between childcare and home. Getting to work on time is concrete. Getting to the dentist on time is concrete. Grocery shopping, phone calls, and errands are "gravel" that can be fit in around the concrete wherever she can squeeze it in.

The woman with AD/HD should be sure that the concrete dates and times are written into her day planner before assigning a place for the gravel. She should learn to develop the habit of saying "let me check my calendar" before she says "yes" to anything, no matter how appealing the invitation. Given the built-in memory difficulties associated with AD/HD, she should always resist her temptation to assume that she remembers her schedule.

The Value of "Yes" Rests on the Quality of "No"

Because most women, with or without AD/HD, want to do everything and do it successfully, saying "no" can be very difficult. There may be six or eight charities that she really believes in, many community activities she wants to participate in, and many opportunities for service through her church. However, it is not possible for her to engage in all of these activities and maintain any balance in her life. If a woman with AD/HD finds that her day planner is wall-to-wall concrete with gravel overflowing, it is time for her to practice saying "no." Well-intended overcommitment is one of the most common pitfalls of the woman with AD/HD.

Learn to say "no" to overcommitment.

Much of one's activity is based on the assumptions one makes in relationships. The woman with AD/HD who feels constantly

overcommitted needs to examine her assumptions and renegotiate, if necessary, to manage her time better. It is natural for her to
do all the laundry and clean the bathrooms when her children are
two and four years old, but a different thing altogether when
they are ten and twelve. If her partner passes a dry cleaner on the
way to work, why not let the partner take care of the dry cleaning? She needs to renegotiate family-related commitments to fit
current reality rather than continue old habits that are no longer
appropriate. In addition, she should carefully consider all current
commitments, and resign from groups that do not fit her present
needs and availability. If the organization is worthwhile, she can
always return in a year or two when she has time to work for
them.

Learning to say "no" may be difficult for the woman with
AD/HD because she will almost certainly meet resistance from
friends, family, co-workers, or organizations she belongs to as
she makes the decision to cut back on her activities. Her professional organizer can serve as a support and reminder that she
needs to "gird up her loins" and be prepared to hang on tightly to
her well-considered no's. As the woman with AD/HD begins to
set limits with others, the organizer can help her to learn that
elaborate explanations or apologies are not required. Life will
become more satisfying and more orderly for her when she is in
control of how her energy is spent.

Straw Does Not Spin into Gold

It is not productive for a woman with AD/HD to spend significant amounts of time working hard at the things that she will
never do well or that are not high on her priority list. She should
take an honest look at her strengths and weaknesses, and find
another way to accomplish those tasks that are not her strong
suit. If she is good at numbers and enjoys it, then she should
balance her checkbook. If she hates to cook, she should buy iced
cupcakes at a bakery for the class party and add the decorations

herself for a personal touch. Overcoming the challenges that AD/HD puts in her path is the battle to be won. She is more likely to win that battle if she spends her time focusing on her strengths.

Focus on your strengths, not on areas of weakness.

Getting Organized Is a Process, Not a Destination

Life changes, people change—women move, have babies, change jobs, send the children off to college, or bring a parent to live with them. Whatever a woman does today sets the stage for tomorrow, but nothing she does can prevent a plot change. Organization, like a good stage set, allows the story to take place while remaining in the background. Whenever one area of life is "fixed," something else in the life of a woman with AD/HD inevitably needs attention.

Organizing is a lifetime process.

The process of organizing allows a shift to that area, using the guidelines and priorities that are already established. It is self-defeating for a woman with AD/HD to think that she can "get organized"—that is, change all her habits as well as her surroundings—in a weekend or two. Organizing is a lifetime process. Each time a woman gets to step five in one area, she goes back to step one for the next challenge.

Whatever the theories about the origin and mechanics of AD/HD, whatever the medical findings and treatments, whatever else is learned about how the brain functions and the biology of AD/HD, the primary battleground will continue to be in the setbacks and victories of daily routines. For a woman with AD/HD, growing in organizational skills is a tangible way of improving her life and her relationships, and the process can be initiated and nourished at any age or stage in life. While perfection is a goal that she should stoutly resist, the ragged, painful edges of her disorganization can be smoothed and shaped, like the polishing of a raw, rare stone, until the color and sparkle shines through for all to see. And that is the best accomplishment of all.

References

American Psychological Association (1994). *Diagnostic and statistical manual of mental disorders. (4th ed.)* Washington, DC: Author.

Hemphill, B. (1996). *Taming the office tiger*. Washington, DC: The Kiplinger Washington Editors, Inc.

Hemphill, B. (1997). *Taming the paper tiger* (4th edition). Washington, DC: The Kiplinger Washington Editors, Inc.

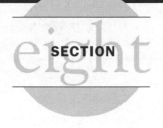
SECTION
eight

CONCLUSION

Future Directions

Patricia O. Quinn, M.D.
and Kathleen G. Nadeau, Ph.D.

A D/HD has long been defined as a behavioral disorder of childhood that primarily affects boys. In recent years, however, all of these defining characteristics have been reconsidered.

The first assumption, that AD/HD is a behavioral disorder, has been challenged by Russell Barkley, who proposes that AD/HD is more appropriately categorized as a developmental disorder. The second long-held assumption, that AD/HD is a disorder of childhood has largely been swept aside as recognition of AD/HD in adults has grown over the past decade.

A third assumption, that AD/HD is a disorder that primarily affects males, is now strongly called into question as a result of recent research that suggests as many females as males may be affected by AD/HD (Walker, 1999; Faraone et al., 2000). Joseph Biederman, one of the leaders in AD/HD research has called the under-diagnosis of females a significant public health concern (Biederman et al., 1999).

Other assumptions about AD/HD have been challenged as well. For example, for many years, hyperactivity was considered to be central to the disorder. This defining characteristic was reassessed a number of years ago when non-hyperactive children were noted to also have significant attentional problems. The recognition of primarily inattentive type AD/HD was one of the factors that has led to increasing identification of girls and women.

Despite these recent changes in how AD/HD is conceptualized, the focus of research is slow to change. The overwhelming majority of AD/HD research continues to focus on the academic and behavioral problems of young boys. The recent MTA study, the largest coordinated study ever undertaken to study the treatment of children with AD/HD, investigated a population that was 83 percent male (The MTA Cooperative Group, 1999). To date, only marginal interest in exploring gender issues has been demonstrated by MTA researchers.

This ongoing emphasis on young males in AD/HD research is not a conspiracy to ignore females or adults, but rather a natural outgrowth of referral patterns. Numerous studies have reported the greater incidence of referral of boys for diagnosis and treatment of AD/HD—the response of parents and teachers to their more noticeable and disruptive academic and behavioral problems.

While AD/HD is the most highly researched childhood disorder, research on AD/HD in females is sorely lacking. Of the several thousand published studies on AD/HD conducted before 1992, only 13 examined gender issues (Gaub & Carlson, 1997). By the year 2000, an additional 23 studies had been added to the literature (Gershon, 2000), a positive trend, but greatly overshadowed by the growing body of research on predominantly male populations.

Research Interest in Gender Issues

The first clear sign that gender issues in AD/HD were being considered was the "Conference on Sex Differences in AD/HD" jointly sponsored by the National Institute of Mental Health (NIMH) Office of Special Populations and the Child & Adolescent Disorders Research Branch of the Division of Clinical & Treatment Research, NIMH in 1994. A broad range of questions were raised (Arnold, 1996):

> ▶ Are the same diagnostic criteria and diagnostic tools equally appropriate for males and females?

> ▶ What are the normal sex differences in attention, impulsivity, and activity level, and how do those differences affect how AD/HD is manifested in girls and boys?

> ▶ How do neurological gender differences affect AD/HD in males and females?

> ▶ Do males and females have different treatment needs?

> ▶ Is the life course of AD/HD the same in males and females?

> ▶ Why are so many more males than females diagnosed with AD/HD?

Considerable debate on these questions led to some areas of agreement. Overall, there was recognition that requiring a lower score on hyperactivity factors was appropriate for girls (implying that girls with AD/HD have the same behavior patterns as boys, but to a lesser degree). Although there was discussion of the need for *self-report* in girls to better assess their internalized symptoms (feelings as opposed to behaviors), no concrete recommendations were made. Standard questionnaires currently used do not adequately address this need.

The conference closed with a long list of proposed research directions. Conference attendees agreed that it was important to explore this disorder in females to discover how AD/HD is manifested and experienced in girls and women, and to explore whether the expression of the disorder, its course, and its prognosis varied according to gender. Research on issues unique to females, such as the impact of hormonal fluctuations, and the challenges of motherhood for women with AD/HD, were recommended. Sadly, however, in the intervening years, little research on gender issues has taken place.

Clinical Interest in Gender Issues

In contrast to the paucity of research on gender issues, there has been a strong and growing interest in gender issues among treatment providers. Two years ago, the contributing editors of this volume coauthored, with Ellen Littman, the first book addressing the issues of girls with AD/HD (Nadeau, Littman, & Quinn, 1999). Now, this companion volume expands the focus to include women. The frequency of workshops and presentations on the issue of AD/HD in women and girls has grown in recent years, with daylong workshops designed for both women with AD/HD and for clinicians treating women offered by both major AD/HD advocacy organizations, CHADD and ADDA, at their national meetings.

Proposed Research Directions

As so often happens, clinical experience and anecdotal evidence precedes research. This body of clinical experience has been described in a growing number of articles, chapters, and books. Such clinical observations can serve as a beacon to guide future research directions.

Research on New Diagnostic Tools

While AD/HD is generally accepted to be a neurobiological disorder, the current diagnostic process is one in which we attempt to infer dysfunctions in the brain through behavioral observations. To date, diagnosis of AD/HD is based largely upon behavioral observation, with self-report used increasingly in adult populations. However, whether self-report or observations by others are used, the diagnosis is dependent upon reported behaviors that conform to the DSM-IV AD/HD diagnostic criteria, a list of behavior patterns that are more typical of boys than girls, and more descriptive of children than adults.

Now, new technologies already under development, may allow us to escape from this "black box," inferential approach to diagnosis that relies upon approximate and subjective behavioral observations. From measures of glucose metabolism, to blood flow in discrete areas of the brain, to precise measures of receptor density—these recent non-invasive measures of brain function make it increasingly likely that the diagnosis of AD/HD will be made in the future by precisely measuring differences in brain structure and function.

Then, with diagnosis established, we can turn our attention to a careful exploration of behaviors and self-reported internal experiences. Differences related to gender, age, comorbidity, and protective factors (among others) can be more clearly delineated. Freed from current preconceptions that result from viewing AD/HD as a childhood disorder of males, we may learn that females manifest symptom clusters to different degrees and at different stages of development than those of males, as well as possibly exhibiting symptom patterns unique to females.

Gender Appropriate Diagnostic Criteria

Perhaps the most critical need is for more gender-appropriate diagnostic criteria and diagnostic tools that are more gender sensitive. Without such gender-appropriate diagnostic criteria, the females included in research studies will continue to be those who most closely resemble males with AD/HD, instead of those most representative of their gender. Barkley has proposed a fresh look at adult patterns, suggesting that AD/HD in adults is different than, not "less-than" AD/HD in children. A similar reassessment of female patterns is needed, in order to consider that AD/HD in females may be different than, not less than AD/HD patterns in males. Ohan and Johnston's study (1999) was one of the first to support the notion that current criteria are more appropriate for males than females.

Gender Differences in Age of Onset

There is growing evidence that symptoms of AD/HD in girls, particularly girls with predominantly inattentive type AD/HD, may not be evident until puberty. Continued adherence to the DSM-IV criterion that requires evidence of AD/HD before age seven, therefore, excludes many girls and women with AD/HD from diagnosis and treatment.

Gender Differences in the Life Course of AD/HD

The course of the disorder for women, throughout their lifespan, has yet to be studied, but clinical evidence suggests that the strong interaction between estrogen levels and AD/HD symptomatology in females would lead to gender-specific patterns throughout the life stages. Huessy (1990) was one of the first to suggest a different life course for girls when he noted a distinct pattern for some girls whose AD/HD worsened at puberty.

Gender Differences in Behavior

Some gender differences in behavior associated with AD/HD are readily observable, and have become well-accepted. Many studies report that girls are less hyperactive and demonstrate fewer impulsive behaviors. Research is needed, however, to explore a range of behavior patterns that may be more typical of females, such as shyness and social isolation or, conversely, hyper-talkativeness, slow processing speed, emotional hyperreactivity, low self-esteem, lack of assertiveness, school anxiety, test anxiety (related to need for approval), messiness, and forgetfulness.

In the self-report questionnaire contained in Chapter Two, the authors have attempted to suggest a range of observable classroom behaviors that may be more characteristic of females with AD/HD.

Cognitive/Neurological Differences

Gender differences in brain development begin in-utero, influenced by sex hormones. Other gender-based brain differences have been described at many stages of development. The sex hormones that have such a profound influence on brain development in-utero have a major impact again at puberty, leading to more gender-linked changes in the brain. It is now understood that the brain is a target organ for estrogen. Cyclical variations in estrogen levels during the menstrual cycle, as well as low-estrogen states during the postpartum period, in perimenopause, and menopause have all been demonstrated to impact the cognitive functioning of women. With this awareness of hormonal impact upon the brain, it reasonably follows that the cluster of cognitive functions associated with AD/HD—including attention, memory, impulse control, planning ability, self-monitoring, persistence and motivation—will also be influenced by gender-related brain differences. Research in such areas is eagerly awaited.

Russell Barkley has already introduced the notion that AD/HD in adulthood may be characterized more by disorders in executive function rather than by hyperactivity and impulsivity. While some research suggests that girls with AD/HD, compared to boys, have higher levels of executive functioning, clinical experience suggests that for women with AD/HD, presenting complaints of executive functioning difficulties are prominent, including problems with planning, organization, prioritization, and decision-making.

Sari Solden, in her book, *Women with Attention Deficit Disorder,* aptly describes this phenomenon, calling AD/HD in women the "disorder of dis-order." Current neuropsychological measures of "executive functioning" seem inadequate to measure the types of executive dysfunction that so often impact the daily lives of women with AD/HD.

Gender Differences in Coexisting Conditions.

There is general agreement that gender-related differences can also be seen in the coexisting conditions that commonly accompany AD/HD. However, these differences have usually been addressed in general terms, with boys described as having more "externalizing" disorders, such as oppositional or defiant behavior, while girls tend to have more "internalizing" disorders such as anxiety and depression. More specific gender-related patterns of coexisting conditions remain to be explored.

Rucklidge and Kaplan's research has found much higher levels of depression in women with AD/HD, compared to women without this disorder (Rucklidge & Kaplan, 1997), but the issue of the coexistence of AD/HD and depression, and even whether depression may be an integral part of the disorder in some women remains to be examined.

Gender Appropriate Treatment Considerations

Treatment approaches specifically designed for girls and women are critically needed. Currently, not only do we use diagnostic criteria based on studies of males, but we also emphasize treatment programs more appropriate for males. For example, most treatment programs for children with AD/HD focus on behavior management—a high priority issue for many boys, but a much less salient issue for most girls.

1. Different motivators

Recent research suggests that children with inattentive type AD/HD are strongly motivated to seek approval, in contrast to children with more hyperactive/impulsive patterns (Booth, Carlson, Shin, & Canu, 2000). Such findings are very important in designing treatment programs or classroom interventions for girls, the majority of whom fall into this inattentive subtype.

2. Different peer issues

Some research suggests that peer problems are more troublesome for girls, but treatment programs to address their problems in social relationships have been slow to develop. There is growing evidence that feelings of differentness and experiences of social rejection are among the most damaging aspects of AD/HD for girls. Interventions in the school environment, such as the use of peers as reinforcing agents, strategic seat assignment, and increased teacher awareness, could be very helpful. Group therapeutic interventions designed to help girls receive acceptance and support while learning better self-awareness and social skills could also reduce the feelings of rejection and low self-esteem that often impact females with AD/HD throughout their lives.

3. Different reactions to academic struggles

Other research has found that for many girls with AD/HD the classroom experience is significantly anxiety provoking. These findings suggest that teachers need to make the classroom feel more safe and supportive for girls with AD/HD. Such an approach is in great contrast to the AD/HD behavior management techniques that currently predominate in the classroom. Jane Adelizzi's research (Adelizzi, 2002) suggests that situations that raise anxiety levels and lead to experiences of shame and humiliation in the classroom, when extreme, can create enduring posttraumatic stress patterns in females with AD/HD. We need to further research this issue, both to prevent classroom trauma in girls growing up today and to treat women with AD/HD who still suffer the consequences of their traumatic classroom experiences.

4. *Hormone regulation in AD/HD treatment*

The interrelationship of female hormones and AD/HD symptoms in females suggests that different treatment regimens should be considered that may involve the use of hormone regulation or replacement, as well as psychostimulants. Studies of the effects of the interactions of estrogen and AD/HD symptomatology in females are needed. We need to investigate such effects at puberty, when a marked increase in AD/HD symptoms in girls has been noted by Huessy (1990) and others, at perimenopause and menopause, when women's AD/HD symptoms may be markedly affected by declining estrogen levels, as well as at different phases of the menstrual cycle. AD/HD patterns, anxiety, and depression can be affected by varying levels of female hormones.

Additional Research Issues

Posttraumatic Stress Disorder

Another important, but unexplored area of research is the relationship between AD/HD and Posttraumatic Stress Disorder. Adelizzi (2002) has conducted exploratory research on this topic in women. It is important, for example, to study the incidence of AD/HD among women who are victims of domestic violence. Could the trauma of living with AD/HD predispose women to seek out or become involved in more abusive relationships?

Is a possible relationship between AD/HD and trauma be gender-linked? Or, could males with AD/HD be trauma-prone as well, but express it in a different manner—through angry altercations, fatal or near-fatal accidents, road rage, or through physical aggression in general? Our focus has been for so long upon children, we need to turn more attention toward the issues of adults, and of adult women in particular.

The Challenges of Motherhood

Another area of research specific to women is the challenge of being a mother with AD/HD. The little research that exists suggests that they are more likely to put their children at risk in a variety of ways. Most parenting books and parenting programs for children with AD/HD don't take a mother's AD/HD into account. Research in this area is badly needed, for the sake of both mothers with AD/HD and their children.

Substance Abuse

The relationship between AD/HD and substance abuse is also a critical issue for females. Biederman and his colleagues (1999) reported that girls with AD/HD are at even higher risk than boys with AD/HD to become substance abusers. Girls with AD/HD are also more likely to take up cigarette smoking and at a younger age, compared to boys with AD/HD. Research is needed on the relationship between AD/HD and substance abuse, exploring whether patterns of abuse and treatment response vary according to gender.

Disordered Eating Patterns

Until recently, obesity, although clearly recognized as a significant public health problem in the U.S., has not been considered in connection to AD/HD. One initial study (Fleming & Levy, 2002), suggests that AD/HD may be a factor among women who are least successful in achieving weight loss using traditional methods. An informal survey of women with AD/HD (Nadeau, 1998) found that a significant number of women report using food on a regular basis as a means of self-calming. Clinical experience suggests that those who are more at risk for addiction are also more likely to have difficulties in controlling eating patterns. Research is badly needed to explore whether women with AD/HD and patterns of compulsive overeating need different treatment approaches that address their obesity and AD/HD in tandem.

Hopes for the Future

AD/HD is a very treatable disorder, but first the diagnosis must be made. Many women with AD/HD remain undiagnosed because the current diagnostic criteria are, in part, gender inappropriate. It is of the utmost importance that this stumbling block be removed. Beyond the diagnosis, treatment approaches focused on the unique concerns of women must be developed. Only when these two critical issues have been addressed will women with AD/HD gain the possibility of leading full and satisfying lives.

In view of the deeply-entrenched pattern in the mental health community of research focused on boys with AD/HD, perhaps the impetus for research on women with AD/HD will emerge from another direction. For example, researchers in the field of women's medicine may more readily appreciate the importance of gender differences in AD/HD, and the potential risk for females if male-derived concepts about AD/HD are not challenged, but assumed to apply equally to females.

It is unlikely, however, that these developments will occur until increasing numbers of women actively advocate for themselves and their daughters with AD/HD. Mothers of children with AD/HD have long been a major force behind the development of accommodations and supports for their children with AD/HD. It is time that women bring this same energy and effort to increase recognition of AD/HD in females, demanding that health care providers and educational institutions turn their attention to girls and women with AD/HD, in order to help them to feel and function at their best.

References

Adelizzi, J. (2002). Posttraumatic stress symptoms. In P. Quinn, & K. Nadeau (Eds.), *Gender issues and AD/HD: Research, diagnosis, and treatment.* Silver Spring, MD: Advantage Books.

Arnold, L. (1996). Sex differences in ADHD: Conference summary. *Journal of Abnormal Child Psychology, 24,* 555-569.

Barkley, R.A. (1997a). *ADHD and the nature of self-control.* New York: Guilford Press.

Barkley, R.A. (1997b). Update on a theory of AD/HD and its clinical implications. *ADHD Report, 5(4),* 10-13.

Biederman, J., Faraone, S., Mick, E., Williamson, S., Wilens, T.E., Spencer, T.J., Weber, W., Jetton, J., Kraus, I., Pert, J., & Zallen, B. (1999). Clinical correlates of ADHD in females: Findings from a large group of girls ascertained from pediatric and psychiatric referral sources. *Journal of the American Academy of Child and Adolescent Psychiatry, 38,* 966-975.

Booth, J., Carlson, C.L., Shin, M., & Canu, W. (2000). Parent, teacher, and self-rated motivational styles in the ADHD subtypes. *ADHD Report, 9(1),* 8-11.

Faraone, S. V., Biederman, J., Spencer, T., Wilens, T., Seidman, L. J., Mick, E., & Doyle, A. E. (2000). Attention-deficit/hyperactivity disorder in adults: An overview. *Biological Psychiatry, 48,* 9-20.

Fleming, J., & Levy, L. (2002). Eating Disorders. In P. Quinn, & K. Nadeau (Eds.) *Gender issues and AD/HD: Research, diagnosis, and treatment.* Silver Spring, MD: Advantage Books.

Gaub, M., & Carlson, C. (1997). Gender differences in ADHD: A meta-analysis and critical review. *Journal of the American Academy of Child and Adolescent Psychiatry, 36,* 1036-1045.

Gershon, J. (2000). *A meta-analytic review of gender differences in AD/HD.* Journal of Attention Disorders, 5, (3), 143-154.

Huessy, H.R. (1990). *The pharmacotherapy of personality disorders in women.* Paper Presented at the 143rd Annual Meeting of the American Psychiatric Association (symposia), New York.

Nadeau, K. (1998). Survey on problem eating patterns - preliminary report. *ADDvance, 2(1),* 26.

Nadeau, K., Littman, E., & Quinn, P. (1999). *Understanding girls with AD/HD.* Silver Spring, MD: Advantage Books.

Ohan, J.L., & Johnston, C. (1999). Gender appropriateness of diagnostic criteria for the externalizing disorders. In M. Moretti (Chair), *Aggression in girls: Diagnostic issues and interpersonal factors.* Symposium conducted at the biennial meeting of the Society for Research in Child Development, Albuquerque, NM.

Rucklidge, J.J., & Kaplan, B.J. (1997). Psychological functioning in women identified in adulthood with attention-deficit/hyperactivity disorder. *Journal of Attention Disorders, 2,* 167-176.

Solden, Sari (1995). *Women with attention deficit disorder: Embracing disorganization at home and in the workplace.* Grass Valley, CA: Underwood Books.

The MTA Cooperative Group. (1999). Moderators and mediators of treatment response for children with attention deficit/ hyperactivity disorder. *Archives of General Psychiatry, 56,* 1088-1096.

Walker, C. (1999). Gender and genetics in ADHD: Genetics matter, gender does not. Paper presented at the ADDA Regional Conference, Chicago.

About the Authors

CHRIS ADAMEC is a professional writer and author of *Moms with ADD*. She writes from a personal perspective as a mother with AD/HD.

BARBARA COHEN, Ph.D., MFT is Director of the Center for Healing the Human Spirit, Inc. in Tarzana, California, where she specializes in working with people, with or without AD/HD, on personal and spiritual growth. She is a Certified Trainer in the Art and Science of Hypnotism and Hypnotherapy and Neuro-Linguistic Programming, and a Diplomate of Certified Sports Counseling. In addition, Dr. Cohen provides AD/HD Coaching and Life Coaching, and conducts a variety of training courses and workshops.

WILMA FELLMAN, M.Ed., LPC has been a Licensed Professional Counselor for over 18 years. She specializes in working with adolescents and adults with attention deficit disorder, learning disabilities, and other challenges with respect to career issues. Ms. Fellman is the author of *The Other Me: Poetic Thoughts on ADD for Adults, Kids and Parents*, and *Finding A Career That Works For You*. She is the co-presenter of the instructional video, *Succeeding in College and Career with ADD*, and has presented workshops at local, state and national levels on the subject of career development decisions for people with special challenges.

DAVID GOODMAN, M.D. is Assistant Professor of Psychiatry and Behavioral Sciences at the Johns Hopkins University School of Medicine. He is also Director of the Adult Attention Deficit Disorder Center of Maryland in Lutherville, MD. His psychiatric commentary has been featured on Baltimore television, PBS and national affiliate stations, national magazines (U.S. News and World Report, Self Magazine, Glamour) and radio interviews around the country. Dr. Goodman has been a Principal Investigator for multi-site Phase II, and III drug trials for the treatment of adult Attention Deficit/Hyperactivity Disorder.

BELINDA GUTHRIE, M.A. is a learning specialist and the Director of Disability and Support Services at Vassar College. Ms. Guthrie also works privately as an academic coach with children with AD/HD. Prior to working at Vassar, Ms. Guthrie held a similar position at Smith College and worked as a learning specialist at New York University's Access to Learning Center for Students with Learning Disabilities and Attention Deficit Disorder. Ms. Guthrie recently coordinated a national conference at Vassar College entitled "Enhancing Academic Excellence at Selective Residential Liberal Arts Colleges."

JONATHAN SCOTT HALVERSTADT, M.S., LMFT has a diverse background which includes an undergraduate degree in the ministry. Jonathan has worked in the mental health field since 1987 and is a specialist in adult Attention Deficit Disorder and other learning disabilities, relationships, recovery, codependency, and shame. He is the author of numerous educational materials, lectures extensively throughout the United States and sees patients at his private practice in northern California.

THOM HARTMANN is an award-winning, bestselling author and psychotherapist who was formerly the executive director of a residential treatment facility for emotionally disturbed and abused children. The founder of The Hunter School for AD/HD children, he is also the parent of three children. A guest faculty member at Goddard College and international relief worker, he has lived and worked among indigenous and aboriginal hunter/gatherer people on four continents, an experience that in part led to his development of the Hunter/Farmer metaphor to describe AD/HD.

JUNE JOHNSON is a native Georgian and a graduate of the University of Georgia with a degree in education. As a Professional Organizer, Ms. Johnson is a recognized trainer in organization, time management, and goal setting. She is a founding member of the Georgia Chapter of the National Association of Professional Organizers. Her interest in AD/HD comes from her practical experience with clients in both corporate and home settings.

JERRY LITHMAN, M.D. has a private practice in Durham, North Carolina and is an Assistant Professor at the Duke University Medical Center, Department of Psychiatry. He was for many years the Co-Director of the Dallas Neurobehavioral Institute, Dallas, Texas.

ELLEN LITTMAN, Ph.D. is a licensed clinical psychologist, educated and trained at Brown and Yale Universities. She has been involved in the field of AD/HD for over 15 years, and teaches, lectures and conducts research on gender issues in AD/HD. Dr. Littman practices in Mt. Kisco, NY, where she specializes in individual, couples, and group treatment for adults with AD/HD.

KATHLEEN NADEAU, Ph.D. is a clinical psychologist and director of the Chesapeake Center for Attention and Learning Disorders in Silver Spring, Maryland. A specialist in AD/HD for over twenty years, she is the author of numerous books on attention deficit/hyperactivity disorder, and lectures frequently on issues related to AD/HD.

JEFFERSON PRINCE, M.D. is on the staff of the Pediatric Psychopharmacology Clinic at Massachusetts General Hospital and an Instructor of Psychiatry, Harvard Medical School. He has authored numerous articles and conducted research in the area of AD/HD for several years.

PATRICIA QUINN, M.D. is a developmental pediatrician in Washington. A graduate of Georgetown University Medical School, she specializes in child development and psychopharmacology. Dr. Quinn has worked for over 25 years in the area of AD/HD and learning disabilities. She gives workshops nationwide and has published widely in these fields.

GAIL RODIN, Ph.D. is a clinical neuropsychologist and Director of the Center for Attention, Learning, and Memory in Raleigh, NC. She specializes in the assessment of children, adolescents, and adults with neurobiologically-based developmental learning disorders, including AD/HD and learning disabilities.

JOAN SHAPIRO, Ed.D. holds a Doctoral Degree and an M.Ed. in Special Education as well as a Masters Degree in Curriculum and Reading from Teachers College, Columbia University. Previously an Associate Professor of Education at Marymount Manhattan College, she co-developed and directed the Ruth Smadbeck Communication and Learning Center and the program for college students with learning disabilities. She is coauthor of *Facing Learning Disabilities in the Adult Years*, Oxford University Press, 1999. Now in private practice, she lives in Manhattan.

TANYA SHUY, B.S. is a Program Specialist, National Institute of Child Health and Human Development (NICHD), National Institute of Health, as well as a Learning Specialist with the SUCCESS Program, (Graduate Assistant), University of Maryland. Tanya R. Shuy is a master's student in learning disabilities, Department of Special Education, University of Maryland. Research interests include reading disabilities, bilingual learning disabilities, and attention deficit hyperactivity disorder.

GAYLE VOIGT was not diagnosed with AD/HD until she was in her mid-thirties. Born and raised in Sydney, Australia, she moved to Baltimore, Maryland, in 1989, where her husband holds a faculty position at the University of Maryland Medical School. She is pursuing a Bachelor of Science degree, and is currently in her final semester. Through raising children with AD/HD, as well as learning to understand her own AD/HD, she has become an active voice in the community on AD/HD issues. Gayle enjoys sharing her personal experience in the hope of helping other women with AD/HD find acceptance and fulfillment.

LYNN WEISS, Ph.D., is a seasoned professional with 30 years of experience as a practicing psychotherapist and counselor. An accomplished author, Dr. Weiss wrote the bestselling *Attention Deficit Disorder in Adults*, *The A.D.D. in Adults Workbook*, *A.D.D. on the Job*, *A.D.D. and Creativity*, *A.D.D. and Success,* and most recently, *View from the Cliff.* She holds a doctorate from the University of Santa Barbara, a master's degree from New York University, and received her clinical training from the Department of Psychiatry, University of Washington Medical School.

TIMOTHY WILENS, M.D. is Director of Substance Abuse Services and the Pediatric Psychopharmacology Clinics at Massachusetts General Hospital. He is an Associate Professor of Psychiatry at Harvard Medical School and the author of numerous writings and research papers on AD/HD and its treatment.

Subject Index